Wright's Behavior Management in Dentistry for Children

# Wright's Behavior Management in Dentistry for Children

Third Edition

*Edited by*

*Ari Kupietzky, DMD, MSc*
*Diplomate of the American Board of Pediatric Dentistry*
*Private Practice*
*Senior Clinical Instructor, Department of Pediatric Dentistry*
*The Hebrew University, Hadassah School of Dental Medicine*
*Jerusalem, Israel*

*Visiting Professor, Department of Pediatric Dentistry*
*Rutgers School of Dental Medicine*
*The State University of New Jersey*
*Newark, New Jersey, USA*

**WILEY** Blackwell

*Edition History*
W B Saunders Co. (1e, 1975); John Wiley and Sons, Inc. (2e, 2014)

*Registered Offices*
John Wiley & Sons, Inc., 111 River Street, Hoboken, NJ 07030, USA
John Wiley & Sons Ltd, The Atrium, Southern Gate, Chichester, West Sussex, PO19 8SQ, UK

*Editorial Office*
111 River Street, Hoboken, NJ 07030, USA

For details of our global editorial offices, customer services, and more information about Wiley products, visit us at www.wiley.com.

Wiley also publishes its books in a variety of electronic formats and by print-on-demand. Some content that appears in standard print versions of this book may not be available in other formats.

*Library of Congress Cataloging-in-Publication Data*

Names: Kupietzky, Ari, editor.
Title: Wright's behavior management in dentistry for children / edited by
  Ari Kupietzky.
Other titles: Behavior management in dentistry for children
Description: Third edition. | Hoboken : Wiley-Blackwell, 2022. | Preceded
  by Behavior management in dentistry for children / [edited by] Gerald Z.
  Wright, Ari Kupietzky. Second edition. 2014. | Includes bibliographical
  references and index.
Identifiers: LCCN 2021028037 (print) | LCCN 2021028038 (ebook) | ISBN
  9781119680840 (cloth) | ISBN 9781119680932 (adobe pdf) | ISBN
  9781119680949 (epub)
Subjects: MESH: Dental Care for Children | Behavior Control | Child
  Behavior | Dentist-Patient Relations | Anesthesia, Dental–methods |
  Child | Adolescent
Classification: LCC RK55.C5 (print) | LCC RK55.C5 (ebook) | NLM WU 480 |
  DDC 617.6/45–dc23
LC record available at https://lccn.loc.gov/2021028037
LC ebook record available at https://lccn.loc.gov/2021028038

Cover Design: Wiley
Cover Image: Wiley

Set in 9.5/12.5pt STIXTwoText by Straive, Pondicherry, India

Printed in Singapore
M106217_130721

*This book is dedicated to the memory of two great leaders of pediatric dentistry who have been both my mentors and colleagues.*

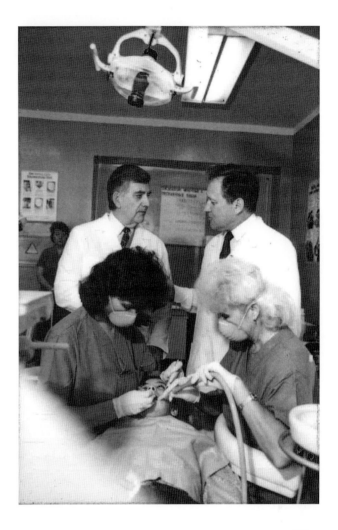

*Professor Gerald Z. Wright (left) at Belarusian State Medical University in 2003. He received an honorary degree for bringing modern dentistry to the children of Belarus, social and medical activities, and mastering of educational process.*

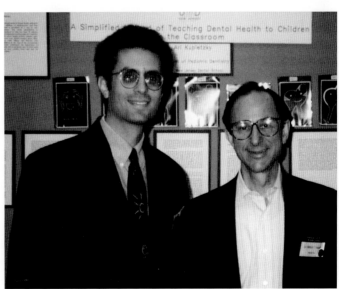

*The editor, Dr. Ari Kupietzky (left) and Professor Milton Houpt (right) presenting "A simplified method of teaching dental health to children in the classroom". American Academy of Pediatric Dentistry, Annual Session, Kansas City, Missouri, 1993.*

# Contents

# About the Editor

**Dr. Ari Kupietzky,** DMD, MSC, is a Diplomate of the American Board of Pediatric Dentistry and served as a member on the Advisory Council of the American Board of Pediatric Dentistry, Sedation and Hospital Section. He teaches part time at the Department of Pediatric Dentistry of the Hebrew University Hadassah School of Dental Medicine in Jerusalem, Israel, and is Visiting Professor at Rutgers School of Dental Medicine in Newark, New Jersey, USA.

# Acknowledgments

## From Gerald Z. Wright (second edition)

Few books are solo efforts, and this one is no exception. If it were not for three people, it would not have been written and published at all. The first to be acknowledged is Professor Anna Fuks. For years, my good friend Anna had been urging me to write another edition to my first book, *Behavior Management in Dentistry for Children*. Urging is probably putting it mildly, but her requests went unheeded for many reasons. Finally, she put me in communication with Dr. Ari Kupietzky.

My co-editor Dr. Kupietzky is a very persuasive and persistent individual. We had several discussions about the need for this type of book, the differing approaches to treating children in dentistry in the world today, and the fact that it would be timely to once more consolidate some of the thinking and writing in behavior management. When he offered to co-edit this book with me, I assented, and we moved forward with this project. Essentially, the second edition is a new work and includes new chapters and contributors. Once the planning and writing was underway, I realized that he is a well-organized person, has an excellent knowledge of the most current literature, and possesses a passion to meet deadlines. He has been a pleasure to work with.

The third person who was influential in this project was my wife, Nancy Wright. She knew that I was unsure about involving myself in this commitment; it was 12 years since my retirement from dental teaching and practice. She urged me to go ahead with this book. Not only did she provide encouragement, but Nancy read and commented upon most of the chapters to which I contributed. Her professional background in psychology was instrumental in creating numerous "book discussions" in our home.

Ari and I enlisted 14 contributors from five different countries to lend their expertise to this book. Each of them provided worthy chapter drafts, met deadlines, and accepted our editing with grace and understanding. Consequently, the book was completed ahead of schedule.

## List of Contributors

**Debra A. Cohen, DDS**
Diplomate, American Board of Pediatric Dentistry
Private Practice
Elmwood Park, New Jersey, USA

**Marcio A. da Fonseca, DDS, MS**
Chicago Dental Society Foundation Professor and Head
Department of Pediatric Dentistry
College of Dentistry
University of Illinois at Chicago
Chicago, Illinois, USA

**Larry Dormois, DDS, MS**
Associate Professor
University of Tennessee Health Science Center
Memphis, Tennessee

**Dimitris Emmanouil, DDS, MS, PhD**
Assistant Professor of Pediatric Dentistry
Athens, Greece

**Anna B. Fuks, DDS**
Professor Emeritus, Department of Pediatric Dentistry
The Hebrew University, Hadassah School of Dental Medicine
Jerusalem, Israel

**Gunilla Klingberg, DDS, PhD**
Professor, Department of Pediatric Dentistry
Faculty of Odontology, Malmö University
Malmö, Sweden

**Ari Kupietzky, DMD, MSc**
Diplomate of the American Board of Pediatric Dentistry
Private Practice
Senior Clinical Instructor
Department of Pediatric Dentistry
The Hebrew University, Hadassah School of Dental Medicine
Jerusalem, Israel;
Visiting Professor, Department of Pediatric Dentistry
Rutgers School of Dental Medicine
Rutgers, The State University of New Jersey
Newark, New Jersey, USA

**Brian D. Lee, DDS, MSD, FACD, FAAPD**
Diplomate of the American Board of Pediatric Dentistry
Private Practice
Foster City, California, USA

**Jonathon E. Lee, DDS, FACD, FAAPD**
Diplomate of the American Board of Pediatric Dentistry
Diplomate of the American Board of Orthodontics
Private Practice
Foster City, California, USA

**Travis Nelson, DDS, MSD, MPH**
Department of Pediatric Dentistry
University of Washington
Seattle, Washington, USA

**Amanda Jo Okundaye, DDS**
Dentist Anesthesiologist
Private Practice Mobile Dental Anesthesiology
Instructor, School of Dental Medicine
University of Nevada Las Vegas, Nevada, USA

**Tammy Pilowsky Peleg, PhD**
Department of Psychology
The Hebrew University of Jerusalem
Mt. Scopus, Jerusalem, Israel
The Neuropsychological Unit
Schneider Children's Medical Center of Israel
Petah Tikva, Israel

**Kenneth L. Reed, DMD**
Associate Program Director, Dental Anesthesiology
Attending in Anesthesiology, Graduate Pediatric Dentistry
New York University Langone Hospital, Brooklyn,
New York, USA;
Affiliate Assistant Professor, Department of
Periodontology, School of Dentistry, The Oregon Health
Science University, Portland, Oregon, USA;
Clinical Instructor, Department of Dentistry, Faculty of
Medicine and Dentistry, University of Alberta, Edmonton,
Alberta, Canada

**Steven Schwartz, DDS**
Staten Island University Hospital
New York, New York, USA

**Barbara Sheller, DDS, MSD**
Chief, Pediatric Dentist and Orthodontist
Department of Dentistry, Seattle Children's Hospital
Affiliate Professor
Department of Pediatric Dentistry and Department of
Orthodontics
School of Dentistry, University of Washington
Seattle, Washington, USA

**Eyal Simchi, DMD**
Diplomate, American Board of Pediatric Dentistry
Montefiore Nyack Hospital
Nyack, New York;
Private Practice, Elmwood Park, New Jersey, USA

**Janice Townsend, DDS, MS**
Chief, Dentistry
Nationwide Children's Hospital
Columbus, Ohio, USA

**Jaap S. J. Veerkamp, DDS, PhD**
Pediatric Dentist, Head
KINDERTAND, Secondary Dental Care Clinics in
Amsterdam and Rotterdam
Amsterdam, Netherlands

**Martha Wells, DMD, MS**
Heber Simmons Jr. Distinguished Professor and Program
Director, Pediatric Dentistry
The University of Tennessee Health Science Center
Department of Pediatric Dentistry and Community Oral Health
Memphis, Tennessee, USA

**Stephen Wilson, DMD, MA, PhD**
Chief Dental Officer
Blue Cloud Pediatric Surgery Centers, Inc.
Scottsdale, Arizona, USA;
Adjunct Professor
Department of Pediatric Dentistry
The Ohio State University/Nationwide Children's Hospital
Columbus, Ohio, USA

**Gerald Z. Wright, DDS, MSD, FRCD (C)**
Diplomate of the American Board of Pediatric Dentistry
Professor Emeritus
Schulich School of Medicine and Dentistry
Western University
London, Ontario, Canada

# Preface

When approached by Wiley to consider editing a third edition of *Behavior Management in Dentistry for Children*, both Professor Wright and I were encouraged to proceed, given the splendid reception to the second edition. Professor Wright asked me to assume the role of leading editor, and a plan was made to improve and expand the third edition, including the selection of new contributing authors and new areas to focus on. It was decided that the third edition would follow rather closely the second, with updated references and new topics.

Sadly, Professor Wright became ill during the early stages of the revision. He was adamant that I continue on with the project without him, and soon after, he passed away. He has been described as being one of the giants in pediatric dentistry and a pioneer in behavior management. He published no less than three textbooks on the subject, laying down the principles of which became the foundation for the teaching and practice of managing children's behavior in the dental setting. As a tribute to him, I decided to rename the title of the third edition in his honor and memory to be called *Wright's Behavior Management in Dentistry for Children*. This is not only a semantic change; the new edition draws on Dr. Wright's other books, listed below, thus merging his theses and monographs into one book. He had requested that case studies from *Managing Children's Behavior in the Dental Office* be included, and many have been added throughout the text. Credit of these additions is given here to his co-editors.

- *Behavior Management in Dentistry for Children*. Editor: Gerald Z. Wright (W.B. Saunders Company, 1975)
- *Managing Children's Behavior in the Dental Office*. Co-editors: Gerald Z. Wright, Paul E. Starkey, and Donald E. Gardiner (The C.V. Mosby Company, 1983)
- *Child Management in Dentistry: Dental Practitioner Handbook*. Gerald Z. Wright, Paul E. Starkey, and Donald E. Gardner (IOP Publishing Ltd., 1987)

At the writing of the second edition, I acknowledged Professor Milton Houpt, who had been an inspiration throughout my professional career. A month after the passing of Professor Wright, Professor Houpt also passed away. Interestingly, they started out together at University of Toronto Dental School as undergraduate classmates and left the profession and this world together. Our specialty has lost two of its great founders of modern pediatric dentistry.

## Aims and Scope of the Third Edition

This book has two main purposes: (1) to introduce current information basic to the understanding of children's behavior, and (2) to describe and discuss many of the techniques and methods, new and old, used for promoting cooperative behavior in children.

Due to numerous clinical approaches, increased research output by behavioral scientists, and growing awareness of the importance of this area, we no longer have one up-to-date source that dentists or dental students can rely on for a comprehensive coverage of the subject. Books dealing with behavior management have come and gone—and that is one more reason for reviving this book with a third edition. It is intended to integrate current pertinent information from research with current clinical practices.

Another aim has been to balance the practitioner's need for some basic knowledge of child psychology with the requirement of practical clinical instruction. Dental teachers and clinicians have expressed the need for such a book, provided that it is relevant to dental practice. Little psychological background on the part of the reader is therefore presumed, but an attempt is made to build a foundation on which a practicing dentist can develop an understanding of the dynamics of children's behavior in the dental environment.

The volume begins by describing the psychological, social, and emotional development of children. What is normal behavior for a three-year-old may be unacceptable for a five-year-old child. There are margins of normality that those treating children should understand. When the first edition of this book was written, maternal anxiety was significantly related to children's cooperative behavior and was the primary focus of a chapter. But there are many types of families nowadays—single-parent families, same-sex families, blended families, to name a few—and they too will be discussed. While the nuclear family is still predominant in society, understanding family environments and how they influence child behaviors is much more complex than in the past. Therefore, much more emphasis has been placed on the study of families of dental patients, and an entire new chapter is devoted to this subject. The chapter dealing with parents offers new material—and is exceptional. It highlights many of these changes in society. As mentioned earlier, not only are there changes in the populations that we serve but also in our dental staffs and dentists' beliefs. All of these changes—diversity, language, and customs—are making life more interesting.

As the reader progresses through the book, a spectrum of techniques for managing the behavior of children is offered. The approach is characterized by eclecticism. It includes clinical management of children using many non-pharmacologic and pharmacologic methods. The subject of hypnosis was not included in either of the two previous books. It keeps coming back and is topical, so it was decided to include it in this third edition.

The non-pharmacologic techniques generally are those which have been time-tested over generations. They still form the basis of behavior management. However, there has been an increase in the use of sedation, and it is obvious that many new pharmacologic methods need to be highlighted. Sedation usage has led to numerous changes in dental practice: new sedation agents—along with optimum drug dosages and new drug combinations, guidelines for patient monitoring, and emergency measures—are only some of these changes.

An entire chapter is devoted to the management of children with disabilities. Most work on this topic have been technique-oriented writings. The present chapter takes a broader approach. A disabled child creates special problems in a family and alters the dynamics of that family. Since the trend today is to maintain the special patient in the community, rather than in an institution, it is apparent that a greater knowledge and understanding of the management of these patients is required. The revised chapter also addresses the home care that is absolutely essential to maintain the oral health of these special children. Additionally, much more is known today about communicating with these children than was known when the first edition of this book was created. Some of these communication methods will be addressed in this chapter.

In the last two chapters, the book covers practical considerations in the office, discussing a myriad of strategies. The dentist plans and has ultimate responsibility for these strategies, while the office personnel implements them. There is abundant evidence that successful behavior management is facilitated by a well-run office, the employment of personnel well-trained in relating to children, and the design and appearance of the dental office. The final chapter is devoted to the office environment. Having an office that appeals to children makes management much easier. An appealing office might be considered a starting point in behavior management.

This book also has a major difference when compared to the original book. To elucidate some of the key points in the writings, cases are presented. The cases provide examples that make the book more clinically relevant. Some of these cases are from the book *Managing Children's Behavior in the Dental Office* (1983) as mentioned earlier. The cases are set apart from the text, appearing in boxes. The scenarios may be used as a teaching aid, allowing for further discussion amongst clinicians and their students during teaching seminars. A few are used to give examples of fallacious arguments, the intention being that the separation from the text in this way will eliminate possible misconstruction of the point.

I acknowledge the following contributors to the second edition:

**Eileen Wood, HBA, MA, PhD**
Professor, Developmental Psychology, Department of Psychology, Wilfrid Laurier University, Waterloo, Ontario, Canada
And **Steven Schwartz, DDS,** of blessed memory.

The editor thanks Mirva Maki, RDA for being a part of the dental team and providing support in behavior management. Many of the clinical photographs throughout the text were taken by Ms. Maki during routine treatment of our patients.

**Ari Kupietzky,
Jerusalem, Israel**

# 1

## The Pediatric Dentistry Treatment Triangle

*Ari Kupietzky and Gerald Z. Wright*

## Introduction

The subject matter "behavior of children in the dental environment" seems unlimited and is timely. Therefore, this new book contains material that has not been included in previous editions. Changes in society are occurring at an extremely fast pace, and the need for revising and adding new information to address these changes is self-evident. Not only are children changing, so are the dentists treating them. For example, during the writing of the first edition of *Behavior Management in Dentistry for Children*, the majority of pediatric dentists were male. This persisted into the twenty-first century with only 18% of all pediatric dentists being female. However, a recent survey conducted by the American Academy of Pediatric Dentistry (AAPD 2017) showed that the percent of female pediatric dentists has tripled, the majority of pediatric dentists being female (51.8%). Additionally, pediatric dentists are young; females in the workforce are, on average, younger (41.6 years) than their male counterparts (49.1 years). Young pediatric dentists, millennial dentists (or *Dentennials*, as coined by Piers in 2018), may not be accepting of the traditional methods to manage their pediatric patients and accompanying parents.

Societal changes in family structure, formal education and the influence of technology and social media on children and adults alike – all require a fresh outlook on how we treat our patients and their parents in our offices. Modern society no longer regards children as "adults-in-the-making" whose lives are determined by their parents who take into consideration their age and stage of development. Rather, modern society recognizes children as active agents, capable of participating and indeed entitled to be involved in the decision-making process and the determination of their well-being. This may explain the avoidance of any aversive techniques which were previously employed by pediatric dentists and the subsequent rise in the usage of deep sedation and general anesthesia for the dental treatment of children. And yet, since the publication of the second edition of *Behavior Management in Dentistry for Children*, the US Food and Drug Administration (FDA) issued a warning with regard to the use of general anesthesia on children under 3 years of age which may affect the neurological development during their toddling age (US Food and Drug Administration 2017). On the other hand, more and more pediatric dentists avoid using invasive restorative techniques in the case of an uncooperative pediatric patient and instead employ techniques such as interim therapeutic restoration (ITR), also referred to as *atraumatic restorative treatment (ART)*, silver diamine fluoride (SDF), and the Hall Technique to manage dental caries. These procedures can be performed without the use of general anesthesia or sedation and do not require expertise in basic behavior guidance. These techniques indeed have a place in the pediatric dentist's armamentarium; however, they should be reserved for use in the case of a pre-cooperative patient and should not be used due to a practitioner's lack of patient management skills.

The primary objective of this book is to help the dental office team manage the behavior of children in the dental environment. Some parts of the text are directed primarily to dentists, while other parts pertain to the roles of dental hygienists, dental assistants, and dental receptionists. It is unusual for a professional book to address all these functions. However, guiding children through their dental experiences requires teamwork; thus, a multidisciplinary approach seems reasonable. If dental teams are to use consistent and effective methods, each member of the dental team must have an understanding of the dynamics of child behavior and appreciate others' roles in behavior management. These thoughts were addressed more than a century ago when a dentist, while writing in one of the professional journals of the day, voiced concern about the behavior of children in his practice (Raymond 1875). It was his opinion that "getting into the good graces of children is almost half the work to be accomplished." This observation opened the gates to a flood of comments on a subject which hitherto had been unrecognized in the dental literature.

Much attention has been focused on shaping children's behavior in the dental environment. Although some dentists have reacted intuitively to the needs of their child patients, others have been more systematic. They have tried to identify children's behavior patterns and to find the best means of coping with them. Practitioners have adopted and adapted the techniques of their dental colleagues. The better methods have been passed from one generation of practitioners to the next. These procedures have stood the test of time. The cumulative effect of this knowledge and experience has been the gradual development of an area known as *behavior management.*

When planning the second edition of this book, the change in nomenclature was an initial stumbling block. Forty years ago, the foremost national specialty organization in the world, the American Academy of Pedodontics, now known as the American Academy of Pediatric Dentistry (*AAPD*), used the term *behavior management.* The AAPD now prefers the term behavior *guidance* rather than behavior *management.* The editor believes that the role of the pediatric dentist remains to be the leader in the dental clinic. The verb "manage" is defined as to be in charge, to administer. Therefore, at the risk of political incorrectness, the term *behavior management* will be used throughout in this book.

The study of behavior management has undergone changes. Early writings on the subject were essentially subjective and anecdotal. Interest matured in the 1970s. The result has been a more scientific approach to behavior management.

The descriptive terms "subjective" and "anecdotal" might be interpreted as a criticism. This was not the intention. Earlier writers on the subject of behavior management were pioneers. They attempted to list the causes of uncooperativeness. They classified behavior patterns. They made accurate observations. They established guidelines for behavior management, some of which are incorporated into the foundation of contemporary practice.

Professional recognition that the behavior of the child patient is the most influential factor affecting treatment outcomes significantly heightened interest in behavior management. As a consequence, dentists began to confer on the subject the same respect and objectivity that they have accorded to other areas of science in dentistry (Teuscher 1973). Collaborations with psychologists and psychiatrists have broadened the theoretical bases of behavior management. The current systematic approach has been referred to as *behavioral science research* in pediatric dentistry. The maturing interest has resulted in a healthy questioning of our earlier subjective considerations. Investigators have explored various hypotheses, new and old, in an attempt to further enhance our relationships with children.

As one would expect, the practice of behavior management has been a dynamic one. Differing treatment techniques have been recommended and debated by pediatric dentists. The choice and acceptability of technique are directly dependent on the societal norms of specific cultures. As a result, today's practitioners have a wide selection of methods which can be used for managing children's behavior.

By now, it should be apparent that this book has been organized to present an overview of an extremely broad field, rather than an investigation of a few topics. It was designed for all members of the dental health team who deal with children. These team members combine their efforts in the management of children's behaviors. Each makes their own unique contribution as a dental professional. Consequently, certain aspects of this book will be more appealing, or more germane, to one or the other team members. It is the sum total of the children's experiences in the dental environment which ultimately determines their cooperative behaviors. All team members have a stake in determining the nature of those experiences: each of the team members should have a mastery of their own profession and an understanding of the roles of office associates.

The fundamentals of behavior management are brought into the focus of clinical reality through an understanding of the pediatric dentistry treatment triangle with true-to-life situations presented alongside in accompanying boxes throughout the book.

## The Pediatric Dentistry Treatment Triangle

The *pedodontic triangle* was first introduced in 1975 in the first edition of *Behavior Management in Dentistry for Children.* The evolution of the concept of the newly named *pediatric dentistry treatment triangle* (Figure 1-1), to some extent, has provided the framework for this entire volume. It pointed out that it is not possible to view any single corner of this triangle in isolation; each interrelates. The child is at the apex of the triangle and is the focus of attention of both the family and the dental team. At the base of the triangle are mainly adults: the child's family and the entire

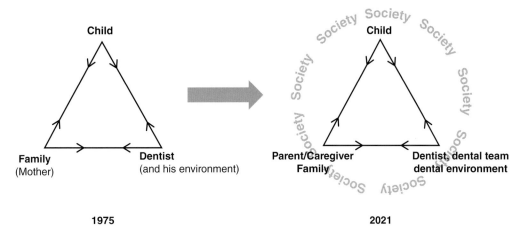

**Figure 1-1** The pediatric dentistry treatment triangle. The illustration shows how things have changed since the first edition of this book.

dental team. A child's family can affect the child's dental behavior. This aspect is discussed in Chapter 4. Obviously, all the dental team, particularly the dentist, participate in guiding the chairside behavior of the child. Throughout the book, the roles of both dentists' and other members of the dental team will be discussed.

The two lines of communication emanating from the dentist's corner emphasize a major difference between children's dentistry and adult dentistry. These lines show that treating children is at least a 1:2 relationship (i.e., dentist:child and parent). Adult dentistry tends to be a 1:1 situation (i.e., dentist:patient). It is extremely important for all dental personnel to communicate in both directions.

---

### Case 1.1

Zara, 4-years-old, was brought to the dental clinic by her father for her first dental visit. While they both waited in the reception room for the appointed time, Zara was calm. The receptionist notified them that it was now their turn. She heard Zara's father say: "Let's go inside, Zara. Nobody will hurt you today. It's just a check-up."

---

***Case 1.1, Discussion:*** The case demonstrates the 1:2 relationship that is distinctive to pediatric dentistry. When pediatric dentists treat children, parents are part of the dental relationship, for better or for worse. Many people in clinical dentistry have heard children introduced to the dental situation in this unthinking way (Figure 1-2).

A much better approach would have been for Zara's father to say, "Let's go inside and show the dentist how well you brush your teeth. I heard that you're going to get a prize!" This situation highlights the influential role parents play in the dental situation. They are an integral part of the triangle. Numerous sections throughout this book will

discuss how both parents and children may be prepared by the dentist and dental team for their visit. A well-prepared parent's messages to the child may be more supportive.

The arrows at the end of the lines indicate that communication is reciprocal. They also signify that the dental treatment of the child patient is a dynamic relationship between the corners of the triangle—the child, the family, and the dentist. The relationships among the three angles of the triangle are not static. They are vibrant and ever-changing. A harmonious situation can exist at one dental visit, which can be subsequently upset by marital strife within a family or a changing school situation for the child. Moreover, communication among the different personalities in the triangle alters relationships; hence, the arrows indicate that the communication is reciprocal. The importance of this unifying concept will become evident as techniques are described in subsequent chapters.

Note the difference in Figure 1-1 between the triangular illustrations in 1975 and 2021: a circle has been added surrounding the original triangle. In 2021, societal expectations have greatly impacted the practice of pediatric dentistry. The pediatric triangle does not represent an isolated environment, but rather exists within and is influenced by the surrounding society, hence the addition of the circle. The diagram has not changed for 2021, but the societal changes within it have been dynamic. Diversity, cultural beliefs, and attitudes of the dentists, their staffs, and the parents of child patients have had a significant impact on pediatric dentistry today and are discussed in Chapter 5.

Perhaps, the utmost societal impact on pediatric dentistry was the law of informed consent. Informing the parent about the nature, risk, and benefits of the technique to be used and any professionally recognized or evidence-based alternative is essential to obtaining informed consent. The impact upon professionals became more widespread in the 1980s. Pediatric dentists became aware that it was far more

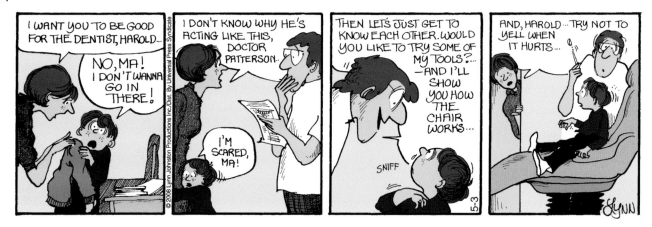

**Figure 1-2** For better or for worse. *Source:* © 1995. Lynn Johnston Prod. Used courtesy of the creator and Universal Uclick. All rights reserved.

difficult to obtain legal consent from a parent on behalf of a child than it was to have consent when dealing with an adult on a dentist–patient (1:1) relationship.

The term *informed consent* first appeared in the United States in court documents in 1957. It was in a civil court ruling for a patient who underwent anesthesia for what he thought was a routine procedure. He woke up permanently paralyzed from the waist down. The doctor had not told him that the procedure carried risks. In a subsequent civil suit, the judge in the case ruled that "a physician violates his duty to his patient and subjects himself to liability if he withholds any facts which are necessary to form the basis for an intelligent consent by the patient to the proposed treatment." Obtaining informed consent for all procedures is now mandatory, and it is an example as to why society has to be considered when illustrating the pediatric dentistry treatment triangle. The evolving and constantly changing nature of the triangle is also reflected in the new requirement of seeking the child's assent in addition to parental consent. As stated by the American Academy of Pediatrics in its 2016 policy statement: "Informed consent should be seen as an essential part of health care practice; parental permission and *childhood assent* is an active process that engages patients, both adults and children, in health care. Pediatric practice is unique in that developmental maturation allows, over time, for *increasing inclusion of the child's and adolescent's opinion* in medical decision-making in clinical practice and research."

Societal norms affect all corners of the triangle individually, as well as the interactions between all three components. The intimate relationship between parent and child has been changed by society. The professional relationships between dentist and child and dentist and parent have also evolved, dictated by societal changes. In 1975, it was widely accepted that a mother's attitude significantly affected her offspring's behavior in the dental office. Roles in families

are changing, and now, the total family environment has to be considered. A father bringing a child for treatment is not unusual. Not infrequently, both parents are working, and the child presents at the dental office with a caregiver. Hence, the new triangular illustration recognizes the change that has occurred in the last 40 years. This book will highlight some of these changes and identify how they have influenced the practice of pediatric dentistry.

## What is Behavior Management?

McElroy (1895) inadvertently provided a definition for behavior management near the beginning of this century. She wrote, "although the operative dentistry may be perfect, the appointment is a failure if the child departs in tears." This was the first mention in the dental literature of measuring the success or failure of a child's appointment on anything other than a technical basis.

The term *behavior management* (or guidance), or its synonym *child management*, has been used repeatedly in dentistry for children. Generally, it has referred to methods used to obtain a child's acceptance of treatment in the dental chair. Considering the frequency with which these terms have been applied, it was somewhat surprising that a precise definition was non-existent when the first edition of this book was produced. For the purpose of that monograph, the term *behavior management* was defined as follows:

> It is the means by which the dental team effectively and efficiently performs treatment for a child and at the same time instills a positive dental attitude.

Let us briefly discuss the definition. Each component is essential to succeed in providing proper behavior management.

*The dental team*: As mentioned above, behavior management involves the entire dental team. Indeed, many dental auxiliaries are invaluable when it comes to dealing with children. Thus, all clinic personnel have a stake in guiding a child through a dental experience.

---

### Case 1.2

Mr. Z brought his 8-year-old daughter to the dental office for a recall appointment. The receptionist was on the phone. Without even glancing at the father and child she instructed them: "Mr. Z., please have a seat with your daughter in the waiting room. The hygienist will call for you shortly."

---

**Case 1.2, Discussion:** The dental team includes all staff members. The receptionist is the first team member that the child will meet and subsequently should also be trained in behavior management techniques. A child's dental experiences begins as soon as he or she enters the dental environment. In the above case scenario, a receptionist properly trained in behavior management would have stopped conversing on the phone and directed her attention to the child and parent. The pediatric dentistry treatment triangle dictates having the child as the focus and center of attention of the entire dental staff. It places the child at the apex of the triangle.

The receptionist should greet the child with a smile first, the parent second. Smiling is critical when greeting a child (Figure 1-3). Even at times that require all staff to wear facial masks such as during the Covid-19 pandemic, staff should be encouraged to smile. Smiling not only affects others but also one's self, lowering stress and improving cardiovascular

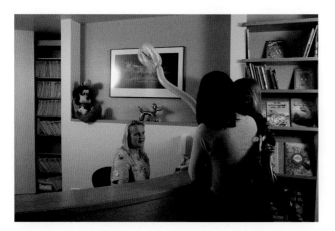

**Figure 1-3** The receptionist should greet the child with a smile first, the parent second. Smiling is critical when greeting a child. A practical tip is to place a mirror behind the reception desk thus reminding the receptionist to always smile while communicating with patients and parents.

function (Kraft and Pressman, 2012). A smiling person perceives others more positively (Alejandra et al., 2015). Positive nonverbal communication includes in addition to smiles, body language, eye contact and tone of voice. Proper body language is essential while communicating with children. Staff members who use a pleasant tone of voice and smile convey a message of the dental office being a non-threatening and calm environment to the child. The rule: "it's not what you say but how you say it" applies particularly with children who are more sensitive to body language than adults. Children encountering negative nonverbal communication might feel rejected and sense a feeling that the staff don't care about their well-being.

As mentioned above, the dental experience begins in the waiting room and so does behavior management. The front desk staff must not ignore poor behaviors displayed by patients. The tasks of setting limits and enforcing office policies are shared by all staff members. A child misbehaving in the waiting room should not be ignored. The dental team must project a degree of firmness when necessary. Children have to realize who is in charge, and they must be aware of what is expected of them. Once again, body language is employed. Speaking in a clear, firm tone while maintaining consistent eye contact with the child will assist in relaying the message. For a more detailed discussion on the dental team's role in patient management see Chapter 17.

Let us now consider the meaning of two key words in the proposed definition: effectively and efficiently. They are important to a contemporary definition.

*Effective* refers to providing high-quality dental care. Treatment should not be compromised to the detriment of the child's oral health. For example, postponing treatment of a 2-year-old with early childhood caries until the child is older is unacceptable. It is not behavior management, and it is not good dentistry. In addition, as mentioned above, non-invasive caries management techniques should be chosen as *part* of the behavior management strategy and not due to a *lack* of clinical behavioral skills that are mandatory for a pediatric dentist to possess and master.

*Efficient* treatment is a necessity in both public and private practices. Giving a child a ride in the chair over a series of appointments to "get used to the environment" without accomplishing any treatment objectives is inefficient. Neither today's busy parents nor the dentist can afford this unnecessary expenditure of time. A proper introduction to dentistry is indeed one of the fundamentals of behavior management and must be followed by necessary treatment in a timely manner. However, in certain situations, for example, while treating a child with autism, repeated visits are indeed *part* of the treatment strategy for these special children, as will be explained in Chapter 8.

Finally, the goal of behavior management is to instill a *positive dental attitude* and not to simply perform dental treatment. Pediatric dentists should be trained to be "dental teachers" and not "dental technicians" (Kupietzky 2004). Reasonable cooperation between child and operator is implicit in the proposed definition of behavior management. What is meant by "reasonable" varies from operator to operator. This will be discussed at length in Chapter 3.

### Case 1.3

Dr. K., the attending dentist at a dental school, observed her second-year graduate resident treating a 5-year-old patient who was undergoing a preventive resin restoration. The child was crying and constantly fidgeting on the dental chair. The resident was engrossed in the procedure and ignoring the child's behavior. Dr. K. interrupted the treatment and questioned the resident with regard to the child's persistent crying and poor behavior. The resident answered: "Oh, the crying doesn't bother me. I'm able to complete the treatment and that's what counts!"

***Case 1.3, Discussion:*** The development of a child's positive attitude is an integral part of the proposed definition of behavior management. That attitude may become positive after a single appointment or over a series of appointments. Indeed, the positive attitude sometimes takes years to develop. "Getting the job done" is not good enough. Many practitioners believe that getting the job done without taking into consideration their child patients' crying is behavior management. This is not good enough. A child who associates dental treatment with crying and whining is not undergoing a positive experience. If the child is expected to exercise preventive measures and continue regular treatments as an adult, a long-term positive attitude is mandatory. Evidence of this type of attitude is demonstrated in several ways. Periodically, a toddler may stroll into the office and hug the dentist or a member of the dental staff. Older children may express interest in becoming a dentist or dental hygienist. Parents may say that their children look forward to the semiannual checkups.

Note that this definition makes no mention of any specific techniques or modalities of treatment. Years ago, discussions with colleagues led to the belief that behavior management was absolutely non-pharmacologic. Some stated that behavior management was not truly practiced when drugs were employed to allay apprehension. There is no mention in the definition of any specific techniques or modalities of treatment. Indeed, behavior management may be defined and visualized as a continuum of techniques (Figure 1-4). Thus, the definition allows the exercise of individuality, and treatment methods are left to the clinician's discretion and direction. The challenge to the dentist is to satisfy the elements of the definition as frequently as possible and as safely as possible for each child in a dental practice. Every dentist must develop or adapt an interpretation for behavior management. This philosophical necessity influences the clinician's total approach to children in dental practice.

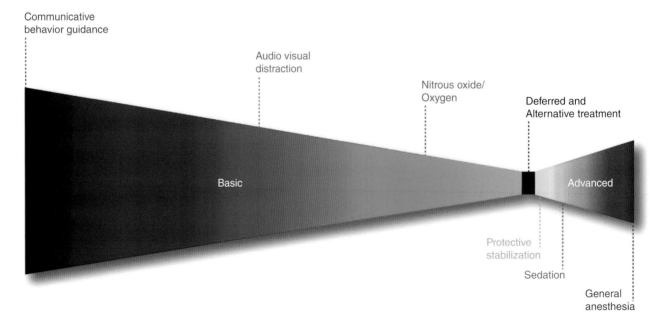

**Figure 1-4** Technique continuum. *Source:* Nelson (2013). © 2013, Elsevier.

Drugs are an adjunct to behavior management. Their use depends upon the philosophy and attitudes of the dentist. Personalities and educational backgrounds tend to influence clinical practice (Wright and McAulay 1973). However, as long as the proposed definition has been satisfied, it is behavior management. Not all techniques advocated in this book will be the reader's personal choice. But they are the means by which some dentists successfully practice behavior management with children.

Since the introduction of the above definition, the AAPD guidelines have stated (AAPD Reference Manual 2019/20):

> Behavior guidance techniques, both nonpharmacological and pharmacological, are used to alleviate anxiety, nurture a positive dental attitude, and perform quality oral health care safely and efficiently for infants, children, adolescents, and persons with special health care needs.

As the reader can see, these goals are very similar to the definition proposed for this book.

## Importance of Behavior Management

If a generalization can be made about dental curricula of the past, it is that the study of human behavior has played a secondary role to the scientific and technical learning. Recognizing this in academia, behavioral sciences now are included as an integral part of a modern curriculum, and behavior management has been a part of this newly developing course of study. It is taught using a multimedia approach. Educators have an array of literature and video films to call upon as effective teaching aids.

Concomitant with expanded teaching in behavior management, there was a surge in behavior management research. It was spurred on by educators like McDonald (1969) who wrote, "Until recently little research has been undertaken to provide answers to even the common problems associated with the guidance of the child's behavior in the dental office." The emphasis on the humanistic aspect in teaching and research had led to many fine studies published in the 1970s into the 1980s. Unfortunately, this research productivity has slowed (Wilson and Cody 2005). This is probably due to practical reasons, such as lack of funding and a greater emphasis on other aspects of pediatric dentistry. Funding has a great impact on research, and behavioral science research primarily is dependent upon government funding.

Considerable effort has been directed toward the question, "Why do people not attend a dentist regularly?" No simple answer has emerged. Indeed, there are so many related variables that it boggles the mind to think of them.

Does public opinion vary geographically? Does ethnic background affect viewpoints? What bearing would socioeconomic status have upon the question? Dentists have been aware of the jibes of humorists, artists and authors in the past. Have these reflected or shaped the public attitude? When studying individual behaviors, there are exceptions to cause–effect relationships. When dealing with large population groups with an increased number of variables, the difficulty in establishing relationships becomes more complex. Despite the difficulties, however, certain variables have cropped up repeatedly as sources of the public's negative attitude. The major variables are economics and dental anxiety or fear.

Investigations into dental utilization have repeatedly demonstrated that many children lack care. In a perfect world, every child would receive routine dental care. However, it is not a perfect world, and many children go uncared for. Why? Many have attempted to answer this question. It is complex, and no single variable can provide the answer. Numerous practical barriers to care have been described, such as a limited availability of dental providers, low reimbursement, and transportation difficulties. The cost of dental care has also been suggested as a chief reason why many do not attend to their dental needs on a regular basis. While this may be a good reason for some, poor attendance at low-income, government-sponsored dental programs discounts the economic factor as a chief barrier. It is apparent that the reasons many people do not seek regular dental care go well beyond the simplistic contention of some that if the economic impediment were removed, then demand and dental care standards would improve. Other factors obviously affect public attitude and utilization.

The importance of behavior management becomes more significant when assessing the effects of dental anxiety. It completely limits, or partially limits, utilization of health care (Berggren and Meynert 1984; Locker 2003). Dental anxiety is certainly associated with avoidance of care and lack of regular dental visits (Nicolas et al. 2007) and remains high and a hindrance to seeking dental treatment (Nermo et al. 2019).

While dental anxiety has been studied to determine its effect on dental care, little attention has been given to the age of onset of dental anxiety, even though it may have a bearing on the origins of dental fear. Locker et al. (1999) studied this variable and concluded that the onset of dental anxiety was overwhelming reported to have occurred during childhood. Considering the variables leading to childhood anxiety, there was a strong association with an aversive incident. Interestingly, half of the participants who had child anxiety onset also reported that they had a mother, father, or sibling who was anxious about dental treatment.

Dental anxiety or fear is not inherited. It is acquired, and it is commonly accepted that genesis occurs in childhood. A reasonable speculation is that these early dental fears shape a patient's attitude in adulthood. Research has demonstrated that adults holding negative dental attitudes can and do convey their feelings to their offspring. Therefore, it can be concluded that negative attitudes tend to be self-perpetuating (Figure 1-5).

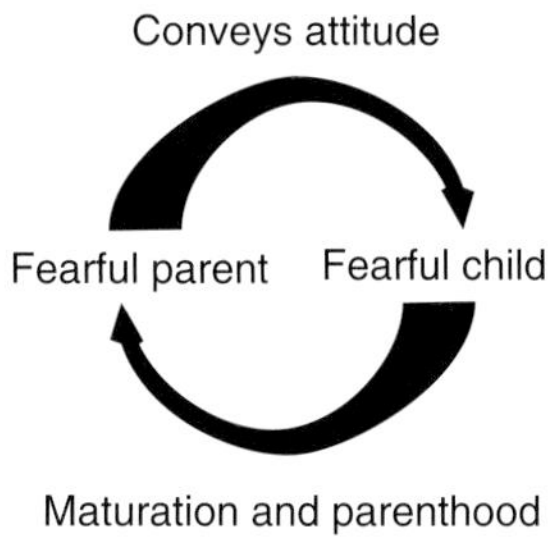

---

**Case 1.4**

Mrs. H. had heard about the importance of bringing her first and only child to the dentist at an early age. She and her husband decided to bring their 3-year-old for her first check-up. They both had negative dental experiences as children and also as adults, and they wanted to avoid similar situations for their daughter.

With her daughter Jessica on her lap, Mrs. H. tells the dentist: "I am so glad we came to see you. Both my husband and I are totally scared of going to the dentist and we don't want our daughter to feel the same. I hate going for my checkups!" Jessica begins to cry.

---

*Case 1.4, Discussion*: The parent should not have shared her dental anxiety with the dentist in the presence of her daughter. The well-trained and experienced pediatric dentist could have guided the parent to allow for a positive first visit if properly alerted before the exam. However, with quick reactions and improvisation, the appointment can be saved. The dentist talks directly to the child: "Oh, don't worry, I am a doctor of teeth not a dentist! My name is Dr. Sue and I would like to show you a special doll. We are going to have a great time and you are going to get a prize!" Later, after the examination, in the waiting room, the receptionist overhears Jessica telling her mother, "I liked going to Dr. Sue, but I am never going to a dentist, only to Dr. Sue." Patient management is all about

**Figure 1-5** Dental attitudes are passed from one generation to another. The illustration is a diagrammatic representation of the circular pattern.

improvising. That's what makes it so challenging and interesting!

The early part of this book focuses on thefamily and the home environment. If the circular pattern is to be interrupted, that is where we must begin. Since dental anxiety and fears are acquired, the most logical place to interrupt these sequential events is in childhood. It is far simpler to start patients with proper dental attitudes than to attempt to change deeply rooted negative ones. The establishment of a dental home as early as the first year of life will be expanded upon in Chapter 6. The early development of a positive relationship with the dentist will help shape the future behavior of both child and parent. It is obvious that in order to accomplish this, early dental exposures must occur with minimum psychological trauma. Thus, the need for continually improving behavior management becomes obvious and extremely important.

Considerable effort has been expended by organized dentistry over the years to improve its image. If we are to promote positive dental attitudes and improve the dental health of the public, then children are logically the keys to the future. No greater compliment can be paid to the dentist than when the parent of a young patient says, "I can't understand it, but my kids really look forward to going to the dentist." That is another reason for this book.

## References

Alejandra, S., Calvo-Merino, B., Tuettenberg, S. et al. (2015). When you smile, the world smiles at you: ERP evidence for self-expression effects on face processing. *Social Cognitive and Affective Neuroscience*, 10(10), 1316–1322. doi:10.1093/scan/nsv009

American Academy of Pediatrics Committee on Bioethics (2016). Informed consent in decision-making in pediatric practice. *Pediatrics*, 138(2), e20161484.

American Academy of Pediatric Dentistry (AAPD) (2017). The 2017 Survey of Pediatric Dental Practice. https://www.aapd.org/globalassets/media/aapd_chws_survey_pediatric_dentistry_final_2017.pdf. Accessed 12-8-19.

American Academy of Pediatric Dentistry (AAPD) (2019). Behavior guidance for the pediatric dental patient. The Reference Manual of Pediatric Dentistry 2019-2020/P, 266–279.

Berggren, U. and Meynert, G. (1984). Dental fear and avoidance. Causes, symptoms and consequences. *Journal of the American Dental Association*, 109, 247–251.

Kraft, T.L. and Pressman, S.D. (2012). Grin and bear it: the influence of manipulated facial expression on the stress response. *Psychological science*, 23(11), 1372-1378. doi:10.1177/0956797612445312.

Kupietzky, A. (2004). Dental teachers or dental technicians? *Pediatric Dentistry*, 15, 235.

Locker, D. (2003). Psychological consequences of dental fear and anxiety. *Community Dentistry and Oral Epidemiology*, 31, 144–151.

Locker, D., Liddell, A., Dempster, L. et al. (1999). Age of onset of dental anxiety. *Journal of Dental Research*, 78, 790–796.

McDonald, R.E. (1969). Dentistry for the Child and Adolescent. St. Louis, C. V. Mosby Co.

McElroy, C.M. (1895). Dentistry for children. *California Dental Association Transactions*, 85.

Nelson, T. (2013). The continuum of behavior guidance. *Dental Clinics of North America*, 57, 129–143. http://dx.doi.org/10.1016/j.cden.2012.09.006

Nermo, H., Willumsen, T., and Johnsen, J.K. (2019). Prevalence of dental anxiety and associations with oral health, psychological distress, avoidance and anticipated pain in adolescence: A cross-sectional study based on the Tromsø study, Fit Futures. *Acta Odontologica Scandinavica*, 77, 126–134. doi: 10.1080/00016357.2018.1513558

Nicolas, E., Collado, V., Faulks, D. et al. (2007). A national cross-sectional survey of dental anxiety in the French adult population. *BMC Oral Health*, 7, 12–17.

Piers, C. (2018). Millennials in dentistry: A journey toward understanding. *California Dental Association Journal*, 46, 355–357.

Raymond, E.H. (1875). Children as patients. *Dental Cosmos*, 17, 54.

Sel, Alejandra et al. "When you smile, the world smiles at you: ERP evidence for self-expression effects on face processing." *Social cognitive and affective neuroscience* vol. 10,10 (2015): 1316-22. doi:10.1093/scan/nsv009

Teuscher, C.W. (1973). *Editorial. Journal of Dentistry for Children*, 40, 259.

US Food and Drug Administration (2017). FDA Drug Safety Communication: FDA approves label changes for use of general anesthetic and sedation drugs in young children. https://www.fda.gov/media/104705/download, Accessed 1-1-2020.

Wilson, S. and Cody, W.E. (2005). An analysis of behavior management papers published in the pediatric dental literature. *Pediatric Dentistry*, 27, 331–337.

Wright, G.Z. and McAulay, D.J. (1973). Current premedicating trends in pedodontics. *Journal of Dentistry for Children*, 40, 185–187.

## 2

# Child Development: Basic Concepts and Clinical Considerations

*Tammy Pilowsky Peleg*

## Introduction

Pediatric patients encompass a wide range of ages and development stages from infants, toddlers, and children to pre-adolescents and adolescents, challenging clinicians in their attempt to communicate with children at different ages and adapt their practice, respectively. A national study of pediatric clinicians, performed in 13 diverse sites in the United States, established that a therapeutic relationship and individualized care significantly contributed to the success of pediatric health encounters, and early recognition of developmental and behavior problems was viewed as a priority to improve pediatric effectiveness (Tanner et al. 2009).

In order to understand child development in relation to dental behavior management, it has been suggested that pediatric dentists be acquainted with psychological development, in the areas of cognitive development, socioemotional and language development, and emotion regulation, including temperament (Bee and Boyd 2003). These will be addressed in this chapter.

## Typical Development

Among the most remarkable characteristics of human beings is how much our thinking changes with age, from the cognitive ability of an infant, to that of a toddler, an elementary school student, and adolescent (Siegler 1994). These changes represent brain development, from neurogenesis to neural migration, maturation, synaptogenesis, pruning, and myelin formation (Kolb and Gibb 2011), which starts from the prenatal period and continues well after birth, through childhood and early adulthood.

Since development has its basis in biology, its course is relatively predictable (Bjorklund and Causey 2017), and most children will acquire particular skills over a certain period of time (Johnson 2012). However, development is non-linear and does not occur at a constant rate, and variability occurs both within one child and across children (Johnson 2012). The brain develops in a complex interplay between genetics and environmental components (Kolb and Gibb 2011). Factors influencing development include biological elements such as hereditary characteristics, epigenetics, gender, prenatal influences, and nutrition, as well as non-biological elements such as nurture, experience, education, parent–child relationships, peer relationships, stress, drugs, and culture (Johnson 2012; Kolb and Gibb 2011; Nelson et al. 2019; Wang 2011).

Thus, development may be described by a series of consecutive accomplishments, as well as a process involving dynamic interactions between a child as an active organism and the physical and social environment (Scarr 1992), and should not be considered outside of its context (Bjorklund and Causey 2017), including characteristics such as demographic group, economic background, gender, culture, and other physiological characteristics (Siegler 2002).

Normal development is the developmental course that the majority of children in a population group will follow (Johnson 2012). Although considered an ideal standpoint or an expected distribution, the frequency distributions of many physical, biological, and psychological attributes, as they occur across individuals, tend to conform, to a bell-shaped curve (see Figure 2-1), named "The Normal Curve," or the Gaussian or Laplace-Gauss distribution (Strauss et al. 2006). As can be seen in Figure 2-1, most cases (68%) fall within one standard deviation of the mean, usually

*Wright's Behavior Management in Dentistry for Children*, Third Edition. Edited by Ari Kupietzky.
© 2022 John Wiley & Sons, Inc. Published 2022 by John Wiley & Sons, Inc.

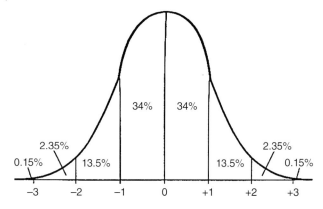

**Figure 2-1** The normal distribution of development.
*Source:* Strauss et al. (2006). © 2006, Oxford University Press.

referred to as *the mean range*, whereas only about 2%, indicating two standard deviations from the mean, are usually referred to as *deviation from the expected norm.*

Albeit expected heterogeneity, characteristic developmental milestones and their typical or average age at which they are achieved can be noted. Examples of typical development according to age are presented in Table 2-1 (Centers for Disease Control and Prevention CDC 2018).

Regarding dental practice, it has been found that mental age (the age level at which the child is functioning) and chronologic age (his/her actual age) influenced children's acceptance of dental treatment: 3-year-olds needed 20% more time to accept treatment than older children, and similarly, children with mental ages of 3 and 4 years needed

**Table 2-1** Developmental milestones by age.

| Age | Social and Emotional | Language and Communication | Cognitive | Motor |
|---|---|---|---|---|
| 2 months | Begins to smile at people, can briefly calm himself (may bring hands to mouth and suck on them), tries to look at parent. | Coos, makes gurgling sounds, turns head toward sounds. | Pays attention to faces, begins to follow things with eyes, begins to act bored (cries, becomes fussy) if activity doesn't change. | Holds head and begins to push up when lying on tummy, makes smoother movements with arms and legs. |
| 4 months | Likes to play with people and might cry when playing stops, copies some movements and facial expressions like smiling or frowning. | Babbles with expression and copies sounds heard, cries differently to show hunger, pain, or being tired. | Lets you know if she is happy or sad, responds to affection, reaches for a toy with hands. | Holds head steadily, may be able to roll over from tummy to back, holds and shakes a toy, brings hands to mouth. |
| 6 months | Knows familiar faces and recognizes if someone is a stranger, responds to other's emotions, likes to look at self in a mirror. | Makes sounds to show joy and displeasure, responds to sounds, likes taking turns while making sounds, responds to own name. | Looks around at things nearby, shows curiosity about things and tries to get things that are out of reach, passes things from one hand to the other. | Rolls over, begins to sit without support, when standing supports weight on legs and might bounce, rocks back and forth. |
| 9 months | May be afraid of strangers, may be clingy with familiar adults, has favorite toys, uses fingers to point at things. | Understands "no," makes a lot of different sounds, copies sounds and gestures of others. | Looks for things he sees you hide, plays peek-a-boo, picks up things like cereal o's between thumb and index finger. | Stands while holding on, sits without support, pulls up to stand, crawls. |
| 1 year | May be shy or nervous with strangers, cries when parent leaves, has favorite things and people, hands you a book when wants to hear a story. | Responds to simple spoken requests, uses simple gestures (nodding, waving "bye-bye"), makes sounds with changes in tone (sounds more like speech), says simple words, tries to copy words you say. | Explores things in different ways (shaking, banging), looks at the correct picture or thing when it is named, copies gestures, puts things in and out of a container. | Pulls up to stand, walks holding on to furniture, may take a few steps without holding on, may stand alone. |
| 18 months | Likes to hand things to others as play, has temper tantrums, may be afraid of strangers, shows affection to familiar people, plays simple pretend play (feeds a doll), may cling to parent in new situations. | Says several single words, points to show someone what he wants or to show something interesting. | Points to one body part, scribbles, can follow 1-step verbal instruction without gestures (sits when you say "sit down"). | Walks alone, may walk up steps and run, drinks from a cup, eats with a spoon. |

**Table 2-1** (Continued)

| Age | Social and Emotional | Language and Communication | Cognitive | Motor |
|-----|----------------------|----------------------------|-----------|-------|
| 2 years | Copies others especially adults and older children, gets excited when with other children, shows defiant behavior (doing what he has been told not to), plays mainly beside other children. | Names items in a picture book or points to things when they are named, knows names of familiar people and body parts, says 2–4 word sentences, follows simple instruction. | Sorts shapes and colors, completes rhymes in familiar books, plays simple make-believe games, might use one hand more than the other. | Stands on tiptoe, kicks a ball, begins to run, climbs furniture without help, walks up and down stairs holding on, makes or copies straight lines and circles. |
| 3 years | Copies adults and friends, shows affection for friends, takes turns in games, shows concern for a crying friend, understands the idea of "mine" or "his," shows a wide range of emotions, separates easily from parent, may get upset with major changes in routine. | Follows 2–3-step instructions, names most familiar things, understands words like "in" or "under," talks well enough for strangers to understand most of the time, carries on a conversation using 2–3 sentences. | Can work toys with buttons and moving parts, plays make-believe with toys and people, completes 3–4-piece puzzles, understands what "two" means. | Climbs well, runs easily, pedals a tricycle, walks up and down stairs one foot on each step, dresses and undresses self, turns door handle. |
| 4 years | Enjoys doing new things, is more and more creative with pretend play, prefers play with others than alone, cooperates with other children, often can't tell what's real and what's make-believe. | Talks about what she likes or is interested in, knows some basic rules of grammar, sings a song or recites a poem from memory. | Understands the idea of counting, starts to understand time, understands the idea of "same" and "different," plays board or card games. | Hops and stands on one foot for 2 seconds, catches a bounced ball most of the time, uses scissors, pours and cuts with supervision, draws a person with 2–4 body parts. |
| 5 years | Wants to please friends and to be like friends, likes to sing, dance, and act, shows concern and sympathy for others, is aware of gender, can tell what's real and what's make-believe, may visit a friend by himself, adult supervision is still needed. | Speaks very clearly, tells a simple story using full sentences, uses future tense, says name and address. | Counts 10 or more things, can draw a person with 6 body parts, can print some letters or numbers, copies a triangle and other shapes, knows about things used every day like money and food. | Stands on one foot for 10 seconds or longer, hops, may be able to skip and do a somersault, uses a fork, a spoon and sometimes a table knife, can use the toilet on her own, swings and climbs. |

*Source:* Adapted from Centers for Disease Control and Prevention (2018).

20% more time to accept treatment than children with higher mental ages (Rud and Kisling 1973). Accordingly, it may be suggested that pediatric dentists should consider age and development appropriate expectations when designing a treatment plan.

## Intelligence

Individual differences in intelligence are a prominent aspect of human cognitive ability and play a substantial role in influencing important life outcomes (Deary et al. 2009), such as predicting educational achievements and occupational and financial outcomes (Gottfredson 2003; Neisser et al. 1996). Intelligence is considered a relatively stable measure within childhood, from childhood to mid-adulthood, across young- to mid-adulthood, and in old age (Deary et al. 2000). Accordingly, Shaw et al. (2006) concluded that children who are adept at any one of the skills of reading, writing, and arithmetic tend to be good at others and grow into adults who are similarly skilled at diverse intellectually demanding activities. Thus, intelligence represents a quality of cognitive ability with predictive and operational implications.

An intelligence test is a standardized test, administered by a psychologist, assessing different cognitive abilities, representing the complex construct of intelligence. Examinees might be asked to explain concepts, to construct patterns, copy designs, etc. Many of the developmental and psychological evaluations, including intelligence tests, are

**Table 2-2** Classification of intelligence level.

| Classification | IQ | Deviation from Average in Z Scores | Lower limit of Percentile Range |
|---|---|---|---|
| Very superior | 130 and above | +2.0 and above | 98 |
| Superior | 120–129 | 1.3–2.0 | 91 |
| High average | 110–119 | 0.6–1.3 | 75 |
| Average | 90–109 | ±0.6 | 25 |
| Low average | 80–89 | −0.6−1.3 | 9 |
| Borderline | 70–79 | −1.3−2.0 | 2 |
| Extremely low | 69 and below | −2.0 and below | – |

*Source:* Adapted from Strauss et al. (2006).

standardized to use similar scales, in order to unify results, enable comparison between different measures available and between assessments (e.g., at different ages and before and after intervention), and to ease communication among clinicians. An individual's performance is compared to age-appropriate norms and converted to standard scores (usually, with a mean of 100, and a standard deviation of 15), allowing comparison of the child's functioning to that expected at his/her age and enabling identification of deviations from the expected development.

As can be seen in Table 2-2, intelligence scores (or intelligence quotient, IQ) are often classified into descriptive categories based on their deviation from the mean (adapted from Strauss et al. 2006). For example, assuming that given test scores are plotted on a normal curve, a child who scores an IQ of 130 is in the 98th percentile compared to his/her age, indicating that 98% of the children obtain lower scores, and only less than 2% will obtain a similar or higher score; thus, his/her performance will be described as very superior to his/her age. He/she will probably speak and reason more similarly to children that are older and might be addressed with more complicated ideas and communication.

## Intellectual Disability

Whereas most individuals' functioning falls into the mean range or above, about 2% of the populations' score of IQ or developmental quotient (DQ), the equivalent measure used in younger children, are significantly lower, at the extremely low end of the normal curve, that is, their IQ score is lower than 70 (see Table 2-2). These children may be described as showing developmental delay in attaining the expected milestones and may be described as having a developmental or intellectual disability.

Intellectual disability (previously referred to as *mental retardation* or *developmental delay*), is a developmental disability that includes both intellectual and adaptive functioning deficits in conceptual, social, and practical domains, that are present prior to the age of 18 years (DSM−5; American Psychiatric Association 2013). Varied degrees of severities exist, reflecting variability in functioning within the range of intellectual disability as well. Deficits in intellectual functioning might include difficulties such as reasoning, problem-solving, planning, abstract thinking, judgment, academic learning, and learning from experience. Deficits in adaptive functioning address difficulties in skills of everyday functioning, such as language and literacy, self-direction, interpersonal skills, and activities of daily living (APA 2013). Thus, children with an intellectual disability will require more care and supervision in life activities, including those related to their oral health (Diéguez-Pérez et al. 2016).

Intellectual disabilities are thought to be largely genetic in origin (Batshaw et al. 2012), and various genetic syndromes are characterized by a phenotype that includes intellectual disabilities (Najmabadi et al. 2011). However, many other etiologies exist, including prenatal risks such as maternal illness, or exposure to teratogens, perinatal complications such as birth injury, or prematurity, and postnatal risks such as malnutrition, or traumatic injury (Carr and O'Reilly 2016). Co-occurring mental, neurodevelopmental, medical, and physical conditions are frequent (APA 2013). For example, lifetime prevalence of epilepsy is 7.6:1,000 persons (Fiest et al. 2017), whereas an estimate of prevalence of epilepsy reached 22.2% in individuals with intellectual disabilities (Robertson et al. 2015).

General opinion is that patients with intellectual disability should be given the same level of dental treatment as those without intellectual disability (Maeda et al. 2005). However, the degree of unmet dental needs amongst this population is high compared to the general population (Waldman et al. 2009). These include poorer oral hygiene, less restorative treatment, and more periodontal problems (Diéguez-Pérez et al. 2016; Petrovic et al. 2011). Moreover, orofacial anomalies are not uncommon in children with chromosomal defects (Charles 2010), and abnormalities in dental development such as, delayed eruption and the presence of wear and abrasions are common (Diéguez-Pérez et al. 2016). Higher incidence of dental trauma was found in children with intellectual disabilities, and bruxism was found in children with cerebral palsy (Diéguez-Pérez et al. 2016). Thus, it would be considered prudent for children with intellectual disability to receive early and regular dental treatment to avert and limit the severity of their dental pathologies (Diéguez-Pérez et al. 2016).

In view of the need for proper care, some challenges necessitate attention. Physical challenges, including cerebral palsy, epilepsy, hearing or vision deficits, and hypotonia, may warrant special considerations. Behavioral aspects may create additional challenges. Patients with intellectual disability might have deficits in language comprehension and expression, attention, motor skills, and learning new tasks. Therefore, difficulty in rendering proper comprehensive treatment arises because it may be harder for individuals with intellectual disabilities to understand dental treatments and therefore cooperate (Maeda et al. 2005). Furthermore, anxiety about new situations is common, resulting in uncooperative behaviors such as crying, aggression, and agitation (Charles 2010). Individuals with intellectual disability may be less aware of dental problems and more dependent on their caregivers for decision-making and support for visiting the dentist and tooth-brushing. Therefore, it has been suggested that caregivers be given training in oral care and the use of dental services and support in dealing with patients who have problems tolerating tooth-brushing (Cumella et al. 2000); for more details, see Chapter 8.

Several recommendations have been suggested for dental practitioners regarding children with intellectual disabilities (Charles 2010). Some children may require significant preparation, with one or two visits to the office prior to treatment or examination to allow the child to become comfortable with the room and office staff. Caregivers are great resources for techniques that have been successful in helping their child's behaviors in the past. They can help the child in anticipating the scheduled visit, answer the child's questions and worries, or bring a favorite toy or blanket to help reduce anxiety. Appointments should be short, and time consideration may be made to reduce waiting time. Knowing the child's functioning level may help with behavioral expectations. For example, a 15-year-old who functions at the level of about 48 months may respond to similar management techniques as a typically developing 4-year-old would. To reduce anxiety and improve cooperation, it has been suggested to make an effort to communicate on the patient's level or through concrete or visual examples, so that the child understands what is going to happen, and to reward cooperative behaviors with frequent verbal reinforcement (see Chapter 8).

## Social Communication

Social skills are a set of learned behaviors that allow one to successfully initiate and perpetuate positive social interactions, such as sharing, helping, and initiating relationships (Gresham and Elliott 1990). Communication includes both verbal and non-verbal communication (Silove 2012): verbal communication includes aspects of execution (expression) and understanding language. *Expressive language* in the early stages includes vocalization, and later, use of spoken language. *Receptive language* refers to the understanding (semantics) of language, e.g., following instructions. *Articulation* refers to the motor aspects of producing language (i.e., how much of what is said is intelligible). *Prosody* refers to the musicality of the expressive language (e.g., intonation, or pitch). *Pragmatics* refers to the communicative aspects of language (e.g., using gestures in communication and using intonation to convey message, taking into account the knowledge of the recipient by saying "Tom, my teacher. . ." when the recipient does not know who Tom is). *Non-verbal communication* refers to gestures and facial expression used to communicate (e.g., smiling appropriately and pointing to request with coordinated eye contact) (Silove 2012). Table 2-3 presents examples of language development by age (Johnson 2012).

Table 2-3  Language development by age.

| Mean Age | Pre-language and Language Skills |
| --- | --- |
| 6–16 weeks | Coos in response to parental interaction and "motherese" (intonations of voice that mothers use when talking to their babies) |
| 4–8 months | Babbles; makes sounds that show early communicative intent in response to parent's verbal responses |
| 9–12 months | Babbling approximates the intonations of language |
| 12–14 months | First single words, pointing to objects |
| 15–24 months | Increase in word vocabulary, up to about 50 words, with a large variability in normal development |
| 2 years | Short two-word phrases |
| 3 years | Full sentences; may have grammatical errors; may not yet grasp concepts like "under" and "behind" |
| 4 years | Complex sentences |

*Source:* Adapted from Johnson (2012).

Through development, social interactions become prolonged, complexed, and abstract. These include face-to-face interactions in early infancy and sharing interest with others such as joint attention to a toy with the mother some months later (sharing and coordinating attention with others; Mundy 2016). Further advanced social interactions include: an emerging understanding of others as intentional beings, whose attention to outside objects may be shared (Carpenter et al. 1998), simultaneous play, pretend play with others, peer friendships, and group participation. Examples of social communication development are presented in Table 2-4.

As suggested for pediatricians (Voigt et al. 2011), different social-emotional motives are typically described through development, hence affecting the clinician's role and management. See Table 2-5.

Table 2-4   Social communication development by age.

| Age | Social Communication |
| --- | --- |
| 6 months | Shows interest in faces, particularly when spoken to; vocalizes differently to indicate happiness and unhappiness |
| 12 months | Copies actions (e.g., clapping hands), anticipates and shares enjoyment playing a game together such as "peek-a-boo" |
| 18 months | Points toward items of interest and back to the adult to show and share the enjoyment |
| 2 years | Communicates primarily with words supported by means such as gestures and pointing, beginning of awareness of their own feelings and the feelings of others |
| 3 years | Plays with other children, more spontaneous pretend play, can take turns in conversations, may find it difficult to stay focused on topic |
| 4 years | Initiates and joins in play with other children, engages in imaginative and role play, shares toys, takes turns in games without assistance, uses language for different reasons such as greeting, commenting, and asking questions |
| 5 years | Chooses friends and begins to develop friendships, takes on different roles within imaginative play |
| 5–11 years | Takes turns in group conversations; begins to understand jokes, sarcasm, and metaphors; adapts language and interaction with different people in different situations with some adult guidance; communicates about their own and others' feelings |
| 11–16 years | Adapts language to suit the situation and/or the listener independently, can negotiate with friends to resolve conflicts, understands sarcasm and uses slang terms |

*Source:* Adapted from Speech and Language Therapy Humber NHS Foundation Trust (2017).

## Emotion Regulation

The ability to effectively regulate emotions is a critical component of early socio-emotional development (Ekas et al. 2013). Emotion regulation describes the ability to respond to environmental stimuli with a range of emotions in a controlled manner (Panfile and Laible 2012), and refers to the processes by which we influence which emotions we have, when we have them, and how we experience and express them (Gross 1998).

The importance of biological foundation of emotion regulation in early years is emphasized by the significance of temperament (Thompson and Goodman 2010). Temperament is biologically based and linked to one's genetic endowment (Rothbart 2007), and is considered a relatively stable trait (Benson et al. 2009). Differences in temperament are evident even in young babies. From early infancy, children show considerable variability in their reactions to the environment—their activity level, biological regulation, adaptability, approach or withdrawal, sensitivity, intensity of emotions expressed, distractibility and attention span, and the amount of positive or negative mood (Thomas and Chess 1977). These reactions, together with the mechanisms that regulate them, constitute the child's temperament (Rothbart 2007). Three phenotypes of temperament are usually described (Chess 1990):

*The easy child* is regular in biological rhythms, adaptable, and approachable; usually adapts to change quickly; and is generally cheerful and expresses distress or frustration mildly.

*The difficult child* may be hard to get to sleep through the night, feeding and nap schedules may change daily, and may be difficult to toilet train because of irregular bowel movements. Typically, fusses or cries loudly at anything new and adapts slowly and often expresses a disagreeable mood and if frustrated may have a temper tantrum.

*The slow-to-warm-up child*, often called shy, has discomfort with the new and adapts slowly, but negative mood is often expressed slowly. Typically, stands at the edge of the group, clinging to the parent when taken to a birthday party. If pressured to join the group, shyness becomes worse, whereas, given time to accustom, can gradually become an active, happy partner.

In addition to innate characteristics, social-emotional contributions are crucial to the development of emotion regulation. Emotion regulation development begins from birth, in the effort of the caregiver to manage the newborn's arousal (Thompson and Goodman 2010). From infancy through adolescence, parents intervene in managing children's emotional reactions by soothing distress, engaging in exuberant play, organizing routines to create manageable emotional demands, and providing reassurance and

**Table 2-5** Communication with children in view of development.

| Age | Development | Practical Implication |
|---|---|---|
| Infant (0–1 years) | Development of a sense of trust; the infant is dependent on the caregiver for a sense of safety, security, and emotion regulation. | A soft tone of voice and gentle handling are important for a sense of trust and comfort; narrating to the infant what will happen during the visit can help both infant and caregiver feel more comfortable. |
| Toddler (1–3 years) | Desire for autonomy, stranger wariness, separation, and individuation; the caregiver serves as a "secure base" enabling to explore an unfamiliar environment and to whom to return when distressed. | Rapport can be built by allowing exploration, being sensitive to the need for "emotional refueling" from caregiver, and indulging the toddler's desire for autonomy and control, "First I will blow wind on your hand so you can feel it, then I will blow wind in your mouth. . .". |
| Preschooler (3–6 years) | Greater verbal and cognitive capacities than the infant and toddler, but often views the world in a very concrete and self-oriented way. | It is often helpful to reassure the child that the medical problem is not their fault or a result of bad behavior, and probe the child's understanding of the problem and the treatment. |
| School-aged (7–12 years) | Advancing verbal and cognitive development; thinking is more logical and organized; better able to understand cause and effect. | Rapport can be facilitated by inquiring about school, hobbies, and friends. Can be more actively engaged in the clinical interview, and assume a greater responsibility in the treatment process. |
| Adolescent (13–21 years) | In the process of gaining autonomy from his/her parents. | It is important to promote alliance with both the adolescent and caregiver, facilitated if communication respects and acknowledges both as independent agents. |

*Source:* Adapted from Voigt et al. (2011).

assistance in uncertain and demanding circumstances (Thompson and Meyer 2007).

The development of emotion regulation evolves throughout life (Cole et al. 2009) and corresponds to general development in other domains of functioning (Ekas et al. 2013). During the first year of life, infants progress from relying on external sources for regulation (e.g., caregivers), to being able to initiate behaviors that facilitate the regulation of emotions (Kopp 1989). Usually, 3-month-old infants are able to engage in behaviors such as self-soothing (e.g., thumb sucking) to regulate their arousal levels, 6-month-olds are able to voluntarily shift their attention away from a distressing stimulus (Calkins and Hill 2007), and 7- to 9-month-olds may discover that seeking out an interesting toy may alleviate distress (Kopp 1989). Socialization of emotional displays also begins, with parents responding differentially to various emotional displays by gender (Zeman et al. 2006).

By the end of their toddler years, children will have acquired an extensive emotion lexicon and an ability to use language to self-regulate by talking to themselves through emotionally challenging situations or expressing their concerns to a person who can help regulate their mood state (Zeman et al. 2006). Preschoolers obtain a repertoire of strategies to manage their emotions to adapt to the demands of the social context, including hiding their feelings

intentionally, such as saying "thank you!" when they receive an ugly sweater as a present. Interestingly, girls tend to substitute one emotional display for another, and boys tend to be more skilled at neutralizing their emotional expressions (Zeman et al. 2006). From middle childhood into adolescence (i.e., 12–18 years), emotion regulation ability increases, and decisions become more differentiated as a function of motivation, emotion type, and social-contextual factors (Zeman and Garber 1996).

Adolescence represents an important developmental period in the maturation of adult emotion regulation skills (Dahl 2001). It is a period of increased emotional reactivity, as well as increased vulnerability to psychopathologies associated with poor emotion regulation, including depression, anxiety, antisocial behavior, and behaviors such as alcohol use and nicotine dependence (Dahl 2001).

A well-known model of the process of emotion regulation (Gross 2002) offers a framework for addressing and assisting emotion regulation by suggesting five points in the emotion generative process that may be regulated:

1) Selection of the situation (e.g., avoiding stressful situations)
2) Modification of the situation (e.g., changing aspects that cause discomfort)

3) Deployment of attention (e.g., not looking at the stress-inducing stimulus such as a syringe while taking a vaccine shot)

4) Change of cognitions (thinking differently with regard to the situation—e.g., thinking of the importance of treatment in the long run, thus reappraising the situation)

5) Modulation of experiential, behavioral, or physiological responses (i.e., changing the reaction after the stimulus happened, hence suppressing the original reaction).

The first four of these are antecedent focused, occurring before the event, and the fifth is response focused, dealing with the response after the event happened. Application of this model to practice might be relevant when encountering a child who refuses treatment or who is expressing tension during the dental visit. Strategies to assist a child who is expressing unease during the dental visit may include enabling him/her to change an aspect (e.g., choosing the color of a handheld mirror) to help him/her gain a sense of control and reduce negative emotions, or distracting him/her from his/her stress by talking, or presenting a video screen to watch during treatment. Reappraisal of the situation might be encouraged through emphasizing positive aspects of the situation. These are usually more effective in emotion regulation than suppression of reaction.

---

### Case 2.1

Billy, a pleasant 4-year-old with no apparent health problems, arrived for his first dental visit. Following a parent–child interview with the dentist, he was separated from his parent without incident and subsequently introduced to the dental operatory environment.

During the clinical examination, the child cooperated but seemed fidgety and had to be reminded repeatedly to open his mouth and remain still. His conversation was limited and at an immature level. When x-rays were introduced, Billy smiled and seemed to be trying to cooperate, although he did not follow instructions. When he was asked to close his mouth on an occlusal film, the mouth remained open. After several frustrating attempts, the dentist realized that there was a problem. It was difficult to determine if Billy was a slow learner or was using an avoidance tactic.

---

***Case 2.1, Discussion:*** The initial interaction with Billy leads to the impression of a calm young boy, who is not stressed by the new situation, gets acquainted easily, and is generally very cooperative with new adults (the dentist and receptionist) and the unfamiliar setting (dental office). Although the novel situation and meeting with a stranger are expected to raise some tension, he presents himself calmly and even separates easily from his caregiver, which is not always the case at his age. His behavior is supported by his parent, who "frees" Billy to enter the treatment room independently, signaling an approval for his ability to manage his behavior properly. These adaptive behaviors, along with the interview with Billy's parent, which records nothing exceptional about his development, language, or communication, result in an impression of a typically developing and well-behaved young boy. In terms of *temperament*, he seems to be the "*easy child*" who is adaptable and approachable.

However, during the examination, several observations were noted. His speech was described as limited and at an immature level, he was easily distracted, and he failed to follow simple one-step instructions, such as to open his mouth, although he seemed to be trying to cooperate. Furthermore, an inconsistency was apparent between his smile and his inability to sit still and misunderstanding of instructions. These raised concerns regarding his *general cognitive development, language and communication abilities, and emotion regulation.*

There seems to be a discrepancy in Billy's behavior. Prior to examination, he displayed more mature behavior by easily being introduced to the clinic and entering the examination independently. Similarly, although not detailed, no exceptions were reported on the clinical interview. His behavior was very different during the examination. It may be suggested that his lower functioning during examination were not reflecting his full abilities, rather affected by temporal factors, such as the situational stress.

During examination, Billy was described as fidgety and needed repeated reminders to open his mouth and to remain still. These might have been attributed to his young age, or to some degree of hyperactivity; however, they were not present prior to the examination. Therefore, it may be that these behaviors reflect his struggle in coping with a higher level of stress and reveal his effort for *emotion regulation*. Nervous fidgeting has indeed been described in 3-year-old children when meeting a stranger, alongside fewer emotion regulation strategies and especially no cognitive emotion regulation strategies. Since cognitive strategies for emotion regulation are more advanced strategies, it has been suggested that the distress of this situation probably has left fewer cognitive resources available for the deployment of more advanced and varied emotion regulation strategies (Zimmermann and Stansbury 2003). This suggestion corresponds with Billy's behavior, who did not succeed in expressing his stress verbally by asking for assistance or calling for his parent.

In order to clarify the picture concerning Billy's development, a specific discussion with his parent might have been useful, as well as continuing the interaction with Billy, after tension reduction, or upon reunion with his parent. For example, most 3-or 4-year-old children know their age. When they are asked, "How old are you?", the reply is sometimes verbal, but frequently children identify their age by holding up the appropriate number of fingers. Another assessment procedure might be to ask youngsters to name the colors of their clothing. Questioning children in this way and noting the responses help the dentist to form an opinion at the initial assessment. Correct responses usually can alleviate some of the dentist's concern, whereas 4-year-old children who do not know their age or the color of their clothing may cause the clinician to question such youngsters' development to proceed with further screening. Ruling out Billy's behavior as being a delaying tactic, the dentist should employ calmer tones, slow and simple instructions, and possibly a shorter visit.

## Summary

This chapter presents basic aspects of child development, focusing on typical development and addressing cognitive, social, and emotional development as manifested in the areas of intelligence, social communication, and emotion regulation. Through these areas of development, it is apparent that biological and neurological foundations interact with environmental experiences to result in the child's growing abilities and competencies. In respect to clinical practice, the knowledge of age-appropriate behavior is beneficial in communication with the young patient contributing to management of behavior through the visit and meeting the specific needs of the young patient.

## References

American Psychiatric Association (APA). (2013). *Diagnostic and Statistical Manual of Mental Disorders (DSM-5®)*. American Psychiatric Pub.

Batshaw, M.L., Roizen, N.J., and Lotrecchiano, G.R. (2012). *Children with Disabilities*. Paul H. Brookes Publishing, Baltimore, MD.

Bee, H. and Boyd, D.R. (2003). *The Developing Child*, 10th ed. Needham Heights: Pearson Higher Education.

Benson, N., Oakland, T., and Shermis, M. (2009). Cross-national invariance of children's temperament. *Journal of Psychoeducational Assessment*, 27(1), 3–16.

Bjorklund, D.F. and Causey, K.B. (2017). *Children's Thinking: Cognitive Development and Individual Differences*. Sage Publications.

Carpenter, M., Angel, K., Tomasello, M. et al. (1998). Social cognition, joint attention, and communicative competence from 9 to 15 months of age. Monographs of the Society for Research in Child Development, i-174.

Carr, A. and O'Reilly, G. (2016). Diagnosis, classification, and epidemiology. In: A. Carr, C. Linehan, G. O'Reilly, P.N. Walsh, and J. McEvoy (Eds.), *The Handbook of Intellectual Disability and Clinical Psychology Practice*. Routledge.

Charles, J.M. (2010). Dental care in children with developmental disabilities: Attention deficit disorder, intellectual disabilities, and autism. *Journal of Dentistry for Children*, 77(2), 84–91.

Calkins, S.D. and Hill, A. (2007). Caregiver influences on emerging emotion regulation: Biological and environmental transactions in early development. In: J.J. Gross (Ed.), *Handbook of Emotion Regulation*. Guilford Press, New York, NY.

Chess, S. (1990). Temperaments of infants and toddlers. In: J.R. Lally (Ed.), Infant/Toddler Caregiving: A Guide to Social-Emotional Growth and Socialization (Second Edition) developed by WestEd, San Francisco.

Centers for Disease Control and Prevention. (2018). CDC's Developmental Milestones. Available at: https://www.cdc.gov/ncbddd/actearly/milestones/index.html

Cole, P.M., Dennis, T.A., Smith-Simon, K.E. et al. (2009). Preschoolers' emotion regulation strategy understanding: Relations with emotion socialization and child self-regulation. *Social Development*, 18(2), 324–352.

Cumella, S., Ransford, N., Lyons, J. et al. (2000). Needs for oral care among people with intellectual disability not in contact with Community Dental Services. *Journal of Intellectual Disability Research*, 44(1), 45–52.

Dahl, R.E. (2001). Affect regulation, brain development, and behavioral/emotional health in adolescence. *CNS Spectrums*, 6(1), 60–72.

Deary, I.J., Johnson, W., and Houlihan, L.M. (2009). Genetic foundations of human intelligence. *Human Genetics*, 126, 215–232. https://doi.org/10.1007/s00439-009-0655-4

Deary, I.J., Whalley, L.J., Lemmon, H. et al. (2000). The stability of individual differences in mental ability from childhood to old age: Follow-up of the 1932 Scottish Mental Survey. *Intelligence*, 28(1), 49–55.

Diéguez-Pérez, M., de Nova-García, M.J., Mourelle-Martínez, M.R. et al. (2016). Oral health in children with physical (Cerebral Palsy) and intellectual (Down Syndrome) disabilities: Systematic review I. *Journal of Clinical and Experimental Dentistry*, 8(3), e337–e343. https://doi.org/10.4317/jced.52922

Ekas, N.V., Lickenbrock, D.M., and Braungart-Rieker, J.M. (2013). Developmental trajectories of emotion regulation across infancy: Do age and the social partner influence temporal patterns. *Infancy*, 18(5), 729–754.

Fiest, K.M., Sauro, K.M., Wiebe, S. et al. (2017). Prevalence and incidence of epilepsy: A systematic review and meta-analysis of international studies. *Neurology*, 88(3), 296–303.

Gottfredson, L.S. (2003). Dissecting practical intelligence theory: Its claims and evidence. *Intelligence*, 31(4), 343–397.

Gresham, F.M. and Elliott, S.N. (1990). *Social Skills Rating Scale: Manual*. AGS Publishing, Circle Pines, MN.

Gross, J.J. (1998). The emerging field of emotion regulation: An integrative review. *Review of General Psychology*, 2(3), 271–299.

Gross, J.J. (2002). Emotion regulation: Affective, cognitive, and social consequences. *Psychophysiology*, 39(3), 281–291.

Humber NHS Foundation Trust (2017). *Social Communication Developmental Milestones*. Humber Teaching NHS Foundation Trust. https://www.humber.nhs.uk/search.htm

Johnson, S. (2012). *A Clinical Handbook on Child Development Paediatrics-E-Book*. Elsevier Health Sciences.

Kolb, B. and Gibb, R. (2011). Brain plasticity and behaviour in the developing brain. *Journal of the Canadian Academy of Child and Adolescent Psychiatry*, 20(4), 265.

Kopp, C.B. (1989). Regulation of distress and negative emotions: A developmental view. *Developmental Psychology*, 25(3), 343.

Maeda, S., Kita, F., Miyawaki, T. et al. (2005). Assessment of patients with intellectual disability using the International Classification of Functioning, Disability and Health to evaluate dental treatment tolerability. *Journal of Intellectual Disability Research*, 49(4), 253–259.

Mundy, P.C. (2016). *Autism and Joint Attention: Development, Neuroscience, and Clinical Fundamentals*. Guilford Publications.

Najmabadi, H., Hu, H., Garshasbi, M. et al. (2011). Deep sequencing reveals 50 novel genes for recessive cognitive disorders. *Nature*, 478(7367), 57–63.

Neisser, U., Boodoo, G., Bouchard, T.J., Jr. et al. (1996). Intelligence: Knowns and unknowns. *American Psychologist*, 51(2), 77.

Nelson, C.A., 3rd, Zeanah, C.H., and Fox, N.A. (2019). How early experience shapes human development: The case of psychosocial deprivation. *Neural Plasticity*, 1676285. https://doi.org/10.1155/2019/1676285

Panfile, T.M. and Liable, D.J. (2012). Attachment security and child's empathy: The mediating role of emotion regulation. *Merrill-Palmer Quarterly*, 58(1), 1–21.

Petrovic, B., Markovic, D., and Peric, T. (2011). Evaluating the population with intellectual disability unable to comply with routine dental treatment using the International Classification of Functioning, Disability and Health. *Disability and Rehabilitation*, 33(19–20), 1746–1754. doi:10.3109/09638288.2010.546934

Robertson, J., Hatton, C., Emerson, E. et al. (2015). Prevalence of epilepsy among people with intellectual disabilities: A systematic review. *Seizure*, 29, 46–62.

Rothbart, M.K. (2007). Temperament, development, and personality. *Current Directions in Psychological Science*, 16(4), 207–212. https://doi.org/10.1111/j.1467-8721.2007.00505.x

Rud, B. and Kisling, E. (1973). The influence of mental development on children's acceptance of dental treatment. *European Journal of Oral Sciences*, 81(5), 343–352.

Scarr, S. (1992). Developmental theories for the 1990s: Development and individual differences. *Child Development*, 63(1), 1–19.

Shaw, P., Greenstein, D., Lerch, J. et al. (2006). Intellectual ability and cortical development in children and adolescents. *Nature*, 440(7084), 676–679. doi:10.1038/nature04513.

Siegler, R.S. (1994). Cognitive variability: A key to understanding cognitive development. *Current Directions in Psychological Science*, 3(1), 1–5.

Siegler, R.S. (2002). Variability and infant development. *Infant Behavior and Development*, 25(4), 550–557.

Silove, N. (2012). Developmental assessment in the young child. In S. Johnson (Ed.), *A Clinical Handbook on Child Development Paediatrics-E-Book*. Elsevier Health Sciences.

Strauss, E., Sherman, E.M.S., and Spreen, O. (2006). *A Compendium of Neuropsychological Tests*, 3rd ed. Oxford University Press, New York.

Tanner, J.L., Stein, M.T., Olson, L.M. et al. (2009). Reflections on well-childcare practice: A national study of pediatric clinicians. *Pediatrics*, 124(3), 849–857.

Thomas, A. and Chess, S. (1977). *Temperament and Development*. Bruner/Mazel, New York.

Thompson, R.A. and Goodman, M. (2010). Development of emotion regulation: More than meets the eye. In: A. Kring and D. Sloan (Eds.), *Emotion Regulation and Psychopathology*. Guilford, New York, NY.

Thompson, R.A. and Meyer, S. (2007). The socialization of emotion regulation in the family. In: J.J. Gross (Ed.), *Handbook of Emotion Regulation*. Guilford Press, New York.

Voigt, R.G., Macias, M.M., and Myers, S.M. (2011). *Child development: The basic science of pediatrics. Developmental and Behavioral Pediatrics*. American Academy of Pediatrics, Elk Grove, IL.

Waldman, H.B., Rader, R., and Perlman, S.P. (2009). Health related issues for individuals with special health care needs. *Dental Clinics of North America*, 53(2), 183–193. doi: 10.1016/j.cden.2008.12.008. Epub 2009/03/10.

Wang, P.P. (2011). *Nature, nurture, and their interactions in child development and behavior.* In: R.G., Voigt, M.M., Macias, and S.M. Myers (Eds.), *Developmental and Behavioral Pediatrics.* American Academy of Pediatrics, Elk Grove, IL.

Zeman, J. and Garber, J. (1996). Display rules for anger, sadness, and pain: It depends on who is watching. *Child Development*, 67, 957–973.

Zeman, J., Cassano, M., Perry-Parrish, C. et al. (2006). Emotion regulation in children and adolescents. *Journal of Developmental & Behavioral Pediatrics*, 27(2), 155–168.

Zimmermann, L.K. and Stansbury, K. (2003). The influence of temperamental reactivity and situational context on the emotion-regulatory abilities of 3-year-old children. *The Journal of Genetic Psychology*, 164(4), 389–409. doi: 10.1080/00221320309597886

**3**

# Children's Behavior in the Dental Office

*Jaap S. J. Veerkamp and Gerald Z. Wright*

## Introduction

This chapter discusses the reactions of children to dental treatment. It is intended to assist the dental health team in raising its perception of children's behavior. The information will hopefully help dental professionals attain a greater sensitivity to the underlying factors which contribute to children's reactions in the dental office. It is this kind of broad understanding that facilitates decisions concerning the management techniques that are likely to be successful for an individual child patient. Although clinical suggestions are offered on fostering positive reactions and dealing with negative ones, this is not the chapter's main purpose: that information receives more attention in Chapter 7.

Historically, early writing on the subject of children's behavior in the dental office began by following two lines of thought. First, a number of techniques for the "containment" of children in the dental environment were suggested. Second, the need for psychological knowledge and its application to children's treatment was realized.

In the 1930s, professionals began to assess and detail children's reactions to dentistry. There was an immediate interest in these writings which has been maintained and has steadily grown. The writings have taken two forms. The early descriptions were, for the most part, based on clinical observations and personal opinion. Collectively, these writings can be highly informative and useful in supporting theoretical guidelines. In the 1960s, controlled data-seeking investigations began to appear in the dental literature. As a result of differing viewpoints and experimental designs, the information gleaned from these studies can sometimes be confusing or contradictory. Nonetheless, they are helpful.

Guidelines are currently research based. The focus is on evidence-based clinical trials (Roberts et al. 2010), which implies the use of randomized clinical trials. Since there has been a deficiency of this type of pediatric dentistry research over the past few decades, evidence often is gathered from other disciplines such as psychology or medicine (Gustafsson et al. 2010; Klingberg 2008).

The writings describing children's behavior in the dental office have centered around three main areas. These areas include (1) classifying children's behavior; (2) describing various forms of behavior, wherein negative behavior patterns have been labeled; and (3) elaborating on factors which affect behavior in the dental environment. Hence, these main areas have served as natural focal points for the organization of this chapter.

## Classifying Children's Behavior

Numerous systems have been developed for classifying children's behavior in the dental environment. The knowledge of these systems holds more than academic interest and can be an asset to clinicians in two ways: it can assist in evaluating the validity of current research, and it can provide a systematic means for recording patients' behaviors. Interestingly, most classification systems that are used in clinical practice nowadays were spawned from research investigations.

When a clinician treats a child patient, the first issue of concern is the child's behavior. The clinician has to classify the behavior (mentally at least) to help guide the management approach. There is wide variation between classification systems. One of the first was described by Wilson (1933), who listed four classes of behavior—normal or bold, bashful or timid, hysterical, and rebellious. During the same year, Sands wrote that children were of five types—hypersensitive or alert, nervous, fearful, physically

*Wright's Behavior Management in Dentistry for Children*, Third Edition. Edited by Ari Kupietzky.
© 2022 John Wiley & Sons, Inc. Published 2022 by John Wiley & Sons, Inc.

unfit, and stubborn. These systems identified behaviors during dental procedures that mainly limited success of treatment. Nowadays, classification systems are often based on principles used in psychological questionnaires. Child behaviors during daily, non-dental situations may be placed into categories that summarize the personality of the child (Klaassen et al. 2002). This provides information on the attitude of the child that is unrelated to treatment situations which may assist the dentist in predicting the way children will react to the dental experience before the actual appointment.

One of the most widely used systems was introduced by Frankl et al. in 1962. It is referred to as the *Frankl Behavioral Rating Scale*. The scale divides observed behavior into four categories, ranging from definitely positive to definitely negative. A detailed description of the scale is provided in Table 3-1.

The Frankl classification method, as seen in Table 3-1, is often considered the gold standard in clinical rating scales, mainly as a result of its wide usage and acceptance in pediatric dentistry research. Its popularity as a research tool has stemmed from three features. First, it is functional, as has been demonstrated through repeated usage. Second, it is quantifiable. Since it has four categorizations, numerical values can be assigned to the observed behavior. Finally, it is reliable. A high level of agreement among observers can be obtained. In fact, many investigations using this tool have shown the level of agreement to be 85% or higher—a very acceptable level in this type of research. These are the criteria for a measurement tool that are necessary for a successful investigation.

Other classification systems similar to the Frankl scale have been developed. Most notable are Likert-type scales,

**Table 3-1** The Frankl Behavior Rating Scale: A four-point scale with two degrees of positive behavior and two degrees of negative behavior.

---

### Categories of Behavior

---

Rating 1: Definitely negative

Refusal of treatment, crying forcefully, fearfulness, or any other overt evidence of extreme negativism.

Rating 2: Negative

Reluctance to accept treatment, uncooperative behavior, some evidence of a negative attitude but not pronounced (i.e., sullen, withdrawn).

Rating 3: Positive

Acceptance of treatment, at times cautious, willingness to comply with the dentist, at times with reservation but follows the dentist's directions cooperatively.

Rating 4: Definitely positive

Good rapport with the dentist, interested in the dental procedures, and laughing and enjoying the situation.

---

which have five levels of response (Rud and Kisling 1973). The studies of Venham et al. (1977) used the five-point scales to measure anxiety and behavior (self-report and proxy-report). Repeating their study, it was found that the two scales correlated so highly that the use of a single scale seemed appropriate (Veerkamp 1995a). Other scales, such as the Houpt clinical rating scale (Houpt 1993) or the self-reporting Wong and Baker (1988) facial scale, are comparable systems. These are also useful in clinical settings, as well as research.

Self-report is the first method of choice when studying pain and/or anxiety. However, children under eight years of age have limited cognitive capacities; to depend on the accuracy of their reporting, ten Berge (2001) offers a greater risk of incorrect information. Young children have a greater tendency to give socially acceptable answers, answers that they perceive will please the person asking the question. To improve the information on self-reporting rating scales for young children, some investigators have used small icons of dentistry-related situations or happy-to-sad faces as clinical endpoints (Chapman and Kirby-Turner 2002; Venham and Gaulin-Kremer 1979; Wong and Baker 1988). An example of such a scale is shown in Figure 3-1. In general, visual analogue scales are the most effective with young children, with "very cooperative" and "uncooperative" as the clinical endpoints.

In her literature review, Aartman (1998) stated that the method of choice is to take two measurements, e.g., a self-report and an independent observer, and base conclusions on a combination of both reports. However, this approach may be useful for some researchers but impractical for clinicians.

Classification procedures have important clinical application. Many general dentists have up to 2,000 patients in their practices. If a fifth of these are children, the practice would contain 400 child patients. It is impossible to recall how each child reacted during former visits. For pediatric dentists, having 2,000 children in a practice and remembering their behaviors is even more daunting. Since the behavior of a child is an integral factor in the treatment planning, noting reactions can be of major assistance. Developing the habit of systematically recording patients' behaviors on their clinical records takes little effort and can result in a big payoff.

Knowledge of the progression of a child's behavior during a series of appointments, or over a period of years, can assist in behavior management. It provides a base for planning. To gather this information, a separate column on the patient chart should be reserved for recording behavior. Figure 3-2 records a child's behavior over several appointments using the Frankl Rating Scale. Note that the scale lends itself to a shorthand form. A child displaying positive cooperative behavior can be identified by jotting down

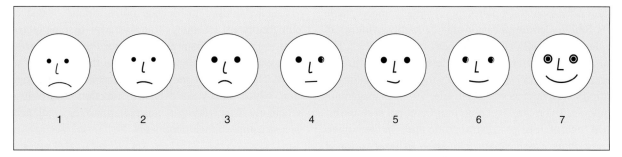

**Figure 3-1** A visual analogue scale using happy and sad faces as its endpoints. *Source:* Chapman and Kirby-Turner (2002). © 2002, Springer nature.

(a)

| PROCEDURE | ANES. | BEH. |
|---|---|---|
| X rays | — | T.S. D<br>— → + |
| d. O Ag | 1.8 Lido 2% | T.S. D<br>+ |
| N.O. Ag | 1.8 Lido 2% | + + |
| | | |

(b)

Initial exam, PA + 2BW, BEH — ---> TSD ---> +

1.8 2% LIDO, 1:100,000 EPI  BEH — ---> VC ---> +

1.8 2% LIDO, 1:100,000 EPI  BEH  + +

**Figure 3-2** A section of a patient's chart showing a child's behavior recorded over a series of appointments (a). A separate column on the chart is reserved for this purpose. Notation of behavior should also be made in computerized patient charts (b). Courtesy of Elaine Schroit.

(+) or (++). Conversely, uncooperative behavior can be noted by (−) or (=). This enables a child's performance to be discerned at a glance. Similar notation of behavior can easily be made in computerized patient charts using appropriate software.

Rating scales, such as the Frankl Scale, have two clear shortcomings. First, they do not communicate sufficient clinical information for uncooperative children. If a child is judged to be (−), the scale does not identify the type of negative behavior. Thus, the dentist using this classification system has to qualify as well as categorize the reaction. An example might be: (−) timid. If behavior ranges from negative to positive during a visit, a simple notation could be (− > +). The management technique can also be recorded. TSD shows that behavioral change was accomplished by the T (Tell), S (Show), D (Do) technique (Addelston 1959). Personal abbreviations can be developed for the various situations such as (−) INJ, which reminds the dental team that behavior was negative at the time of injection or VC indicating the use of voice control. Second, a behavioral scale represents a child's performance during the actual treatment. It has no prognostic value. Nonetheless, it helps clinicians to prepare for the child's future behavior, based on past performances, and to guide the behavior during treatment instead of simply reacting. If a demanding parent claims an emergency appointment

for her son and the secretary is able to notice at a glance the negative behavior of the child displayed during earlier sessions, it might help her reserve a proper time slot instead of squeezing the child between two other appointments. Simple, direct rating scales show a high inter- and intraobserver reliability (Rud and Kisling 1973). Studies have shown substantial correlations between observations of child behaviors during sequential treatment sessions as well as within parts of each treatment appointment (Veerkamp 1995b). Thus, it would be extremely beneficial for dentists to learn and make use of one of the classification systems on child behavior. A few digits are read more easily than a long, detailed report on a child's behavior.

Before leaving this subject, it is important to note that all clinicians do not perceive behavior in precisely the same way. It follows, therefore, that some dentists feel compelled to develop their own classification consistent with their views of children's reactions to dentistry. Furthermore, not only do clinicians perceive children's behavior in different ways, but they also tolerate children's behavior differently (Alwin et al. 1994). As long as the dentists train the staff to understand the notation, every system works.

The interesting concept of the clinician's "tolerance level" was introduced by Wright (1975) in his original behavior management book. Consider children who present with borderline cooperative-uncooperative reactions to dentistry.

What is acceptable to Dr. Jones may be totally unacceptable to Dr. Smith. Certain behavior may be highly irritating to one dentist but only slightly bothersome to another. The dentists have different tolerance levels. They withstand stress differently, and this influences their classifications of children's behaviors as well their selection of management techniques. Tolerance level is an important but seldom-discussed concept. It helps to explain differences in the numerous descriptive classifications. Moreover, an appreciation of this concept points out the necessity for educators to train dentists in a variety of management techniques or advise them to focus on specific patient categories and refer the others to avoid disappointments during treatment.

## Descriptions of Behavior

In describing child behavior, the interest or emphasis in the literature has been on behaviors that dentists find difficult to deal with or are inappropriate in some way. However, there are other aspects of behavior that sometimes can be important, and dentists may need to consider these as well. Questionnaires that appear in Chapter 7 can be used to investigate children's environments, how children react to different situations, and how they express fears prior to and during aversive situations. Children's methods of play and oral habits are forms of behavior. Astute receptionists can observe children playing in the waiting room and often provide important information to the clinician.

When a dentist examines a child patient, one type of behavior—the cooperative behavior—is always assessed because a key to the rendering of treatment is cooperative ability. Most clinicians, consciously or not, characterize children in one of three definable ways (Wright 1975):

1) Cooperative,
2) Lacking in cooperative ability, or
3) Potentially cooperative.

Knowing the clinical aspects of these distinctive child behaviors is important to behavior management and treatment planning.

### Cooperative Behavior

Most children seen in dental offices cooperate. This is substantiated by dental office experiences, as well as indirect data from behavioral science studies (ten Berge 2001). Cooperative children are reasonably relaxed. They have minimal apprehensions. They may be enthusiastic. Further description of their reactions appears in Frankl's positive groupings (Table 3-1).

Children judged to be cooperative can be treated by a straightforward, tell-show-do and behavior-shaping approach (see Chapter 7). When guidelines for their behavior have been established, they perform within the provided framework. These children present a "reasonable level" of cooperation, which allows the dentist to function effectively and efficiently. They seldom require pharmacologic adjuncts to help accomplish their treatments.

### Lacking Cooperative Ability

In contrast to the cooperative child is the child lacking cooperative ability. This could include very young children (less than three years of age) with whom communication cannot be established. Comprehension cannot be expected. If their treatment needs are urgent, they can pose major behavioral problems. Pharmacologic adjuncts may be required for their treatment. McDonald (1969) referred to these children as being in the *pre-cooperative stage*. For these children, time usually solves the behavior problems. As they grow older, they develop into cooperative dental patients and treatment is provided with behavior shaping.

Another group of children who lack cooperative ability are those with specific debilitating or handicapping conditions. The severity of their conditions often prohibits cooperation in the usual manner. Obtaining information on their intellectual development can give the dentist valuable information about the expected level of cooperation. To avoid painful questions, the dentist can ask the child about school ("By the way, aren't you at school now? In which class are you?") and relate the school level to the child's biological age. At times, special behavior management techniques, such as body restraints or sedation, are employed to control body movements. While the treatment is accomplished, major positive behavioral changes cannot be expected.

In most Western societies, thrust in intellectual impairment services is community-oriented, and as large institutions for the mentally challenged are phased out, more children with special needs are being treated in dental offices today. More and more, these children and adults are living in group and private homes within residential communities. Many dental faculties have recognized this societal change, and programs have been established to prepare undergraduate and postgraduate students to meet the foreseeable demand. Chapter 8 provides a more complete description of the disabled patient.

### Potentially Cooperative Behavior

Until recently, the nomenclature applied to a potentially cooperative child was "behavior problem." The child may be healthy or disabled. However, there is a difference between the potentially cooperative child and the child lacking cooperative ability. The potentially cooperative child has the capability to behave well. It is an important distinction. When characterized as potentially cooperative, the judgment is that the child's behavior can be modified: the child has the age-related cognitive capacities to learn to deal with dentistry and can become cooperative.

Perhaps one of the most challenging issues for the clinician is to determine what behavior can be expected from a new patient. There are those children who may approach the dental office crying or screaming. Their behavior is apparent. Conversely, there are children who are quiet, shy, or withdrawn. These children can be hard to read. They may or may not be difficult to treat. Behavioral science researchers in dentistry and allied professions have made efforts to predict children's behaviors before their arrival at a dental clinic. Since the 1990s, the Children's Fear Survey Scale-Dental Subscale (CFSS-DS) has received considerable attention. Initially presented by Cuthbert and Melamed (1982), the CFSS-DS has been used worldwide. Indeed, it has been translated and tested in various cultures and nations such as Finland, the Netherlands, Bosnia, India, and Japan (Bajric et al. 2011; Nakai et al. 2005; Singh et al. 2010; ten Berge et al. 1998). All venues had similar positive findings when rating fear/anxiety.

The CFSS-DS scale has been used in large patient samples between 4 and 14 years of age. It is considered to work well on a group basis and has been evaluated as a diagnostic tool on an individual level. In a report comparing properties of different self-report measures, it was concluded that CFSS-DS was preferred, as it has better psychometric properties measuring dental fear more precisely (Aartman 1998). The psychometric properties were further analyzed and found appropriate for children from 4–14 years (ten Berge 2001). The test consists of 15 items that are shown in Figure 3-3. Each item has five different scores, ranging from one (not afraid at all) to five (very afraid). Thus, there is a possible total score range from 15–75. Scores below 31 suggest an absence of dental anxiety, or low anxiety, whereas those between 31 and 39 are at risk for developing dental anxiety. Above 39, the dental anxiety definitely needs to be taken into account. Children in this group have extremely high anxiety that is undoubtedly due to more than a single bad experience or some age-related apprehension. In general, this group needs special attention, treatment time, and a protocol, likely involving pharmacotherapeutic approaches. Today, the test is mainly used in two versions, one to be answered by the child who reads (about eight years or older) and a proxy (parental) version.

The proxy version of CFSS-DS is used most frequently. It is especially applicable when children cannot read. How accurate are the parental reports? In an attempt to answer the question, Krikken et al. (2013) assessed the accuracy of parents reporting their children's dental fears. The study was conducted with 326 children, 7–11 years old. The children completed the child version of the dental subscale and their parents filled out a questionnaire about their children's dental fears. The two groups' responses were

**I. How afraid Is your child of ..........**

| | Not afraid at all | A little afraid | A fair amount afraid | Pretty much afraid | Very afraid |
|---|---|---|---|---|---|
| | 1 | 2 | 3 | 4 | 5 |
| 1. Dentists .................................................. | O | O | O | O | O |
| 2. Doctors .................................................. | O | O | O | O | O |
| 3. Injection (shots) ..................................... | O | O | O | O | O |
| 4. Having somebody examine your mouth ....... | O | O | O | O | O |
| 5. Having to open your mouth ...................... | O | O | O | O | O |
| 6. Having a stranger touch you ................... | O | O | O | O | O |
| 7. Having somebody look at you ................... | O | O | O | O | O |
| 8. The dentist drilling ................................. | O | O | O | O | O |
| 9. The sight of the dentist drilling .............. | O | O | O | O | O |
| 10. The noise of the dentist drilling .............. | O | O | O | O | O |
| 11. Having somebody put instruments in your mouth | O | O | O | O | O |
| 12. Choking ............................................. | O | O | O | O | O |
| 13. Having to go to the hospital ..................... | O | O | O | O | O |
| 14. People in white uniforms ........................ | O | O | O | O | O |
| 15. Having the nurse clean your teeth ......... | O | O | O | O | O |

**Figure 3-3** Items on The Child Fear Survey Schedule-Dental Subscale (CFSS-DS). *Source:* Based on Krikken et al. (2013); Milgrom et al. (1995).

compared, and the results suggested that a great majority of parents are able to rate the dental fear of their children. If there were discrepancies, parents generally tended to estimate the dental fears of their children slightly higher than their children.

In the Dutch population, an estimated 14% of children suffer from dental fear (ten Berge et al. 2002). Hence, there has been considerable interest and research on the subject of dental fear and anxiety at the Academic Center for Dentistry Amsterdam, and it is recognized that the CFSS-DS is a one-dimensional measure of dental fear. It could help clinicians predict the behavior of children. In the Netherlands, children whose dental anxiety scores are between 31 and 39 are considered to be in the potentially cooperative category. Knowing that they are anxious—and not simply withdrawn or shy—the important issue is to develop strategies to prevent potentially cooperative children from developing serious behavior problems. Research tells us that dental anxiety is related to painful procedures, so avoiding that is the first step (Dahlander et al. 2019). From a general point of view, repeated exposure is the most beneficial technique to increase cooperation. However, busy parents may be reluctant to allow the dentist to advance slowly. Dentists should discuss this approach with the parent and how valuable this approach is for their child (see Chapter 7).

The dental literature is saturated with anecdotal descriptions of potentially cooperative patients. Moreover, their adverse reactions have been given specific tags or labels that conveniently convey to dentists, in as few words as possible, the essence of the clinical problem. The following are some of the more common labels that have been attached to potentially cooperative behaviors. While it is recognized that almost all negative behaviors are caused by a form of anxiety or rejection of dental treatment, the descriptions only relate to the observed behaviors. However, the dentist must keep in mind that behavior might change during sequential sessions. It is also dependent on situational or personal aspects of the child, the parent, and the dentist. Since the initial behavior is the starting point of the contact with the operating dentist, we need to focus on that to start with.

**Uncontrolled Behavior**

When an uncontrolled behavior reaction is observed in a potentially cooperative patient, it usually occurs in a child of three–six years of age on the first dental visit. The reaction, a form of tantrum, may start in the reception area or even before the child enters the outer office. It is characterized by externalized behavior—tears, loud crying, physical lashing out, and flailing of hands and legs. All are suggestive of anxiety and an extroverted personality type. This heightened state is usually seen in preschoolers, but acute stress can cause a five- or six-year-old to regress to an earlier form of behavior and act in this way.

Because of the furnishings in most dental clinics, the child must be dealt with expeditiously to prevent personal physical harm. If any success is anticipated, a line of communication must be established with the patient. In most cases, a time-out will help. If there is no behavior control, it is impossible to explain procedures. Some form of restraint or sedation may be needed to begin any form of treatment. However, most children can comprehend the situation, and their behavior can be controlled. Thus, the potentially cooperative child can become a cooperative patient.

---

**Case 3.1**

Identical twin girls, aged eight years, were referred to a pediatric dentist. One girl was described as a "behavior problem." Jane had the first appointment. Her behavior during the examination was acceptable. Judy, her twin sister, demonstrated out-of-control behavior in the reception area. Once separated from her parent, her cooperation improved. Later, the parent was questioned about these two vastly different reactions. It seemed that Jane had always been the leader – better in school, better in sports, and helpful at home. She was used as a model for Judy. As a consequence of the discussion, at the first scheduled operative dentistry appointment, their appointment sequence was reversed. Judy was the model and she responded admirably.

---

*Case 3.1, Discussion*: School-age children tend to model their behavior after that of adults or older siblings. Out-of-control, immature behavior, which usually occurs with younger children, would not be consistent with their self-concept. If out-of-control behavior does occur in the older child, there are likely deep-rooted reasons for it. An attempt to understand the reasons for this behavior often reveals unusual situations and can lead to a solution.

In this case, where the lack of control occurred in an eight-year-old girl, the pediatric dentist realized that it was unusual and took the time to try and understand the situation. Why was Judy acting in this way? Was she really afraid? Was she rebelling? One reason might be that she was tired of always being second. Another reason might be that she was fulfilling her family's expectations. Whatever the reason, the dentist solved the problem by reversing the expected protocol in the family. This solution would not have come about without a post-clinic interview by the dentist.

### Challenging or Defiant Behavior

Although challenging behavior can be recognized in children of all ages, it is more typical of those in the public school age group. It is one way that some children deal with aversive situations. To some extent, defiant behavior is controlled behavior. It is distinguishable by shouts of "I don't want to" or "I won't." This is not the constructive coping style that facilitates dental care.

Children who react this way often perform similarly in their home environments. Their parents may not provide sufficiently strict guidelines for their behavior. When brought to the dental office against their will, they protest as they would at home. Children exhibiting this type of behavior have been referred to as "stubborn" (Lampshire 1970). While it is generally acknowledged that there is a relationship between the home environment and behavior in the dental environment, it could be fallacious to make this connection. Using the Eyberg Child Behavior Inventory (ECBI), Dunegan et al. (1994) found that a child's disruptive or non-disruptive behavior at home was not a reliable predictor of behavior within the dental setting. The study used a small sample, so the relationship still is debatable.

Challenging or defiant children often have a robust self-esteem. They tend to be strong-willed children who are sufficiently extroverted to express their disagreement. Asking parents how they do at home with things like cutting nails and washing hair or their first visit to school can often create an image of a child without fears. However, it is possible that the child may have been frightened by a single intrusive treatment creating a solid state (situational) anxiety (Spielberger 1973). A straightforward, firm approach often changes their behavior dramatically. After their cooperation has been obtained, their behavior should be goal-directed. Definitive guidelines for their behavior have to be established. By challenging the dentist, an adult authority, defiant children show some courage. With proper techniques, this courage can be used to affect reciprocal behavior. Once won over, these children have the potential to be highly cooperative and can become some of the dentist's best patients.

### Timid Behavior

If timid children are managed incorrectly, their behavior can deteriorate to uncontrolled behavior. This can occur if the dentist is unable to detect the child's timidity. These children are likely highly anxious and can be difficult to treat. The dentist must proceed slowly and gain the child's confidence. If the dentist hurries to start treatment, it might jeopardize the complete treatment alliance that is needed for consecutive sessions. Compared to those behavioral forms already described, timidity is a more introverted type of behavior. Some children may shield themselves behind a parent, but they often fail to offer great physical resistance to the separation procedure. Some may stall when given directions. These children do not always hear or comprehend instructions. Therefore, the dental health team should understand that guidelines presented to them often must be repeated because of their emotional state.

Many reasons may exist for timid reactions. Currently, it is mainly seen as an aspect of the child's personality. Another assumption is that the child's behavior reflects that of the parent. One child may come from an overprotective home environment. Another may have little contact with strangers. Other children may be awed by strange surroundings. Information obtained from office questionnaires may help to guide these children through their early dental experiences (see Chapter 7).

---

**Case 3.2**

Dr. A was seeing four-year-old Jimmy for his initial visit. The following conversation took place:

| | |
|---|---|
| Dr. A: | Do you go to kindergarten? |
| Jimmy: | Silent |
| Dr. A | Turns to mother, "Does Jimmy go to kindergarten?" |
| Mother: | Yes, he does. |
| Dr. A: | Well, let's see your teeth, Jimmy. Open your mouth. |

---

***Case 3.2, Discussion:*** The first step in successful behavior management is to establish communication. By involving a child in conversation, the dentist not only learns about the patient but may also relax the child. There are many ways of initiating verbal communication, and the effectiveness of these approaches differs with the ages of the child. In this case, Jimmy demonstrated timid behavior. He did not respond to the question and was not actively engaged in the communication. Dr. A. was in a hurry to "get to the mouth." He readdressed the question to the mother. Generally, verbal communication is best initiated for younger children with complimentary comments, followed by questions that elicit an answer other than "yes or "no."

| | |
|---|---|
| Dr A: | (To dental assistant) Wow! Jane, look at Jimmy's sneakers. They are so cool! |
| Dr A: | (to Jimmy) Hey, Jimmy, you have great sneakers. Are they new? I wish I could get a pair like yours. Did you pick them out all by yourself? |
| Jimmy: | My mom helped me pick them out. They won't fit you. |
| Dr. A: | You are so lucky. Your mom is great, she helped you get the best sneakers! |

Children are generally proud of their new clothing and like to be asked about it. Observing anything unique about a child offers the opportunity to ask questions and involve the child in conversation. In the above case, the dentist accomplished two goals. He opened a line of communication and also praised the child's mother. Both the child and mother are experiencing a positive feeling.

Children are often shy and reluctant to talk when they are first exposed to a new experience and to new people. When they have gained confidence and are comfortable in the new environment, they will usually begin to speak more freely.

In establishing effective communication, the dental team must take care that it is not "overdone." Some children may realize that by controlling conversations they can exert considerable influence over their environment. They know that if they remain busy talking, little dentistry can be done. Some will use repetitive questions and a lot of talk to avoid treatment. In such instance, the dentist should inform the patient that is time to proceed with the task ahead, thus regaining control of the situation.

### Tense-Cooperative Behavior

The behavior of some tense-cooperative children could be judged as borderline positive-negative. Typically, these children accept treatment. They do not exhibit violent physical misbehavior, nor can they be suitably classed as timid. They are, however, extremely tense. The dentist should realize that these patients are probably quite afraid of the dental treatment. In most cases, a friendly word or a positive remark from the dentist and encouragement by the dental staff can reduce the stress considerably.

The term "tense-cooperative" was coined by Lampshire (1970) specifically for this type of behavior. It should be considered as a positive sign when children are tense-cooperative. They are probably not the most excellent communicators who express their anxiety in eloquent sentences but, without words, they try to control their emotions. Their tension is often revealed by body language. Some patient's eyes may follow the movements of both dentist and dental assistant. These children can be considered in an introverted anxiety group.

When considering the latter portion of the behavior management definition proposed in the introductory chapter referring to the importance of a positive dental attitude, one can recognize that these children are easily mismanaged. Because they accept treatment, the busy or unobservant practitioner fails to see a problem. There are two possible results: (1) the child will either suddenly burst out in distress behavior or (2) the child will develop an attitude detrimental to future dental health. Younger children, toddlers, and preschoolers frequently accept their first restorative treatment in this way, and at a second session, the clinician suddenly finds that there is a major behavior problem. Older children may grow up accepting dentistry, but voicing dislike out of proportion to their personal experiences.

### Crying and Whining

Crying can be considered a manifestation of stress in the dental environment. Some children cry with tears and some without tears. Consider this case.

---

#### Case 3.3

During local anesthesia, eight-year-old Michelle cried loudly, without any tears, and squeezed the hands of the assistant. She had no other signs of stress, before or during the treatment. But, when local anesthesia was administered, she cried. The dentist learned from the intake questionnaire that she developed the crying habit when she was about four years of age, and the crying had continued ever since that time.

After the injection, the dentist asked if it was possible for her not to cry. He explained that the loud crying hurt his ears. He also inferred that it disturbed others in the waiting room, worse yet, he said, it makes some children nervous. Michele pondered this. Finally, she confessed, "You know, I just like to scream, it makes me feel good. But OK, I've grown up now, so next time I'll help you and try not to cry."

---

*Case 3.3, Discussion*: Some view crying as coping—a positive sign. When asked to stop crying, some children may remark that "they can't." Fortunately, that was not the situation in Case 3.3, which is almost laughable. But it happened. Maybe the child cried for attention or to release her tension. We don't know the reason. The important thing is that once the dentist presented the problem to Michelle, she replied in a mature manner and wanted to help the dentist. In many cases, children will alter their behaviors if they are given a forthright, logical explanation.

Few studies have dealt with crying in pediatric dentistry. One interesting investigation, however, by Zadik and Peretz (2000), inquired about parents' attitudes toward their children's crying in the dental environment. Zadik and Peretz asked 104 parents accompanying their children to dental treatment to complete a questionnaire assessing the tendency of their children to cry and how they, the parents, perceived their own role in such a case. The investigators learned that 53% of the parents assessed their children as having a tendency to cry and 73% preferred that the operator cease the treatment and calm the crying child before resuming. They opined that the successful completion of dental treatment of a crying child is a partnership of the dentist and the parent. If parents hold this opinion, it is important that the dentist inform the parent about the method to be used and have their consent.

In the past, some children have been called whiners. When children whine, it could be regarded as an acceptance of the treatment situation, but an expression of serious discomfort at the same time. Since whining plays a prominent part in their performance, their behavior is described as a distinct entity.

It is difficult to describe a child's behavior by aural perception alone. The whining child is, nevertheless, identifiable. The child's emoting is not particularly loud—it is controlled and the sounds are constant. Great patience is required when dealing with whining children. They allow the dentist to proceed, but whine throughout a major part of the procedure, despite encouragements. Their whining may be a part of a developing coping style in line with the tense-cooperative children. Local anesthesia administration may have been repeated because they frequently complain of pain. It can be hypothesized that their apprehensions lower their pain thresholds. Their continuing reactions are a source of frustration and irritation to those involved with the treatment. It is part of the professional attitude of the dentist to accept the whining child's behavior. Although this may be difficult, it will ultimately lead to the best results. With a firm approach, there is a risk of being too directive, overruling the child, and losing the fragile contact that always exists in these situations.

### Passive Resistance

A totally different style, often seen in adolescents, is known as *passive resistance*. Picture the youngster who solemnly slumps in the dental chair. The patient does not respond verbally. When the dentist attempts to involve the child in the procedure, communication fails. When an intraoral examination is attempted, the patient may reject the situation by clenching his teeth. Body language can cue this behavior. The tight grip on the dental chair may turn knuckles white. Eye contact is frequently avoided.

This coping style is a symptom of problem behavior caused by a bundle of reasons. It may be anxiety, a general feeling of dislike, or lack of interest in the situation. These children may act in a similar manner at home if they are not allowed to choose their own clothing or go to movies with their friends. When brought to the dental office unwillingly, they are forced into a situation which has violated their freedom. When treated as juveniles, their self-images are affected. They rebel. Modifying their behavior is a challenge not only for the dentist but for every adult involved. In time, behavior will modify for the better when

the adolescent becomes interested in oral health. If pharmacological support helps them to relax and it is accepted by the patient, it can be an asset with these children. Every attempt should be made to motivate the child to accept the support of the dental team.

Lists of potentially cooperative behaviors exhibited in dental environments could go on ad infinitum. Generalized descriptions lack specificity, and children are individuals. Their behavior is too highly variable to allow accurate pinpointing. However, the foregoing labeled descriptions of negative behaviors are those most commonly observed. They should be adequate for an understanding of clinical situations when they are referred to in later chapters.

## Factors Underlying Children's Cooperation

During the child's first dental visit, the dentist needs to assess behavior in the dental environment. Behavior is the key to treatment. Some children are robust and tolerant in stressful situations and are unlikely to present uncooperative behavior. Other children are vulnerable and may need more attention and time in order to feel at ease and to cooperate with dental treatment. The question is, who are these vulnerable children and what might be the underlying factors which contribute to their behavior in the dental office?

It is axiomatic that an anxious child who anticipates an unpleasant experience is more likely to have such an experience, whereas a child who has a low level of fear or anxiety is likely to have a pleasant dental visit. But what is anxiety? And what is fear? The various psychological schools agree that anxiety is a personality trait that can be assessed based on the child's behavior (Achenbach and Rescorla 2001). Anxiety describes an emotional state of human personality. It is referred to as a construct; that is, it is an abstraction composed of ideas and concepts. One of the difficulties is that anxiety takes on various meanings depending on the operational criteria employed by different researchers or clinicians (Ruebush 1963). Hence, there are many varied definitions of anxiety that have been used by social scientists.

The crux of the problem in defining anxiety is its similarity to fear. There are theoretical differences, but for practical purposes, they can be indistinguishable (Levitt 1967). Both are constructs of social scientists with no clear physical existence themselves. Anxiety and fear are defined in words. For a definition to be operational and clinically applicable, it should be defined in terms of acts. Nonetheless, these terms are frequently used in behavioral science research in dentistry and other areas without operational definitions. If this is the case, any measurement of the construct is open to question.

The distinction between fear and anxiety is difficult to ascertain in dental situations, except for extreme circumstances. If a child has had several extractions without profound anesthesia, then any uncontrollable future behavior could legitimately be attributed to fear. This is one extreme. The opposite is the mildly concerned but cooperative child, about to have a first dental appointment. The concern could be attributed to anxiety. The two are vastly different situations, but it is the "gray zone," the zone between the extremes where fear and anxiety become indistinguishable.

Another way of looking at fear and anxiety is by examining the source or stimulus. Think about the four-year-old who has uncontrollable behavior at the first dental visit. Is the uncontrolled behavior fear or anxiety? Since the child has not seen a dentist previously, by some definitions, the behavior is attributable to anxiety. On the other hand, someone at school or at home may have frightened the child with stories about dentistry. Did this cause the fearful negativism? We don't know. Again, the fact remains that fear and anxiety can be difficult to tell apart.

Now, returning to the child who is vulnerable, the behavior may be due to internal factors stemming from chronic fear and anxiety. Psychologists refer to those aspects of the individual's personality that are innate, rather than learned, as the *temperament*. Since the 1950s, many scientific studies have shown that temperament influences children's health and development. The realization that many behavioral tendencies are inborn—and not the result of poor parenting—is one of the most important insights parents (and dentists) gain from learning about temperament. Internal factors like fear and anxiety can be difficult to clarify at times, but some of the resultant child characteristics that may be in need of special attention include somatic complaints such as gagging or nausea when the child becomes anxious; overactive or impulsive behaviors (Arnrup et al. 2002); or aggressive behaviors such as noncompliance with dental procedures.

On the other hand, some of the behavior may be due to factors relating to the child's perception of the dental office, or perhaps to a prior medical experience. These can be termed *external factors*. At the time of the first appointment or patient intake, if appropriate questions are asked, the child's history may reveal important external factors (see Chapter 7 for questions).

From 1970 to 1985, there was great interest in behavioral science research in pediatric dentistry. The focus for much of this research was to assess external factors to determine which ones influenced children's behaviors. Unfortunately, this type of research is less popular today, and much information is gleaned from older studies. However, a wide variety of variables were identified that still can be useful. Some of these include the following.

## Medical History

The quality of past medical visits was found to be important. If they were unpleasant, this could have a bearing on a child's attitude toward future dental visits. Pain from previous procedures is often reported by a parent, and although it may be inaccurate, this aspect of the medical history ranks high on possible sources of misbehavior. Other aspects of the medical history, such as frequency of medical visits or even hospitalization, have not been found to be consistently related (Bailey et al. 1973; Wright 1975).

## Maternal Anxiety

Historically, using an anxiety scale to assess maternal anxiety, it was found that an anxious mother has a greater likelihood of having a child that will be uncooperative in the dental environment. This variable was studied in depth in the 1970s and repeatedly found to be significant (Wright et al. 1973). Indeed, a recent study confirmed there is evidence of the coexistence of dental fear in parents and their children (Dahlander et al. 2019). However, other studies did not find that relation (ten Berge 2001; Wu and Gao 2018). The latter reported that anxiety was higher in children with siblings (Wu and Gao 2018). However, family environments have changed with increased single parenthood, blended families, and same sex marriages. Mothers do not always accompany their children to dentists. Sometimes, fathers, both parents, or caregivers bring children to the dentist. Further study of this variable is a fertile area for future research.

## Need for Treatment

If a child is aware that a dental problem exists, there is a greater likelihood that anxiety will be heightened (Wright and Alpern 1971). This variable has received current attention from Yang et al. (2011). Examining 195 children aged three–seven years, they found a significant correlation between children with dental caries and uncooperative behavior. One advantage of the Dental Home concept (see Chapter 6) is that children usually do not arrive at the dental office in need of treatment.

Attempts have been made to relate other external factors that clinicians have suggested may have a bearing on children's behavior. While some of these factors have not been significantly related or withstood repeated testing, they cannot be completely discounted. It has to be remembered that research establishes relationships with large population samples, and dentists treat individuals.

When interpreting responses to questionnaires, the clinician should exercise caution. Evaluating external factors in relation to a child's behavior as a cause-and-effect relationship can be misleading. While there is undoubtedly some interaction between factors, no clear agreement exists on the relative importance of factors in relation to one another. Few studies have offered information concerning these relationships.

Once there is an understanding of the underlying factors that can influence a child's behavior, a treatment plan can be developed. Some child patients might need extra time in preparing them for what is to come, especially those with chronic fears and anxieties. Patients with aggressive behaviors may need expectations clearly explained and a highly structured approach throughout their dental visits. Understanding the child's needs in treatment planning should enhance the possibility of a successful outcome.

---

### Case 3.4

Mohammad (six years old) was referred to a pediatric dentist due to his dental anxiety and advanced dental caries. The first visit and subsequent restorative sessions were successful, and Mohammad was asked to return in a half a year for a recall exam. One year later, he returned and was found to be in need of further restorative treatment. At the restorative session, Mohammed appeared with his father and the treatment failed. The child freaked out completely, was unable to communicate, and screamed, bit, and kicked during local anesthesia. Treatment was stopped, and his father got very angry at him. An additional appointment was scheduled. At the next session, the same happened: his father told him to be brave and Mohammad blocked completely. The dentist advised the father to have Mohammad's mother accompany him at the next visit. Next session, Mohammad was afraid but able to control his temper, and the treatment was given successfully.

---

***Case 3.4, Discussion***: Sometimes, small things can tip the balance when guiding a child. In the family situation, many things occur that may have an influence on a child's behavior. Sometimes, the way children react in a specific situation is based on their personality, and it takes knowledge or just intuition from the dentist to find the right code to help them move in the right direction, e.g., to support an anxious patient and to avoid a tense cooperative child turning into an uncontrolled angry bird. In the above case, one parent was just too direct where Mohammad needed a more friendly easy-going type of support. For this, there are no fixed rules, except the knowledge that we should take into account that differences might occur.

The rules of how children react in the presence of adults is supported with all kinds of different studies. For instance, Achenbach's Child Behavior Checklist (Rey et al. 1992), one of the leading psychological questionnaires, has separate versions for toddlers and preschoolers but also for parents and teachers, since children can behave completely different in situations where different adults are in charge. Differences are most clear in externalizing behaviors, where the internalizing behaviors are more difficult to read. In another study, *social referencing* (SR) refers to the process wherein infants use the affective displays of an adult to regulate their behaviors toward environmental objects, persons, and situations. SR represents one of the major mechanisms by which infants come to understand the world around them. Via SR, signs of parental anxiety can lead to infant anxiety. In the study, infants had to crawl over a glass surface covering a visual cliff, and even at that very young age, their reactions were dependent on the parent's support differing between the mother and father's support and encouragement which was related to the degree of paternal anxiety displayed (Moller et al. 2014). This indicates that children are not "machines"; they interact with other people from a very young age and modify their behavior accordingly.

## Summary

Advances in clinical practice are developed by building small portions of information on existing knowledge. Nowhere is this more evident than in this chapter, for it illustrates how clinical observations can lead to objective investigations, which ultimately have implications for dental practice. The chapter highlighted three topics related to children's behavior in dentistry: (1) classification procedures, (2) forms of behavior, and (3) the importance of learning about underlying factors influencing children's cooperative behavior.

Some dentists are intuitive and "get along" with children. All dentists can recall fellow students who coped extremely well with their patients without any theoretical study of children's behavior. Others are less fortunate. They require information to a greater degree. Regardless of individual successes with children, all clinicians should strive to maximize a positive effect on child patients. There are many ways of achieving this effect. Learning about the dynamics of child behavior is one of these ways.

## References

AAPD (American Academy of Paediatric Dentistry). (2008). Clinical Affairs Committee, Guideline on behavior guidance for the paediatric dental patient. *Pediatric Dentistry*, 29, 115–124.

Aartman, I.H.A., van Everdingen, T., Hoogstraten, J. et al. (1998). Self-report measurements of dental anxiety and fear in children: A critical assessment. *ASDC Journal of Dentistry for Children*, 65, 252–258.

Achenbach, T.M. and Rescorla, L.A. (2001). *Manual for the ASEBA School-Age Forms and Profiles*. Burlington, VT: University of Vermont, Research Center for Children, Youth, and Families.

Addelston, H.K. (1959). Child patient training. *Fortnight Review. Chicago Dental Society*, 38(7–9), 27–29.

Alwin, N., Murray, J.J., and Niven, N. (1994). The effect of children's dental anxiety on the behaviour of a dentist. *International Journal of Paediatric Dentistry*, 4, 19–24.

Arnrup, K., Broberg, A.G., Berggren, U. et al. (2002). Lack of cooperation in pediatric dentistry—the role of child personality characteristics. *Pediatric Dentistry*, 24, 119–128.

Bailey, P.M., Talbot, M., and Taylor, P.P. (1973). A comparison of maternal anxiety with anxiety levels manifested in the child patient. *ASDC Journal of Dentistry for Children*, 40, 253–258.

Bajric, E., Sedin, K., and Juric, H. (2011). Reliability and validity of the Dental Subscale of the Children's Fear Survey Schedule (CFSS-DS) in children in Bosnia and Herzegovina. *Bosnian Journal of Basic Medical Science*, 11, 214–218.

Chapman, H.R. and Kirby-Turner, N. (2002). Visual/verbal analogue scales: Examples of brief assessment methods to aid management of child and adult patients in clinical practice. *British Dental Journal*, 193, 447–450.

Cuthbert, M.I. and Melamed, B.G. (1982). A screening device: children at risk for dental fears and management problems. *ASDC Journal of Dentistry for Children*, 49, 432–436.

Dahlander, A., Soares, F., Grindefjord, M. et al. (2019). Factors associated with dental fear and anxiety in children aged 7 to 9 years. *Dentistry Journal*, 7, 68–77.

Dunegan, K.M., Mourino, A.P., Farrington, F.H. et al. (1994). Evaluation of the Eyberg Child Behavior Inventory as a predictor of disruptive behaviour during an initial pediatric dental examination. *Journal of Clinical Pediatric Dentistry*, 18, 173–179.

Frankl, S.N., Shiere, F.R., and Fogels, H.R. (1962). Should the parent remain with the child in the dental operatory? *ASDC Journal of Dentistry for Children*, 29, 150–155.

Gustafsson, A., Broberg, A., Bodin, L. et al. (2010). Dental behaviour management problems: the role of child personal characteristics. *International Journal of Paediatric Dentistry*, 20, 242–253.

Houpt, M. (1993). Project USAP the use of sedative agents in pediatric dentistry. 1991 update. *Pediatric Dentistry*, 15, 36–40.

Klaassen, M.A., Veerkamp, J.S., Aartman, I.H. et al. (2002). Stressful situations for toddlers: Indications for dental anxiety? *ASDC Journal of Dentistry for Children*, 69, 297–305.

Klingberg, G. (2008). Dental anxiety and behaviour management problems in paediatric dentistry: A review of background factors and diagnostics. *European Archives of Paediatric Dentistry*, 9, 11–15.

Krikken, J.B., van Wijk, A.J., ten Cate, J.M. et al. (2013). Measuring dental fear using the CFSS-DS. Do parents and children agree? *International Journal of Paediatric Dentistry*, 23, 94–99.

Lampshire, E.L. (1970). Control of pain and discomfort. In: Goldman, H. et al. (Eds.), *Current Therapy in Dentistry*, Vol. IV, 489–525. C.V. Mosby Co., St. Louis.

Levitt, E.E. (1967). *The Psychology of Anxiety*. Bobbs-Merrill Co. Inc., Indianapolis.

McDonald, R.E. (1969). *Dentistry for the Child and Adolescent*. C. V. Mosby Co, St. Louis.

Milgrom, P., Mancl, L., King, B. et al. (1995). Origins of childhood dental fear. *Behaviour Research and Therapy*, 33, 313–319.

Moller, E.L., Majdandžić, M., and Bögels, S. (2014). Fathers' versus mothers' social referencing signals in relation to infant anxiety and avoidance: A visual cliff experiment. *Developmental Science*, 17, 1012–1028.

Nakai, Y., Hirakawa, T., Milgrom, P. et al. (2005). The children's fear survey schedule—dental subscale in Japan. *Community Dentistry and Oral Epidemiology*, 33, 196–204.

Rey, J.M., Schrader, E., and Morris-Yates, A. (1992). Parent–child agreement on children's behaviours reported by the child behaviour checklist (CBCL). *Journal of Adolescence* 15, 219–230.

Roberts, J.F., Curzon, M.E., Koch, G. et al. (2010). Review: Behaviour management techniques in paediatric dentistry. *European Archives of Paediatric Dentistry*, 11, 166–174.

Rud, B. and Kisling, E. (1973). The influence of mental development on children's acceptance of dental treatment. *Scandinavian Journal of Dental Research*, 81, 343–352.

Ruebush, B.K. (1963). Anxiety. In: H.W. Stevenson, J. Kagan, and C. Spikes (Eds.), *Child Psychology*. The 62nd Year Book of the National Society for the Study of Education. University of Chicago Press, Chicago.

Sands, R.A. (1933). The mental aspect of pedodontics. *Dental Items of Interest*, 5, 927–929.

Singh, P., Pandey, R.K., Nagar, A. et al. (2010). Reliability and factor analysis of children's fear survey schedule—dental subscale in Indian subjects. *Journal of the Indian Society of Pedodontics and Preventive Dentistry*, 28, 151–155.

Spielberger, C.D. (1973). *Manual for the state–trait anxiety inventory for children. Consulting Psychologists Press*. Palo Alto, CA.

ten Berge, M. (2001). Dental fear in children: Prevalence, aetiology and risk factors. PhD Thesis, *University of Amsterdam, The Netherlands*.

ten Berge, M. Hoogstraten, J., Veerkamp, J.S.J. et al. (1998). The Dental Subscale of the Children's Fear Survey Schedule: A factor analytic study in The Netherlands. *Community Dentistry and Oral Epidemiology*, 26, 340–343.

ten Berge, M., Veerkamp, J.S., Hoogstraten, J. et al. (2002). Childhood dental fear in the Netherlands: prevalence and normative data. *Community Dentistry and Oral Epidemiology*, 30, 101–107.

Veerkamp, J.S.J., Gruythuysen, R.J., Amerongen, W.E. et al. (1995a). Dentists rating of child patient dental anxiety. *Community Dentistry and Oral Epidemiology*, 23, 356–359.

Veerkamp, J.S.J., Gruythuysen, R.J.M., Hoogstraten, J. et al. (1995b). Anxiety reduction using nitrous oxide: A permanent solution? *ASDC Journal of Dentistry for Children*, 62, 44–48.

Venham, L., Bengston, D., and Cipes, M. (1977). Children's response to sequential dental visits. *Journal of Dental Research*, 56, 454–459.

Venham, L.L. and Gaulin-Kremer, E. (1979) A self-report measure of situational anxiety for young children. *Pediatric Dentistry*, 1, 91–96.

Wong, D.L. and Baker, C.M. (1988). Pain in children: Comparison of assessment scales. *Pediatric Nursing*, 14, 9–17.

Wilson, C.W. (1933). Child Management. *Journal of the American Dental Association*, 20, 890–892.

Wright, G.Z. and Alpern, G.D. (1971). Variables influencing children's cooperative behavior at the first dental visit. *ASDC Journal of Dentistry for Children*, 38, 126–131.

Wright, G.Z., Alpern, G.D., and Leake, J.L. (1973). A cross-validation of the variables affecting children's cooperative behavior. *Journal of the Canadian Dental Association*, 39, 268–273.

Wright, G.Z. (1975). *Behavior Management in Dentistry for Children (Chapter 3)*. W.B. Saunders Co., Philadelphia.

Wu, L. and Gao, X. (2018). Children's dental fear and anxiety: Exploring family related factors. *BMC Oral Health*, 18(1), 100. https://doi.org/10.1186/s12903-018-0553-z

Yang, C., Zou, H., and Zou, J. (2011). Analysis of dental cooperative behaviors of the first-visit in children's clinic. *Hua Xi Kon Qiang Xue Za Zhi*, 5, 501–504.

Zadik, D. and Peretz, B. (2000). Management of the crying child during dental treatment. *ASDC Journal of Dentistry for Children*, 67, 55–58.

# 4

# Influence of the Family

*Barbara Sheller*

## Introduction

The family is critical to a child's nurturing and development. A child's sense of self-worth develops from being cared for, loved, and valued. Along with meeting basic physical needs, families provide children with emotional support, socialization, coping methods, and other life skills. The purpose of this chapter is to review aspects of the relationship between children and their families which may influence their ability to cooperate for dental treatment. Some parent and family factors, which may be manipulated by the dental team, are identified, and sample strategies are outlined to identify and shape key family factors to enhance child coping and cooperation. To provide the greatest value for the clinician, there is a summary of important learning concepts at the end of each section, translating theory and research into the clinical dental practice with children. Dentistry does not stand alone in its interest in promoting child coping and cooperation skills, or in its recognition that parents and family can affect a child's responses during a dental appointment. Thus, this chapter includes selected research from pediatric medicine, developmental psychology, sociology, and neuroscience to supplement the dental evidence base.

Families influence children's oral health in daily life through eating behaviors and oral hygiene practices. Parents decide when their children should see a dentist, choose the office or clinic and dentist, arrange the visit, and often accompany their children to the appointments. Before stepping into the dental office, parents are invested in the quality of their child's dental experience. Families directly and indirectly influence a child's ability to cooperate during dental treatment.

## Family Structure

A family is a network of interconnected relationships. Over the last several decades, social and cultural changes have expanded the concept of what comprises a family. Dental practices worldwide serve a multicultural population with a wide range of family structures. Family diversity includes, but is not limited to, parental status (married, divorced, separated, single, step, biological, adoptive, and foster), along with differing racial, ethnic, linguistic, spiritual, religious, sexual, social, and inter-generational aspects. Parent age can vary widely—maternal age may extend from pre-teen into late middle age due to advanced fertility treatments and surrogacy, and there is no clear upper limit for paternal age. Family size and composition may range from a small family of one parent and one child to a large and complex multi-generational, multi parent, multi-child, multi-household family with varying relationships among children and parents. Important variations within these diverse family structures are parenting style, parenting behaviors and practices, communication style, roles of family members, use of time within the family, commitment to individual family members, type and quality of childcare, connection to the community, economic and social resources, and methods of responding to challenges of life (American Academy of Pediatrics Task Force on the Family 2003).

A child's well-being is closely linked to physical, emotional, and social health; social circumstances; and behavior of the parents. Children do best when raised by two caring, cooperative parents with adequate social and financial resources providing a secure, supportive, and nurturing environment. The family stress model proposed by Conger et al. (2000) recognizes that parents become emotionally

*Wright's Behavior Management in Dentistry for Children*, Third Edition. Edited by Ari Kupietzky.
© 2022 John Wiley & Sons, Inc. Published 2022 by John Wiley & Sons, Inc.

depleted by financial hardships, health problems, marital discord, fatigue, employment difficulties, lack of social support, and other traumatic life events. Parents' emotional distress can lead to family conflict, instability, and disrupted, poor-quality parenting.

A growing body of research consistently links family structure to child well-being. The Fragile Families and Child Wellbeing Study is a longitudinal cohort study of 4,898 children born between 1998 and 2000 in 20 large cities in the United States. Approximately three-quarters of the children were born to unmarried parents (Reichman et al. 2001). Data collection included interviews with parents shortly after birth, and at child ages 1, 3, 5, 9, and 15 years. In-home, childcare, or teacher assessments and interviews with the child were done at child ages 3, 5, 9, and 15 years.

Compared to married parents, unmarried parents are more likely to be teens, less likely to have lived with both biological parents growing up, more likely to have children with other partners, more likely to be poor, more likely to suffer from depression, report substance abuse, and have spent time in jail. Nearly 40% of all unmarried mothers formed at least one new partnership and 14% had a child with the new partner (Kalil and Ryan 2010; McLanahan and Beck 2010; Waldfogel et al. 2010; Wildeman and Westren 2010).

The findings regarding children's behavioral problems may be directly relevant to the dentist. Children living with unmarried parents exhibit more externalizing problem behaviors. Children who do not live in a stable and secure environment may feel insecure, anxious, and aggressive and exhibit more behavior problems. The co-parenting relationship is critical for child well-being when families undergo change. Each break-up or new relationship for parents in a fragile family has been found to result in negative effects upon children's behavior and upon school performance. The research shows similar effects of relationship transitions on children's aggressive, depressive, and withdrawal behaviors.

Single mothers and mothers in unstable partnerships engage in harsher parenting practices and fewer literacy activities with their child than married mothers. Family instability also reduces children's cognitive test scores and increases aggressive behavior, particularly in boys.

It is now understood that social environments characterized by adversity and stressful events which occur early and result in long-lasting disruptions in a child's care and nurturing lead to worse outcomes for children (Boyce 2014). However, no particular family structure makes poor outcomes for children inevitable (American Academy of Pediatrics 2003). Family risk factors such as a single parent household, a parent's ill health, financial hardship, and community violence adversely impact parents' attitudes and behaviors and reduce their ability to positively socialize, support, and guide their children during dental treatment.

Family characteristics of 230 children and adolescents aged 8–19 years who were referred to pediatric dentistry specialists for behavior management problems were compared to 248 controls without behavior management issues. Striking differences in life and family situations were found between the groups. The uncooperative children more often lived in families with low socioeconomic status, had parents who were not living together, reported fewer leisure-time activities, performed poorly in social interactions, had personal professional support, and had received interventions by social agencies. The "burdensome life and family situation" was suggested as a factor explaining some of the patients' non-cooperation (Gustafsson et al. 2007).

Disparities in utilization of dental care and parent-reported child oral health have been linked to caregiver's age and education, family income, race/ethnicity, and parent's depressive symptoms (Edelstein and Chinn 2009; Kruger et al. 2015). Social support of mothers (reciprocal help, support, and trust in the neighborhood) was positively associated with children's utilization of dental care in a large, population-based survey reported by Iida and Rozier (2013). In a study of mothers who had high dental caries, availability of someone to talk to about problems (appraisal support) was associated with lower odds of their children having high dental caries (Burgette et al. 2019).

## Application in Dental Practice

The dentist has no control over a child's family situation, but knowledge of family circumstances is critical for optimal clinical decision-making. A constructive partnership between the dentist and the parent and/or key caregiver lays the foundation for a positive and satisfying child–dentist relationship over the child's lifetime.

The dentist should know who is most involved in the care and nourishment of the child, as well as the primary caretaker's oral health perspective and preferred style of interaction. Other information to consider includes identity of family members living in the home and in the second home when applicable, custody arrangements, childcare setting and primary caregivers, family disruptions such as marital strain or divorce, severe illness of a family member, moving, refugee status, military deployment, social support, parent employment status, and financial security.

Understanding this information will guide the dentist's communication with parents and/or other key family members whose understanding and "buy in" is essential for promoting a child's positive attitude about healthy diet, oral hygiene behaviors, and cooperation for dental treatment.

For families experiencing difficult circumstances (e.g., single parent, divorce, unemployment, moving to a new city, or death of a family member), the dentist can express appreciation for the effort that has been made to bring the child to the appointment and should understand that recommendations for changes in diet or oral hygiene may not be actualized until the family situation improves.

## Attachment

The bonding of an infant with a parent or other caregiver is one of the key developmental tasks of infancy. Infants become bonded, or attached, to caregivers with whom they have significant amounts of interaction. They develop a hierarchy of preferred attachment figures, having a most-preferred caregiver, a next most-preferred, etc. Infants have limitations in their capacity for attachments, and serious attachment disturbances have been reported among children raised in settings with large numbers of caregivers. Children who are institutionalized or maltreated may have no definite attachments to anyone (Zeanah and Fox 2004). Preferred attachments can develop at any time after infants reach cognitive ages of 7–9 months if the new caregivers have substantial involvement with them. Young children adopted out of foster care or institutions form attachments to their new caregivers, but in some cases, the quality of the attachment is compromised (O'Connor et al. 2000).

Researchers observing securely attached and insecurely attached children have found that those with secure attachments are more likely to actively engage with their environment. Theoretically, successfully attached infants have learned to trust the outside world as a welcoming place and to trust adults. A secure parent–child attachment appears to prepare a child to be receptive to and cooperative with parental socialization influences (Kochanska 1995). Conversely, infants whose emotional needs have not been consistently or adequately met come to view the world as unpredictable and learn that adults are not to be relied upon. For poorly attached children, discipline is experienced as rejection and disapproval, and they overreact to the negative feelings caused by routine childhood rules and restraints. They are at risk for chronic anxiety or distrust, less able to cope with challenging or adverse life experiences, and are more likely to exhibit behaviors that result in adverse experiences (Bowlby 1982). Understandably, children with insecure attachments are more likely than securely attached children to feel threatened by new or stressful situations (McKernon et al. 2001).

Most research on attachment has focused on the child's bond to the mother. Recent investigations indicate the importance of the father–child bond. "Double-insecure" (insecure attachment to both parents) six to eight-year-old children had high levels of behavior problems at school as rated by teachers and by the children themselves. A secure attachment with one parent offsets risk for poor behavior, but having a secure attachment with two parents did not confer additional benefit to the child (Kochanska and Kim 2013).

### Application in Dental Practice

The dentist should assess the child patient's social history regarding risk factors for disrupted attachment, such as extended hospitalization during infancy or toddlerhood, early life in an orphanage with multiple caregivers, history of foster care—particularly with multiple foster home placements, adoption after infancy, history of physical abuse or neglect, or a parent with substance addiction or mental health issues. In the dental setting, a child disadvantaged by an insecure attachment may show extreme fear and reluctance (retreat from an unsafe and unpredictable world) or be defiant and uncooperative (battle against an unsafe and unpredictable world). Either response should elicit the compassion, patience, and understanding of the dentist and dental team. Time, consistency, and patience must be invested when working with an insecurely attached child, using positive and incremental efforts to form a relationship and earn the child's trust. A long-term perspective should be paramount when the dentist meets a child with an attachment disorder. An insecure attachment does not make poor psychosocial outcomes inevitable for a given child or adolescent; it is more useful to think of attachment quality as a risk factor or protective factor in a child's life experience. The advantage and psychological protection resulting from a secure attachment enhances a child's ability to listen, relate, and respond to the dentist, and then to cooperate during dental treatment. The young child will do best if introduced to the dental environment and dental team in the presence of their preferred attachment figure.

## Genetic and Epigenetic Contribution to Child and Parent Interactions

The answer to the question "Does behavior result from nature or nurture?" is now understood to be "both." Genes and epigenetics (modifications to the DNA that do not alter the sequence of the DNA) are both determinants of behavior. The structure and function of the developing brain are strongly influenced by experiences such as social interactions in infancy and early childhood. Recurrent, active, and long-term engagement in behavioral sequences (cultural tasks) shape and modify brain pathways. Connectivity and functions of areas of the brain change as a result of experience in general, and particularly by repeated experiences (Kitayama and Park 2010).

Epigenetic research as applied to human behavior is in its infancy. An area of behavioral epigenetics of particular relevance to this book is the study of effects of early-life experiences and stresses upon emergence of child behaviors. The epigenetic mechanism most studied in humans is DNA methylation, occurring when a methyl molecule is added to a cytosine preceding a guanine. Depending upon the location of methylation, gene expression may be blocked or stimulated. As this chapter is updated in 2021, it is thought that DNA methylation is one of the major mechanisms that links stress in early life to a child's behavioral reactivity and self-regulation (Conradt 2017). Behavioral epigenetics research is expected to clarify the mechanisms of interactions between different aspects of a child's family life experience and the developing brain.

### Application in Dental Practice

Scientific knowledge of genetics, behavior, and the bi-directional influence of genetics upon human behavior and human behavior upon genetic expression is increasing rapidly. Today's partial picture of genetic and epigenetic influences on parent and child behavior should become clearer and more relevant to dental practice than is currently appreciated; increased knowledge in this area is likely to influence some diagnostic and treatment decisions.

## Family Influences on Child Behavior

The family serves as the child's connection to the world and has a critical role in preparing a child for life outside of the home. Socialization, the process by which an individual learns and accepts the established ways of a particular social group or society, may be viewed as the "nurture of nature," whereby the family transmits cultural values, expectations, and behavioral standards to the child. The family is considered the major arena for social growth. Although socialization and resocialization can occur throughout life, childhood is viewed as a uniquely malleable period when social skills, personality attributes, and values are established. Examples of socialization include learning to share toys, obey adult requests, and behave politely (Maccoby 1991). Socialization can also determine a child's response to dental treatment. It can influence behavioral standards, attitude toward adult

authority, how much discomfort justifies complaint, and how to express distress.

### Parenting Styles

A viewpoint or philosophy toward the child is reflected by the parenting style. It creates the emotional climate and context in which parents' socialization behaviors occur. Parenting style classifications consider the balance between (1) parental warmth and affection and (2) parental behavioral controls. The first version of a widely used parenting style typology was proposed by Baumrind in 1973. The degree of parent responsiveness (affection and attentive responsiveness to the child's needs) was considered with the level of parental control (demandingness for developmentally appropriate, prosocial, and responsible behaviors) to classify an individual's parenting style as Authoritative, Authoritarian, or Permissive. Maccoby and Martin (1983) modified Baumrind's groupings, renaming "Permissive" as "Indulgent" and adding "Neglectful." Most research examining parenting styles and child behavior cited in this chapter employs the typology of Baumrind, as well as Maccoby and Martin. The four parenting styles and a brief description of their characteristics are Authoritative (high responsiveness + high behavior control), Authoritarian (low responsiveness + high behavior control), Permissive (high responsiveness + low behavior control), and Neglectful (low responsiveness + low behavior control).

Parents with an Authoritative parenting style set up a collaborative home environment that is democratic, flexible, and supportive of the child, with guidelines aimed at enabling the child to become self-regulating. These parents may be warm and involved, yet still firm and consistent in establishing limits. Rules are not simply set in place but are supported through age-appropriate rationales.

Authoritarian parents clearly take charge, may be more autocratic, rigid, and use punishment as needed to enforce a high degree of structure, expecting obedience from the child. Parents shape and control their children in accordance with a set of standards and rules. The rules are not to be discussed or arrived at by argument and interaction. On the contrary, rules are imposed upon the child as mandatory, and the child or adolescent is not consulted. Authoritarian parents discourage verbal give-and-take between parent and child.

Authoritarian and Authoritative parents share their high expectations for the child's self-control. Parents with a Permissive parenting style indulge the child's wishes and agenda, placing the child in the power position with an appeasing, nondirective, lenient approach without clear rules or guidelines. Permissive parents are considered more responsive than demanding. The Permissive parenting style has more negative than positive effects on the social outcome and is associated with aggressive, impulsive children lacking independence and a sense of responsibility.

Neglectful parents are less involved in their child's lives than parents within any of the other three categories. The passive, emotionally removed, lax, or indifferent attitude exhibited by neglectful parents leaves the child to negotiate the world without structure, assistance, rules, or guidelines. Indifferent parents tend to be cold and uninterested in the needs of their children and adolescents, reflecting a desire to keep them at a distance. They try to minimize time and interaction with their children. This type of parent is characterized as uninvolved, meaning that they have a low degree of commitment to their role as a parent. There is a risk of a child or adolescent being neglected by this type of parent. Both Permissive and Neglectful parents have low expectations for the child's self-control.

## Parenting Practices

Parenting style is expressed through behaviors or "parenting practices." Parenting practices are mechanisms through which parents directly help their child attain socially valued outcomes such as development of a conscience, cooperation, compliance with societal rules, and academic success. Parenting practices include both specific goal-directed behaviors (time-out, physical punishments, and shaming) and non-goal-directed behaviors (gestures, tone of voice, and emotional expression) (Darling and Steinberg 1993). Children become accustomed to their own parent's practices and behaviors and develop the ability to read their parent's internal state. A typically developing child can accurately and rapidly perceive if her parent is pleased or displeased, comfortable or anxious, or calm or distressed by interpreting the parent's tone of voice and body language.

## Cultural Influence on Parenting Style

Culture has a pervasive influence on family life, including the way in which parents socialize their children. Parenting styles and practices hold psychological and cultural meanings and vary between cultures. For example, parental harshness (hostile behavior and/or physical punishment) carries a message of care and concern within a culture valuing strict behavior controls and high expectations for children's behavior. However, in a less strict culture holding lower expectations for children's behavior, it carries a message of unsympathetic criticism (Ho et al. 2008). It was initially suggested that Authoritative parenting likely would result in good psychosocial outcomes for children from all ethnic and cultural groups. Some studies, however, have found better outcomes associated with the Authoritarian parenting style, depending on family context and culture (Deater-Deckard et al. 1996; Ho et al. 2008). No investigation in any culture has reported consistent positive social outcomes for children of any age with the Permissive or Neglectful parenting style; this may be due to lack of rules and limits upon the child's conduct, which communicate which child behaviors are desired and expected and which actions are unacceptable.

The prevalence of parenting style types varies by culture. Sociologists and educators have noted an increase in the Permissive parenting type in many countries, including the United States (Long 2004). In traditional parenting models (Authoritarian, Authoritative), the adult determines, communicates, clarifies, and enforces rules for the child. In families with the Permissive parenting style, children question adult authority and a "the child should feel good" ethos permeates family life and parent decisions. Permissive parents are generally well-intentioned, want to be nice, and would like their children to be happy doing what they want to do. In some cases, the Permissive parent attempts to become a friend to their child, abrogating the traditional parental role of socialization.

The term "helicopter parent" (see also Chapter 5) is employed in the popular lexicon to describe a parent who is attentive, hovering, and available to rescue their child from the consequences of any poor decisions or actions (Cline and Fay 1990). Ubiquitous cell phones have made it inexpensive and simple for parents to stay continuously connected to their child, even when physically separated. It is theorized that the extension of the usual time period of parent–child close connection may prolong the child and young adult's dependence upon parent and family resources.

The disparate cultural views of proper parenting style and practice between Western-European and Eastern-Asian cultures was illustrated for the public consciousness by Chua in the book *Battle Hymn of the Tiger Mother* (2011), which recounts the strict methods she used to promote the academic success of and mastery of musical instruments by her daughters. Chua's behavioral controls over her children, such as limiting access to the bathroom, requiring many daily hours of homework and musical instrument practice, forbidding television viewing, and emotional tactics of ridicule and shame, engendered extensive commentary supporting and criticizing of this parenting style. Those embracing the predominantly Western philosophy that children are fragile and require protection and nourishment of their self-esteem called Chua's strict methods cruel and abusive. In contrast, those with a predominantly

Eastern viewpoint assume that the child has inner strength and the parent's job is to override the child's preferences because "to enjoy anything you have to be good at it, to be good at it you have to work, and children on their own never wish to work" (Chua 2011).

Interactions between culture, parenting, and child behavior are complex and challenging to thoroughly describe and study. Existing research is primarily cross-sectional with varying methodologies, focuses nearly exclusively on mothers, and heavily relies on subjective data such as parent reports on behavior practices rather than on observation of parents' behavior (Paulussen-Hoogeboom et al. 2007). Parenting behaviors appropriate at a developmental stage and in a specific social context will predictably differ depending on a child's developmental stage. A simple example is crossing a street with traffic: parents carry or hold the hand of a young child (high behavioral control) but do not need to hold the hand of a school-age child who has mastered the social task of safely crossing the street (low behavioral control).

There is no single "best" parenting style universal to all children. It is believed that a child's internal state of fear, arousal, and anxiety is integral to their receptiveness to social learning; the best child outcomes appear to result when a parent's style is in harmony with the child's temperament. For example, gentle, low-power discipline has been found to create the optimal anxiety arousal for social learning for temperamentally fearful children. Negative, punitive, and other types of power-assertive parenting have been found to be detrimental for temperamentally fearful children with a low anxiety threshold. In contrast, for relatively fearless children, gentle parental discipline does not capture the child's attention. For low-fear children, high parental pressure results in child anger and disregard for parent messages. Preliminary evidence suggests that reciprocal positive parent–child interactions are more effective in achieving social learning for children with low-fear temperaments (Kochanska et al. 2007).

**Application in Dental Practice**

Dentists should be aware of the parent's style of interacting with their child. To an experienced clinician, the parenting style may be obvious after a short observation of the parent and child. The less seasoned dentist may wish to include questions in the social history to indicate the parent's philosophy and style. Sample questions are presented in Table 4-1.

Children raised by Authoritative or Authoritarian parents who expect and demand appropriate, responsible behavior will understand that the dentist and staff members establish the rules and will guide their child through a

**Table 4-1** Parenting style questions.

1. **Which best describes your family's style of making decisions?**

   Parent in charge    Democracy–shared control    Child in charge

2. **It is best to give children choices instead of telling them just what to do.**

   Disagree    Neutral    Agree

3. **When acting with love, you can never do too much for a child.**

   Disagree    Neutral    Agree

4. **My child interrupts my conversations often.**

   Disagree    Neutral    Agree

5. **I generally need to ask more than once to get my child to do something.**

   Disagree    Neutral    Agree

dental visit. These children have been socialized to follow the lead of adults. The dentist can expect that most Authoritative or Authoritarian parents will endorse and support the rules, structure, and behavior guidance that the dentist presents to the child.

Children raised by Permissive parents have been conditioned to view adults in a more egalitarian manner. They may expect the dentist and staff to offer them the same degree of choices and control that they are accustomed to in their home environment. Since a dental appointment is not a situation where the child should or can lead, he may become unsettled, disappointed, or frustrated with a role of diminished power and react negatively. Permissive parents may take offense at firm, clear structure provided for their child by the dentist and dental staff and advocate for their child's preferences to be accommodated. Research illustrating implications of parenting style on child cooperation during dental treatment is presented later in this chapter in the section "Parental Influence on Child Cooperation in Dental Settings."

## Coping Socialization

The term "coping socialization" is defined as the parental and familial factors that may affect children's coping (Kliewer et al. 1996). Attaining maturity and acquiring social competence occur as a child grows from toddlerhood through childhood, adolescence, and into adulthood. A typically developing toddler is easily frustrated, emotionally labile, and lacks the ability to shift her attention away from sources of stress and toward positive stimuli or thoughts; a socially competent adolescent has developed internal resources and strategies to meet the demands of life outside the home. In the child development, psychology, and medical literature, the term "coping" is used to describe the thoughts and behaviors that an individual uses to manage and respond to environmental or internal stresses and demands. An individual who is cooperative with dental treatment is exhibiting "coping behaviors." Coping behaviors allow a child to handle the demands of dental treatment and accept care.

## Emotional Expression Within the Family

The family is most commonly the initial place for children to experience and learn to cope with negative emotions. The emotional climate of the family results, in part, from the way that parents express their own emotional feelings. Emotional expression is both verbal and nonverbal and has been classified by Valiente et al. (2004) as positive (e.g., praising and demonstrating admiration), negative dominant (e.g., expressing anger and displaying threatening emotions), or negative submissive (e.g., sulking and/or crying). Multiple investigations have found that children of emotionally positive parents are happier, more socially competent, and have lower rates of behavior problems than those of parents with low expressions of positive emotions and/or high levels of negative emotional expression. Parental expression of anger, whether or not it is directed toward the child, is associated with decreased amounts and quality of playtime and exploration with the child; child's avoidance of the parent; increased periods of the child's negative emotions (e.g., sadness, fear, and anger); and deterioration of child's behavior (Teti and Cole 2011).

A majority of answers in the left column indicates a parenting style with high behavioral controls. A majority of answers in the right column indicates a parenting style with low behavioral controls.

Children are strongly influenced by their parents' methods of emotional expression (Thompson 1994). The type and intensity of parent emotional expression provides a model for a child to imitate. Constructive, optimistic expressivity, and support from the parents have been found to relate positively to children's constructive coping with daily stress. Mothers with negative dominant expressions have children with lower levels of constructive coping. Witnessing or being the target of hostile negative emotions is stressful at any age, and children have limited life experience and capacity to withstand, process, and cope with such stress. Evidence that children's constructive coping is positively related to parental supportive strategies is mounting. It is possible that parents who express emotion

in positive ways are more likely to insist that children manage and control their emotions in socially appropriate ways in stressful situations and/or teach them constructive ways of coping (Valiente et al. 2004).

Parental responses to their children's emotions influence and teach them strategies for self-regulation. Effective parent responses have been found to be problem- and emotion-focused and express encouragement. Unhelpful parent behaviors include minimizing, punitive, and distressed responses to their children's emotions. High levels of family chaos have been found to be associated with lower levels of effective parent responses (Valiente et al. 2007).

The terms "emotional contagion" and "emotional attunement" describe the observation that a person's emotions are highly influenced by the emotions expressed by those around them, and there is a tendency for individuals in proximity to emotionally converge. Emotions are shared in multiple ways, subtly and overtly, verbally and non-verbally. Research using functional magnetic resonance imaging has found that observing another individual's emotions and facial expressions activates regions of the brain which (1) experience similar emotions and (2) produce facial muscle activation and mimicry (Morrison et al. 2004). A simple example is that when someone smiles at us, we reflexively smile back. Due to the bias of the human brain to detect potential threats, it is easier to become upset and distressed by someone else's negative emotional expression than it is to become happy and relaxed by someone else's joy and contentment. Emotional contagion theory explains how ambient mood states of both parties influence parent–child interactions. A child in a positive mood is more likely to comply with a mother's requests (Lay et al. 1989). A mother who is angry, even for reasons unrelated to her child, is more likely to believe that interactions with her child will be unpleasant and require a stern approach (Dix 1991).

### Child Influence on the Parent

Children are not passive recipients of adult influence. The parent–child relationship is reciprocal, with each influencing the other's thoughts, feelings, and behavior. Parents and children develop a long history of interaction; each acquires a set of expectations concerning the other's behavior and establishes a method of interpreting the other's reactions. The relationship is unique in the asymmetry of knowledge, power, control, and physical strength, and the balance of power in the relationship changes as the child develops. Disruptive behavior in a toddler holds less consequence, risk to the child, and threat to the parent than disruptive behavior in a teenager. Parenting affects children's behavior most strongly during early childhood (Slagt et al. 2012), while problematic adolescent behavior strongly affects parenting (Reitz et al. 2006). Parental sense of competence is defined as a parent's opinion of their ability to positively influence the behavior and development of their child (Coleman and Karraker 1998).

Social relations theory views children as active agents in their interactions with parents and assumes that disagreements, conflicts, and changes occur frequently. It is developmentally normal for children to resist some of the socialization demands of their parents (Goh and Kuczynski 2009). A parent's philosophy of parenting (style) and behaviors (parenting practices) will determine the degree of parent accommodation and submission to the natural resistance of the child. It has been observed that a child's status and power is higher in single-child homes. China introduced its One-Child Policy in 1979, resulting in a generation of children and young adults without siblings or cousins. Most of these solitary children are the focus of interest for six adults: two parents and four grandparents (Goh and Kuczynski 2009). Chinese parents and teachers have used the term *xiao huangdi*, meaning "little emperor," to describe pampered and entitled children who have inflated views of their own status and importance. Both teachers and employers have observed that many One-Child-Policy babies never learned how to cope with disappointment and frustration in ways that would best prepare them for life outside the home (Cameron et al. 2013).

### Application in Dental Practice

The dentist and staff should continually monitor the ambient emotional tone in the office and quickly intervene in cases of negative emotional expression by parents. A parent who verbally or non-verbally expresses the stress of a bad day is not emotionally available to help his child and may unintentionally sabotage that child's dental appointment. If the dentist or staff member's sincere and respectful attempt to redirect the parent to the intended positive purpose of the dental appointment is unsuccessful, the parent should be offered the opportunity to reschedule at a time when they are more in control.

## Sibling Influences

Throughout life, the sibling relationship may be cooperative, ambivalent, or antagonistic. The child grows and develops within a dynamic and variable family context across time. Multiple studies have confirmed that families differentially distribute such resources as parental time, attention, money, nurture, and love among the children in a family. Parents tend to concentrate resources on some children and not on others. Parent resource inequity between siblings has been examined based on birth order, child gender, sibling gender, birth spacing, and birth intention (wanted versus unwanted pregnancy). Unintended children have been found to receive fewer parent resources than intended siblings (Barber and East 2009). Unwanted children are more likely to receive critical, punitive, abusive, and/or neglectful parenting (Barber et al. 1999). Inequitable treatment by parents has been found to have significant long-term negative effects on the adjustment and self-esteem of the slighted child (McGuire et al. 1995; Volling and Elins 1998).

The sibling relationship is known to be a key part of the developmental context of a child's socialization, yet the complex interactions between siblings are only partially understood. The birth or adoption of a brother or sister is a normal life event for many children. Freud and others have proposed that the changes in home environment, family composition, family function, and parental attention resulting from a new baby (or newly adopted child) cause a developmental crisis for many children. Some are extremely jealous, have behavioral regressions, or display tantrums or disruptive behaviors; other children display minimal behavioral changes. A review of studies considering first-born children's reactions to the birth of a sibling found that the child's developmental level contributes to psychological adjustment during the transition to siblinghood. Skills newly acquired in the weeks and months immediately preceding a sibling's birth (e.g., toilet training, weaning from bottle) appear more vulnerable to regression than behaviors that are better established and part of the child's routine (Volling 2012).

Children in the same family do not experience identical environments. Common variations are the state of the parent relationship, parent–child temperament fit or misfit, family social and economic circumstances, and parent–child interactions. Sibling rivalry begins early. Twelve-month-old infants and young children are sensitive to maternal attention directed toward a newborn infant, sibling, or unfamiliar peer (Volling et al. 2002). Arrival of an infant has been found to adversely affect mother–older-sibling interactions with decreased maternal attention, positive affection, and attachment security, and often results in confrontations with the older child. It is theorized that increased behavior problems of the older child are mediated through changes in the mother–child relationship, particularly through increases in the mother's use of physical discipline (Volling 2005).

## Application in Dental Practice

It is important for the dentist to recognize the disruption and stress caused by new sibling(s) in the home and to realize that the transition of a child to the role of "big brother or big sister" comes at the cost of diminished parental attention. The child patient may show signs of stress in their new role and behave in a negative way to capture their parent's attention. The goal should be to keep the focus and nurturing of the dental team directed toward the child patient, rather than toward the newest family member and parent. The child patient can be invited to introduce his new sibling to the dentist or staff member. Examples of child-focused responses are "It is nice to meet your new sister, but today, you are the special one!" and "This is a very lucky baby to have you for their own big brother!"

When the dentist is caring for children from a family with inequitable distribution of parent resources, the dental team can advocate for the less-favored child. The attention and nurturing of the team should be directed entirely toward the child patient. Comments such as "Parents with more than one child continually need to shift attention between them. Right now, I'd like both of us to focus on (name of child), and decide together how we can (give compliment), (describe concern), (request resource allocation)" will nudge the parent's attention toward the more overlooked child. When the dentist is successful in proactively directing the parent's attention toward the habitually slighted child, the child patient will not need to escalate behavior during the appointment to capture and sustain their parent's interest.

## Family Functioning Models

When treating a child, it is important to understand the family environment. Family systems researchers readily acknowledge the many limitations inherent in describing, quantifying, and evaluating the network of relationships within any family. Family functioning models are the work of many and have evolved over time. One frequently used model of family functioning includes three common family profiles to classify the emotional and relational qualities of the family. These family functioning typology and child security outcomes, as summarized by Davies et al. (2004), are as follows:

- *Cohesive family.* Warm, close, and harmonious family relationships. Discrete but flexible boundaries separate relationships and family members. Autonomy of family members is respected.

- *Enmeshed or chaotic family.* High levels of conflict and hostility. Discordant and/or weak boundaries within and across family relationships. Enmeshed family processes emotionally pull children into adult family problems.

- *Disengaged or separate family.* Emotionally cold relationships with high levels of adversity and low levels of support. Rigid boundaries between and within parent–co-parent and parent–child relationships.

Child security and psychological functioning have been examined in the context of family functioning by many investigators. Children in cohesive families exhibit high levels of attachment security, constructive coping, and psychological adjustment and are thought to be at lower risk for psychological adjustment problems. In a one-year study of kindergarten-aged children and their families, children from both enmeshed and disengaged families had decreased security and were at increased risk for psychological difficulties and maladjustment when compared to children from cohesive families (Davies et al. 2004).

## Application in Dental Practice

The dentist should realize that children from dysfunctional families are unlikely to have experienced positive behavior models in the home and are thus less likely to have developed and practiced methods of constructive coping. These children have increased risk for dental anxiety and poor cooperation with dental treatment. Positive, warm, and supportive habituation to the dental environment is a good practice for any child, but is disproportionately expected to benefit children from dysfunctional families.

## Parental Influence on Child Coping and Cooperation in Medical Settings

Dentists have much to learn from parent–child research from colleagues in pediatric medicine. In pediatric medicine, patient- and family-centered care is based on the understanding that the family is the child's primary source of support and that their perspectives and information are important in clinical decision-making. Family inclusion has become the standard for pediatric medical practice for procedures ranging from venipuncture to anesthesia induction and cardiopulmonary resuscitation (American Academy of Pediatrics Policy Statement 2012). In recent decades, areas of research which have explored the influences exerted by the social environment on children undergoing painful medical treatment include impact of parental presence versus absence, interviews with children regarding their preferences for help during stressful medical procedures, and efforts to assess the impact of adult behaviors on children's coping or distress reactions. Some of these findings can be applied to the dental situation. Separation of the child from the parent during a painful medical procedure is unacceptable to most parents, and most children indicate a preference for parents to be present (Gonzalez et al. 1993). Family presence during medical procedures decreases anxiety for both the child and the parents. When parents have been prepared, they do not prolong the procedure or make the provider more anxious (Blesch and Fisher 1996; Dingeman et al. 2007; Powers and Rubenstein 1999; Wolfram and Turner 1996). In a systematic review by Piira et al. (2005), multiple studies confirmed that parents were more positive about treatment when they were with their children during invasive procedures. Blount and various coauthors have developed, revised, and created a shortened form of a Child–Adult Medical Procedure Interaction Scale (CAMPIS; Blount et al. 1989; Blount et al. 1991; Blount et al. 2001). The CAMPIS scales include categories for both child and adult behaviors, and each participant is scored separately. The child's procedural distress and coping, and the various adults' behaviors that significantly influence the distress of children, are included in the CAMPIS measures. Adult actions or comments which improve child coping and cooperation are termed "Coping-Promoting" and adult actions or comments which worsen the child's coping and cooperation are termed "Distress-Promoting."

Research using the CAMPIS, CAMPIS-R (Revised), and CAMPIS-SF (Short Form) leads to the conclusion that the number of adult Distress-Promoting behaviors exceeds the number of Coping-Promoting behaviors, and that many of the most common parent behaviors are counterproductive in helping the child to accept and cope with an uncomfortable medical procedure. Examples of Distress-Promoting behaviors are:

- *Uninformative reassuring comments*: "I won't let them hurt you." "Don't worry."
- *Informative reassuring comments*: "You're almost done." "Just two more minutes."
- *Giving control to child*: "Do you want to put this mask on?" "Can we start now?"
- *Criticism*: "You are in a bad mood today." "Why can't you be like your sister?"
- *Apology*: "I'm sorry this is taking so long." "I wish they didn't have to hurt you."
- *Empathy*: "I know it hurts." "You must be getting tired."
- *Suggestions or demands to the healthcare provider*: "He does better when he knows what is going to happen."

"When she gets upset, if you'll stop for a moment, she'll calm down."
- *Intimidation*: "I'm going to slap you." "You are seriously going to harm yourself."
- *Inappropriate or confusing comments*: "You can do anything but move." "He's going to try to not hurt you."

Investigations have repeatedly found that parents who displayed a high proportion of Distress-Promoting behaviors had children who were more distressed, fearful, experienced more pain, and were less approachable, less cooperative, and harder to help (Blount et al. 2007; Chorney et al. 2009; Mahoney et al. 2010; Pedro et al. 2010).

Reassurance is a particularly common but unhelpful parental behavior during painful procedures, yet parents likely provide reassurance believing it will comfort their child. Children may perceive that their parents are fearful when they reassure. The facial expression, vocal tone, and verbal content of adult-to-child messages are influential but incompletely understood for children during these procedures. Reassurance may tell the child that the situation is concerning and may direct attention to unpleasant aspects of the procedure (Chorney et al. 2009; McMurtry et al. 2010). Four independent, randomized, controlled trials with differing methodologies have confirmed increased amounts of child distress associated with adult emotion-focused behaviors including reassurance, empathy, and empathic touch during painful stimuli ranging from injections, to cold-pressor, to abdominal pain (Chambers et al. 2002; Walker et al. 2006).

Children displaying a high proportion of coping behaviors have been found to be less distressed, less fearful, experience less pain, and be more approaching, cooperative, and easily helped. Child coping and cooperation is positively related with the proportion of parent Coping-Promoting behaviors, although the association is much weaker than the relationship of parent Distress-Promoting behaviors to a child's lack of coping. Examples of parent actions and comments found to be Coping-Promoting behaviors are:

- *Non-procedural conversation with the child which redirects their attention to something pleasant*: Conversation about pets, toys, food, movies, television, friends, the child's plans or desires, and familiar and well-loved stories.
- *Prompt or command for child to use a coping strategy*: "Use your deep breathing now." "Squeeze my hand as hard as you can."
- *Humor directed to engage the child and improve their mood*: Silly jokes, such as "What is gray, weighs two tons, and puts people to sleep? A Hypnopotamus!" Any statement

that suggests outrageous ideas or emphasizes humorous aspects of a situation—although not at the child's expense. (See Chapter 7 for further use of humor in the dental setting.)

- *Reframing and reinterpreting the situation, equipment, and procedures*: Presenting procedures and equipment as something fun, positive, manageable, and understandable. "Let's play the astronaut game" is an example of reframing presentation of an oxygen mask.

Parents' happy facial expressions and rising vocal tones were interpreted positively by children in one study (McMurtry et al. 2010). Giving parents training improves their effectiveness in helping their child to cope (Blount et al. 1989). Parent coaching is a component of the cognitive behavior therapy package currently considered a "well-established treatment" to manage procedure-related pain in children and adolescents.

In summary, both parent's and healthcare provider's behaviors have been linked to children's levels of distress and coping during painful medical procedures. Providers may be able to directly affect parent's behavior by modeling desirable Coping-Promoting interactions with the child. Adult behaviors which direct the child's attention to their emotions promote distress and poor coping; adult behaviors which distract the child have the opposite result. Distress of the child is more strongly correlated with parent's behavior than with the behavior of the healthcare provider. Coping by the child is more strongly influenced by the healthcare provider's behavior than by their parent's behavior (Chorney et al. 2009; Cohen et al. 2002; Mahoney et al. 2010). Children are best supported during a painful procedure when both parents and providers use Coping-Promoting strategies.

### Application in Dental Practice

Not all strategies are readily transferred from a medical context into a dental context. For example, a child receiving dental restorations isolated with a rubber dam is not able to freely participate in a conversation with either their parent or the dentist. Box 4-1 summarizes information for parents about how to promote the coping and cooperation of their child during a dental appointment.

---

**Box 4-1   How Can I Best Help My Child?**

*Tips for Parents of Dental Patients*
Feelings shape our actions. Your child looks to you when deciding how to feel about a dental appointment. The advice included here is the result of more than 25 years of research on how parents can best help children cooperate for medical and dental treatments. Some of these ideas may surprise you. Thank you for your help in creating a great dental experience for your child.

*Parent Actions and Comments that Help Children Cooperate:*
Calm, relaxed, and upbeat parent attitude and body language. Happy facial expressions.
1) Positive stories or comments about your own dental experiences.
2) Showing no doubt that your child will enjoy the dental visit and make your proud.
3) Parent stays silent when dentist and staff is talking to the child and allows their child to answer questions from the dentist and staff.
4) Bringing something small that your child likes to the appointment (stuffed toy to hold, music, and headphones).
5) Before- and after-appointment talk which directs the child's attention to something pleasant. (Talk about pets, toys, stories, food, movies, television, friends, nd child's plans or desires.)

6) Bring a joke or silly riddle to tell the dentist. (Laughing will relax everyone.)
7) Planning a small reward for your child after a successful appointment.
8) Take a picture of the smiling child after the appointment and send to the grandparents.

*Parent Actions and Comments that Upset Children and Interfere with Cooperation:*
1) Stressed, hurried, or anxious parent attitude or body language.
2) Negative or scary stories and comments about dental treatment or appointments.
3) Uninformative reassuring comments. ("Don't worry.")
4) Informative reassuring comments. ("You're almost done.")
5) Criticism. ("Why can't you be like your sister?")
6) Apology. ("I'm sorry this is taking so long.")
7) Empathy. ("You must be getting tired.")
8) Suggestions to the dentist. ("He does better when he knows what is going to happen.")
9) Intimidation. ("You are seriously going to harm yourself.")
10) Inappropriate or confusing comments. ("He's going to try to not hurt you.")

# Parental Influence on Child Cooperation in Dental Settings

Dental research focusing on correlations between parent and family factors and child cooperation has included the topics of parent's dental anxiety, parent's presence or absence in the operatory during appointments, influence of parenting styles on child dental anxiety and cooperation, parent's behavior during the appointment, and parent's satisfaction. There are few studies of parent and/or family characteristics and cooperation of children that meet the highest standards of scientific evidence, with randomized subject allocation, presence of a control group, inclusion of both mothers and fathers, use of standardized and validated measurement tools, and outcomes measured at multiple time points by blinded observers.

## Parents' Dental Anxiety

Fear of dentistry is common—an estimated 11–20% of the general adult population experiences severe dental anxiety. In contrast to reported increases in general anxiety, the prevalence of dental fear in adults remained stable in studies conducted in the United States between 1954 and 2000 (Smith and Heaton 2003). Child dental anxiety is associated with the parent's own anxiety. Social learning theory predicts that siblings and other family members may create or feed dental anxiety via overt or subtle means. Negative attitudes toward dental care in the family are reportedly common reasons for developing dental fear. Some fearful adults report that their anxiety started in childhood, and in some instances, the anxiety preceded their first dental visit (Berggren and Meynert 1984; Locker and Liddell 1991).

In theory, a parent with dental anxiety could avoid instilling dental fear in their child. The parent could be prepared with education about the safety and comfort of modern dentistry and coached to consciously, continuously, and carefully monitor their emotional expressions and comments about dentistry. Methods for parental education are provided in the pre-appointment behavior modification section in Chapter 7. Ideally, actions of the dentally anxious parent would be ameliorated by the influences of another parent or family member without dental fear.

## Parent Presence or Absence in the Dental Operatory

Family inclusion has become the standard in pediatric medicine, and dental surveys examining parent presence and absence during treatment reflect a similar cultural change in pediatric dentistry (Adair et al. 2004). A clear majority of parents, 66–97%, prefer to stay with their child during dental treatment, as reported by investigators in the United States, India, Ireland, Israel, and Saudi Arabia (Arathi and Ashwani 1999; Crowley et al. 2005; Kamp 1992; Peretz and Zadik 1998; Shroff et al. 2015). A large study of fathers and mothers in Saudi Arabia found that parents most strongly wanted to be present in situations where their child expressed fear prior to the dental visit (Abushal and Adenubi 2009).

Advantages associated with parent presence in the operatory have been reported for the child, parent, and dentist. The proximity of a parent apparently offers the child increased emotional security and support. Parents report higher satisfaction and peace of mind that they are verifying their child's safety, supporting their child, and are presumed to benefit from hearing the dental health messages given to their children by caring dental providers. The dentist may benefit from improved cooperation from the emotionally supported child and their ability to build a trusting relationship with the parent as they provide care to the child (American Academy of Pediatric Dentistry 2019; Feigal 2001; Marcum et al. 1995; Pinkham 1991; Venham et al. 1978; Wright 1983).

Disadvantages of parental presence in the operatory have also been reported. Most problems are created due to division of attention. The child's attention is split between parent and dentist, and they may not know which adult to listen to. No investigator has found that a parent's repetition of a dentist's instructions improves child cooperation. When the parent contradicts the dentist, the child will become confused. Wright observed that parents who take an active and verbal role in the operatory disrupt the interaction between the child and the dentist, increasing potential for more child non-cooperation (1983). The dentist may become distracted or annoyed by a talkative parent, feeling compelled to simultaneously attend to child behaviors and parent concerns and behaviors while performing a procedure. If the parent has high dental anxiety, being in the dental operatory can amplify their negative emotions, which are then transmitted to the child. Fearful parents may directly interfere with dental treatment of their child by interrupting treatment, questioning the dentist's techniques, or relating their own negative experiences. Klingberg et al. (2009) observed that an anxious parent serves as a live and powerful negative model of dental anxiety to their child. Some dentists may be reluctant to use accepted behavior management techniques in the presence of a parent (American Academy of Pediatric Dentistry 2019; Marcum et al. 1995; Wright 1983).

A randomized, controlled trial examining the effect of parent presence in the operatory, patient age, and patient dental anxiety was conducted in a pediatric dentistry clinic in the Netherlands. In all, 90 patients aged four to eight years, had a habituation dental appointment followed by a treatment session on another day. Dentists found that the child's behavior was significantly better during habituation appointments when parents were not present in the operatory. Parents and dentists agreed that dentally anxious children cooperated better during treatment when the parent was not present. Dentists in the study reported disadvantages when parents of anxious children were present in the operatory. Parental presence or absence did not significantly affect the child's perception of the treatment (Cox et al. 2011).

If a parent is to be in the operatory, it is important that she does not disrupt the relationship between the child and dentist or distract the dentist. An investigation in the United States evaluated parents' compliance with instructions to remain silent in the operatory while their four- to nine-year-old children received restorative dentistry. Thirty-nine parents were randomized into two groups: written instruction only or written and verbal instruction. Most parents (82%) remained silent, and there were no significant associations found between the modality of the request to be silent and parent compliance. A few parents (10%) interrupted the appointment multiple times; in all of these cases, the child had a history of previous dental restorations (Jain et al. 2013).

*The American Academy of Pediatric Dentistry's Recommendations: Best Practices: Behavior Guidance for the Pediatric Dental Patient* includes parent presence or absence in the operatory among the methods for establishing effective dentist–child communication. A total of 239 parents of children aged 1–15 years completed surveys at the beginning and end of their children's appointments for preventive, restorative, or oral surgery or orthodontic care. Parents who showed consistency in their desires to be either present or absent and their actual experience during the appointment were more satisfied and positive about their child's appointment than parents who showed inconsistency. As patients were younger, the desire of parents to remain with their children increased (Kim et al. 2012).

Kupietzky et al. (2013) introduced and validated a Parent Cooperation Scale (PCS) to categorize parent behaviors and assess a parent's ability to be a constructive, supportive influence on their child during dental treatment. The PCS is analogous to the Frankl scale for rating child behaviors, with four groups of parent behaviors:

- *PCS 1.* Definitely negative (refusal of treatment plan, suspicious of dentist, overprotective of child);
- *PCS 2.* Negative (some evidence of negative attitude, needs to see caries on radiographs, acts as liaison between patient and dentist);

- *PCS 3.* Positive (accepting of treatment plan, cautious behavior at times, reluctantly allows child to be alone with dentist);
- *PCS 4.* Definitely positive (trustful, expresses confidence in dentist, allows patient to be alone with dental staff).

A study of 244 children and parents found a significant association between parent PCS scores and the Frankl scores of their children. Parents with negative behavior were more likely to present with children who had negative dental behavior, and positive parents were more likely to have cooperative children.

In summary, a negative, distrustful, or intrusive parent is a disruptive influence in the dental operatory, even when the parent is well-intentioned. The child's awareness of and attunement to their parent's negative emotional state undermines their ability to listen, relate, and respond to the dentist positively. For each child–parent pair, the risk and benefit of parent presence during treatment should be considered, and a proactive decision should be made and respectfully explained to the parent.

## Influence of Parenting Style

Pediatric dentists surveyed in 2001 perceived a change in American parenting styles during the last decades of the twentieth century. Families shifted away from traditional family hierarchies with the parent in charge, moving toward a more permissive and democratic family style. In families with permissive parenting styles, child misbehavior does not necessarily result in negative consequences for the child. The dentists also reported increases in single-parent families, family mobility, and dual-income families. The vast majority of dentists believed that these family changes had resulted in somewhat or much worse child patient cooperation during dental treatment. Simultaneously with declining patient cooperation, parent expectations (e.g., no crying) for their child's dental appointments were often inflated and not achievable (Casamassimo and Wilson 2002).

An investigation of many variables relating to child cooperation for dental treatment found that parent-reported frequency of difficult child behaviors in 3–12-year-olds outside the dental setting did not predict the child's disruptiveness during treatment. Young patient age was the best predictor of uncooperative behavior. Uncooperative behavior during the dental appointment also correlated with parents who set few limits and were relaxed and supportive of their child (Allen et al. 2003).

A study of the relationships between parenting style, parent's behavior during the appointment, child's cooperation with dental treatment, and behavior management techniques used was reported by Aminabadi and Farahani (2008) with a follow-up study including validated measures of child temperament and child anxiety (Aminabadi et al. 2015). Both studies included healthy children aged four to six years and their parents. The children, their parents, and the dentist were videotaped while the child received an inferior alveolar block and amalgam restoration of a mandibular molar. Parent style was classified by using typology of Baumrind, as well as Maccoby and Martin, which was described earlier in this chapter.

Parents with an Authoritative style (high warmth and firm behavior controls) primarily observed the treatment, and also rewarded, verbally encouraged (e.g., your teeth are going to be more beautiful"), and explained. The children of Authoritative parents readily tolerated the treatment without any negative reactions; dentists employed basic behavior shaping during treatment. Authoritative parenting style was significantly related both positively to cooperative child behavior and negatively to child's anxiety. Expression of effortful control temperament trait was found in the children of authoritative parents.

Parents with a Permissive style (high warmth and low behavior controls) exhibited vastly different behaviors: physical contacting their child, stopping treatment at least once, questioning the efficacy of the local anesthesia (e.g., "I guess he is suffering from what you do"). Very few Permissive parents observed without participating further. All children were uncooperative with negative responses including crying and/or hand and foot movements. Behavior management techniques involved voice control, immobilization, and separation from the parents. Permissive parenting style significantly increased child negative affectivity.

Fewer parents had an Authoritarian style (low warmth and high behavior control), and all of these parents took aggressive physical control of their child. All children of Authoritarian parents reacted negatively, with most trying to escape. Behavior management techniques of physical restraint and voice control were used for this patient group. Children of Authoritarian parents had significantly higher levels of anxiety.

There were no parents with the Neglectful style (low warmth and low behavior control) in either studies.

These studies provide support for the view that parent behaviors which distract the child from the dentist or undermine the authority of the dentist are destructive to the dentist–child relationship. It provides additional support for the concept of the parent's role as a "silent observer" when in the dental operatory with their child.

In the Netherlands, 100 children aged 4–12 years who were referred to a specialized pediatric dentistry clinic due to uncooperative behavior were analyzed with their parents for the relationship between child dental anxiety,

level of cooperation for treatment, and their parents' style of parenting. Pre-treatment parent expectations of the dentist's effectiveness in managing their child's behavior significantly differed based on the parenting style. Authoritarian parents more strongly expected that their child's behavior could be managed by the dentist; Permissive and Neglectful parents had less confidence in the dentist. In this study, parents were not present in the dental operatory during treatment. Parenting style was not found to be related to the child's pre-treatment dental anxiety or to the child's cooperation during the treatment. Highly anxious children were more disruptive than less anxious children. Parents showed more confidence in the child–dentist relationship after the completion of their child's dental treatment and expressed a lower need to accompany their child into the dental operatory (Krikken and Verrkamp 2008).

A survey of parents of 4–12-year-old children examined association between child dental anxiety and parenting style. Parenting style was categorized for 331 parents of children referred to specialty pediatric dentistry clinics due to non-cooperation, and for 120 parents whose children had not been referred. Child age and child dental anxiety were also examined. Parenting style did not correlate to a child's referred versus non-referred status. No correlation was found between children's dental anxiety and their parents' styles of parenting. Referred children were significantly younger than non-referred children and had significantly more dental anxiety (Krikken et al. 2012).

A study exploring parenting style, sociodemographics, caries status, and cooperation during the first dental visit for 132 children aged three to six years and their parents found that children with authoritative parents exhibited significantly more positive behavior and less caries compared to children with authoritarian or permissive parents. Attending daycare was also associated with improved cooperation during the first dental visit (Howenstein et al. 2015).

## Parent Prediction of Child Cooperation

A parent's ability to predict their child's cooperation for dental treatment is of interest. A study of 273 three-year-old children found that parents were accurate in predicting a negative reaction from their child to introductory dental procedures such as sitting in the dental chair and allowing the explorer against the fingernail and a tooth. The child's anxiety when meeting new people also predicted cooperation (Holst et al. 1993).

A study of 184 parents and their children aged 6–10 years assessed how parents' and children's fear assessments correlated with behavior during dental treatment. There was inconsistency between parents' assessment and child's self-assessment of dental fear. Parents' assessment of their children's dental anxiety was at best a fair predictor for cooperation, and the children's self-assessments were fair to good. Parents overestimated dental anxiety for low anxious children, and parents of highly anxious children underestimated their child's anxiety. The child's dental fear score best predicted cooperation (Klein et al. 2015).

### Application in Dental Practice

Most dentists learn about the child from the parent, but less frequently do they ask parents to predict how well the child will cooperate for treatment. Parents will readily share information about their personal dental attitudes, parenting styles, and desires to be present or absent during their children's treatment if they are asked about these factors in a private, thoughtful, and respectful conversation with the dentist. For school-aged patients, both the parent and child should be questioned about dental fear and anxiety.

## Dentist and Parent Communication

Over the past several decades, the nature of health care delivery has shifted from a paternalistic "doctor is the authority" model to a more egalitarian model where patients and families expect to participate in treatment decisions and health care delivery. The health and welfare of the child should be the primary focus for both parent and dentist. The role of the dentist is to provide parents with the risk and benefit information needed to make an informed decision and to correct any misinformation the parent may have. The role of the parent is to receive and process this information and make a choice for the child. Dentists may need to accept decisions they disagree with if those decisions are not likely to be harmful to the child (Diekema 2005).

The dentist should listen attentively and respectfully to the parent's concerns, recognizing that parents may not use the same decision criteria as the dentist. One dentist will not be an ideal match for every child and family. When distrust develops or significant differences in philosophy of care exist, the child and family should be directed to another dentist and/or clinic.

Wright and Stigers (2011) suggest incorporating a "functional inquiry" about child behaviors into the initial patient health history. Brief questions about the child's past cooperation in the medical setting, the child's perception of his dental health or dental problem, the parent's own dental anxiety, and the parent's prediction of child cooperation for dental care will guide the dentist toward understanding both the child and her parent. Knowledge of the child and parental concerns allows the dentist to more accurately predict a child's ability to cooperate. The functional inquiry is discussed in greater detail in Chapter 7.

It is natural for dentists and parents to take their cues from each other as they interact with the child during a dental appointment. Therefore, even brief interventions which prepare the parent to support their child without disrupting the child–dentist relationship may be beneficial. Educational materials for parents and families explaining the different types of coping strategies with brief examples can be posted on the office website and made available in the office. Box 4-1 offers helpful hints for parents.

## Summary

Families establish styles of interacting between family members and with the world outside the family long before reaching a dental office. Social circumstances and family patterns of behavior may prepare a child to be more or less accepting of dental treatment. The dentist should mindfully assess the dynamics between new patients and their parents or caregivers before deciding how best to guide them through the dental appointment. Early attention to a family's situation, style, and preferences will allow the dentist to gain the trust of the parent and earn the opportunity to form a positive, long-term relationship with the child.

## Acknowledgment

The author thanks Dr. Bryan J. Williams, whose advice helped translate research and theory into clinical dental practice.

## References

Abushal, M. and Adenubi, J.O. (2009). Attitudes of Saudi parents toward separation from their children during dental treatment. *Saudi Dental Journal*, 21, 63–67.

Adair, S.M., Waller, J.L., Schafer, T.E. et al. (2004). A survey of members of the American Academy of Pediatric Dentistry on their use of behavior management techniques. *Pediatric Dentistry*, 26, 159–166.

Allen, K.D., Hutfless, S., and Larzelere, R. (2003). Evaluation of two predictors of child disruptive behavior during restorative dental treatment. *Journal of Dentistry for Children*, 70, 221–225.

American Academy of Pediatric Dentistry. (2019–2020). Behavior guidance for the pediatric dental patient. *The Reference Manual of Pediatric Dentistry*, 266–279.

American Academy of Pediatrics. (2003). Family pediatrics: Report of the task force on the family. *Pediatrics*, 111, 1541–1571.

American Academy of Pediatrics. (2012). Policy statement. *Patient- and family-centered care and the pediatrician's role. Pediatrics*, 129, 394–404.

Aminabadi, N.A. and Farahani, R.M. (2008). Correlation of parenting style and pediatric behavior guidance strategies in the dental setting: Preliminary findings. *Acta Odontologica Scandinavia*, 66, 99–104.

Aminabadi, N.A., Deijavan, A.S., Jamali, Z. et al. (2015). The influence of parenting style and child temperament on child-parent-dentist interactions. *Pediatric Dentistry*, 37, 342–347.

Arathi, R. and Ashwani, R. (1999). Parental presence in the dental operatory—Parent's point of view. *Journal of Indian Society of Pedodontics and Preventive Dentistry*, 17, 150–155.

Barber, J.S., Axinn, W.G., and Thornton, A. (1999). Unwanted childbearing, health, and mother-child relationships. *Journal of Health and Social Behavior*, 40, 231–257.

Barber, J.S. and East, P.L. (2009). Home and parenting resources available to siblings depending on their birth intention status. *Child Development*, 80, 921–939.

Baumrind, D. (1973). The development of instrumental competence through socialization. In: A.D. Pick (Ed.), Minnesota Symposium on Child Psychology, Vol. 7, 3–46. Minneapolis: University of Minnesota Press.

Berggren, U. and Meynert, G. (1984). Dental fear and avoidance: Causes, symptoms, and consequences. *Journal of the American Dental Association*, 109, 247–251.

Blesch, P. and Fisher, M.L. (1996). The impact of parental presence on parental anxiety and satisfaction. *Association of Operating Room Nurses. AORN Journal*, 63, 761–768.

Blount, R.L. Bunke, V.V., Cohen, L.L. et al. (2001). The Child-adult medical procedure interaction scale-short form (CAMPIS-SF): Validation of a rating scale for children's and adults' behaviors during painful medical procedures. *Journal of Pain and Symptom Management*, 22, 591–599.

Blount, R.L., Corbin, S.M., Sturges, J.W. et al. (1989). The relationship between adults' behavior and child coping and distress during BMA/LP procedures: A sequential analysis. *Behavior Therapy*, 20, 585–601.

Blount, R.L., Landolf-Fritsche, B., Powers, S.W. et al. (1991). Differences between high and low coping children and

between parent and staff behaviors during painful medical procedures. *Journal of Pediatric Psychology*, 16, 795–809.

Blount, R.L., Simons, L.E., Devine, K.A. et al. (2007). Evidence-based assessment of coping and stress in pediatric psychology. *Journal of Pediatric Psychology*, 33, 1021–1045.

Bowlby, J. (1982). Attachment and loss: Retrospect and prospect. *American Journal of Orthopsychiatry.* 52, 664–678.

Boyce, W.T. (2014). The lifelong effects of early childhood adversity and toxic stress. *Pediatric Dentistry*, 36, 102–108.

Burgette, J.M., Polk, D.E., Shah, N. et al. (2019). Mother's perceived social support and Children's dental caries in Northern Appalachia. *Pediatric Dentistry*, 41, 200–205.

Cameron, L., Erkal, N., Gangadharan, L. et al. (2013). Little emperors: Behavioral impacts of China's One-Child Policy. *Science*, 339, 953–957.

Casamassimo, P.S. and Wilson, S. (2002). Effects of changing US parenting styles on dental practice: Perception of diplomates of the American Board of Pediatric Dentistry. *Pediatric Dentistry*, 24, 18–22.

Chambers, C.T., Craig, K.D., and Bennett, S.M. (2002). The impact of maternal behavior on children's pain experiences: An experimental analysis. *Journal of Pediatric Psychology*, 27, 293–301.

Chorney, J.M., Torrey, C., Blount, R.L. et al. (2009). Healthcare provider and parent behavior and children's coping and distress at anesthesia induction. *Anesthesiology*, 111, 1290–1296.

Chua, A. (2011). Battle Hymn of the Tiger Mother. Penguin Press.

Cline, F.W. and Fay, J. (1990). Parenting with Love and Logic: Teaching Children Responsibility, 23–25. Pinon Press.

Cohen, L.L., Bernard, R.S., Greco, L.A. et al. (2002). A child-focused intervention for coping with procedural pain: Are parent and nurse coaches necessary? *Journal of Pediatric Psychology*, 27, 747–757.

Coleman, P.K. and Karraker, K.H. (1998). Self-efficacy and parenting quality: findings and future applications. *Developmental Review*, 18, 47–85.

Conger, K.J., Rueter, M.A., and Conger, R.D. (2000). The role of economic pressure in the lives of parents and their adolescents: the family stress model. In: L.J. Crockett and R.J. Silberesisen (Eds.), Negotiating Adolescence in Times of Social Change, 201–233. Cambridge, England: Cambridge University Press.

Conradt, E. (2017). Using principles of behavioral epigenetics to advance research on early-life stress. *Child Development Perspectives*, 11, 107–112.

Cox, I.C.J., Krikken, J.B., and Veerkamp, J.S.J. (2011). Influence of parental presence on the child's perception of, and behaviour, during dental treatment. *European Archives of Paediatric Dentistry,* 12, 200–204.

Crowley, E., Whelton, H., O'Mullane, D. et al. (2005). Parents' preference as to whether they would like to accompany their child when receiving dental treatment—results from a national survey. *Journal of the Irish Dental Association*, 51, 23–24.

Darling, N. and Steinberg, L. (1993). Parenting style as context: An integrative model. *Psychological Bulletin*, 113, 487–496.

Davies, P.T., Cummings, E.M., and Winter, M.A. (2004). Pathways between profiles of family functioning, child security in the interparental subsystem, and child psychological problems. *Development and Psychopathology*, 16, 525–550.

Deater-Deckard, K., Dodge, K.A., Bates, J.E. et al. (1996). Physical discipline among African American and European American mothers: Links to children's externalizing behaviors. *Developmental Psychology*, 32, 1065–1072.

Diekema, D.S. (2005). Responding to parental refusals of immunization of children. *Pediatrics*, 115, 1428–1431.

Dingeman, R.S., Mitchell, E., Meyer, E. et al. (2007). Parent presence during complex invasive procedures and cardiopulmonary resuscitation: A systematic review of the literature. *Pediatrics*, 120, 842–854.

Dix, T. (1991). The affective organization of parenting: Adaptive and maladaptive processes. *Psychological Bulletin*, 110, 3–25.

Edelstein, G.L. and Chinn, C.H. (2009). Update on disparities in oral health and access to dental care for America's children. *Academic Pediatrics*, 9, 415–419.

Feigal, R.J. (2001). Guiding and managing the child dental patient: A fresh look at old pedagogy. *Journal of Dental Education*, 65, 1369–1376.

Goh, E.C.L. and Kuczynski, L. (2009). Agency and power of single children in multi-generational families in urban Xiamen, China. *Culture & Psychology*, 15, 506–534.

Gonzalez, J.C., Routh, D.K., and Armstrong, F.D. (1993). Effects of maternal distraction versus reassurance on children's reactions to injection. *Journal of Pediatric Psychology*, 18, 593–604.

Gustafsson, A., Arnrup, K., Broberg, A.G. et al. (2007). Psychosocial concomitants to dental fear and behavioural management problems. *International Journal of Paediatric Dentistry*. 17, 449–459.

Ho, D., Bluestein, D.N., and Jenkins, J.M. (2008). Cultural differences in the relationship between parenting and children's behavior. *Developmental Psychology*, 44, 507–522.

Holst, A., Hallonstan, A.L., Schroder, U. et al. (1993). Prediction of behavior-management problems in 3-year-old children. *Scandinavian Journal of Dental Research*, 101, 110–114.

Howenstein, J., Kumar, A., Casamassimo, P.S. et al. (2015). Correlating parenting styles with child behavior and caries. *Pediatric Dentistry*. 37, 59–64.

Iida, H. and Rozier, R.G. (2013). Mother-perceived social capital and children's oral health and use of dental care in the United States. *American Journal of Public Health*, 103, 480–487.

Jain, D., Mathu-Muju, K., Nash, D.A. et al. (2013). Parental compliance with instructions to remain silent in the dental operatory. *Pediatric Dentistry*, 35, 47–51.

Kalil, A. and Ryan, R.M. (2010). Mother's economic conditions and sources of support in fragile families. The Future of Children; Princeton, 20, Issue 2.

Kamp, A.A. (1992). Parent child separation during dental care: a survey of parent's preference. *Pediatric Dentistry*, 14, 231–235.

Kim, J.S., Boynton, J.R., and Inglehart, M.R. (2012). Parents' presence in the operatory during their child's dental visit: A person-environmental fit analysis of parents' responses. *Pediatric Dentistry*, 34, 407–413.

Kitayama, S. and Park, J. (2010). Cultural neuroscience of the self: Understanding the social grounding of the brain. *Social Cognitive and Affective Neuroscience*, 5, 111–129.

Klein, U., Manangkil, R., and DeWitt, P. (2015). Parent's ability to assess dental fear in their six-to 10-year-old children. *Pediatric Dentistry*, 37, 436–441.

Kliewer, W., Fearnow, M.D., and Miller, P.A. (1996). Coping socialization in middle childhood: Tests of maternal and paternal influences. *Child Development*, 67, 233–2357.

Klingberg, G., Raadal, M., and Arnup, K. (2009). Dental fear and behavior management problems. In: G. Koch and S. Poulsen (Eds.), Pediatric Dentistry: A Clinical Approach, 2nd ed., 32–43. Blackwell Publishing Ltd.

Kochanska, G. (1995). Children's temperament, mothers' discipline, and security of attachment: Multiple pathways to emerging internalization. *Child Development*, 66, 597–615.

Kochanska, G., Aksan, N., and Joy, M.E. (2007). Children's fearfulness as a moderator of parenting in early socialization: Two longitudinal studies. *Developmental Psychology*, 43, 222–237.

Kochanska, G. and Kim, S. (2013). Early attachment organization with both parents and future behavior problems: From infancy to middle childhood. *Child Development*, 84, 283–296.

Kochanska, G., Philibert, R.A., and Barry, R.A. (2009). Interplay of genes and early mother-child relationship in the development of self-regulation from toddler to preschool age. *Journal of Child Psychology and Psychiatry*, 5, 1331–1338.

Krikken, J.B., van Wijk, A.J., ten Cate, J.M. et al. (2012). Child dental anxiety, parental rearing style and referral status of children. *Community Dental Health*. 29, 89–92.

Krikken, J.B. and Veerkamp, J.S.J. (2008). Child rearing styles, dental anxiety, and disruptive behavior; an exploratory study. European Archives of Paediatric Dentistry. 9 supplement 1, 23–28.

Kruger, J.S., Kodjebacheva, G.D., Kunkel, L. et al. (2015). Caregiver financial distress, depressive symptoms and limited social capital as barriers to children's dental care in a mid-western county in the United States. *Community Dental Health*, 32, 252–256.

Kupietzky, A., Tal, E., and Vargas, K.G. (2013). Parental cooperation scale in the pediatric dentistry setting: Reliability and criteria. *Journal of Clinical Pediatric Dentistry*, 37, 157–161.

Lay, K., Waters, E., and Park, K.A. (1989). Maternal responsiveness and child compliance: The role of mood as a mediator. *Child Development*, 60, 1405–1411.

Locker, D. and Liddell, A.M. (1991). Correlates of dental anxiety among older adults. *Journal of Dental Research*, 70, 198–203.

Long, N. (2004). The changing nature of parenting in America. *Pediatric Dentistry*, 26, 121–124.

Maccoby, E.E. (1991). The role of parents in the socialization of children: An historical overview. *Developmental Psychology*, 28, 1006–1017.

Maccoby, E.E. and Martin, J.A. (1983). Socialization in the context of the family: Parent-child interaction. In P. Mussen and E.M. Hetheringon (Eds.), Handbook of Child Psychology, Volume IV: Socialization, Personality, and Social Development, 4th ed., 1–101. New York: Wiley.

Mahoney, L., Ayers, S., and Seddon, P. (2010). The association between parent's and healthcare professional's behavior and children's coping and distress during venipuncture. *Journal of Pediatric Psychology*, 35, 989–995.

Marcum, B.K., Turner, C., and Courts, F.J. (1995). Pediatric dentists' attitudes regarding parental presence during dental procedures. *Pediatric Dentistry*, 17, 432–436.

McGuire, S., Dunn, J., and Polmin, R. (1995). Maternal differential treatment of siblings and children's behavioral problems: A longitudinal study. *Development and Psychopathology*, 7, 515–528.

McKernon, W.L., Holmbeck, G.N., Colder, C.R. et al. (2001). Longitudinal study of observed and perceived family influences on problem-focused coping behaviors of preadolescents with spina bifida. *Journal of Pediatric Psychology*, 26, 41–54.

McLanahan, S. and Beck, A.N. (2010). Parental relationships in fragile families. The Future of Children; Princeton, 20, Issue 2.

McMurtry, C.M., Chambers, C.T., McGrath, P.J. et al. (2010). When "don't worry" communicates fear: Children's perceptions of parental reassurance and distraction during a painful medical procedure. *Pain*, 150, 52–58.

Morrison, I., Lloyd, D., di Pellegrino, G. et al. (2004). Vicarious responses to pain in anterior cingulate cortex: Is empathy a multisensory issue? *Cognitive & Affective Behavioral Neuroscience*, 4, 270–278.

O'Connor, T.G., Rutter, M., and the English and Romanian Adoptees Study Team. (2000). Attachment disorder behavior following early severe deprivation: Extension and longitudinal follow-up. *Journal of the American Academy of Child and Adolescent Psychiatry*, 39, 703–712.

Paulussen-Hoogeboom, M.C., Stams, G.J.J.M., Hermanns, J.M.A. et al. (2007). Child negative emotionality and parenting from infancy to preschool: A meta-analytic review. *Developmental Psychology*, 43, 438–453.

Pedro, H., Barros, L., and Moleiro, C. (2010). Brief report: Parents and nurses' behaviors associated with child distress during routine immunization in a Portuguese population. *Journal of Pediatric Psychology*, 35, 602–610.

Peretz, B. and Zadik, D. (1998). Attitudes of parents toward their presence in the operatory during dental treatments to their children. *Journal of Clinical Pediatric Dentistry*. 23, 27–30.

Piira, T., Sugiura, T., Champion, G.D. et al. (2005). The role of parental presence in the context of children's medical procedures: A systematic review. *Child: Care, Health, and Development*, 31, 233–243.

Pinkham, J. (1991). An analysis of the phenomenon of increased parental participation during the child's dental experience. *Journal of Dentistry for Children*, 58, 458–463.

Powers, K.S. and Rubenstein, J.S. (1999). Family presence during invasive procedures in the pediatric intensive care unit. *Archives of Pediatrics and Adolescent Medicine*, 153, 955–958.

Reichman, N.E., Teitler, J.O., Garfinkel, I. et al. (2001). Fragile families: Sample and design. *Children and Youth Services Review*, 23, 303–326.

Reitz, E., Dekovic, M., and Meijer, A. (2006). Longitudinal relations among parenting, best friends, and early adolescent problem behavior. *Journal of Early Adolescence*, 26, 272–295.

Shroff, S., Hughes, C., and Mobley, C. (2015). Attitudes and preferences of parents about being present in the dental operatory. *Pediatric Dentistry*, 37, 51–55.

Slagt, M., Decović, M., de Haan, A.D. et al. (2012). Longitudinal associations between mothers' and fathers' sense of competence and children's externalizing problem: The mediating role of parenting. *Developmental Psychology*, 48, 1554–1562.

Smith, T.A. and Heaton, L.J. (2003). Fear of dental care. Are we making any progress? *Journal of the American Dental Association*, 134, 1101–1108.

Teti, D.M. and Cole, P.M. (2011). Parenting at risk: New perspectives, new approaches. *Journal of Family Psychology*, 25, 625–634.

Thompson, R.A. (1994). Emotion regulation: A theme in search of definition. *Monographs of the Society for Research in Child Development*, 59, 25–52.

Valiente, C., Fabes, R.A., Eisenberg, N. et al. (2004). The relations of parental expressivity and support to children's coping with daily stress. *Journal of Family Psychology*, 18, 97–106.

Valiente, C., Lemery-Chalfant, K., and Reiser, M. (2007). Pathways to problem behaviors: Chaotic homes, parent and child effortful control, and parenting. *Social Development*, 16, 249–267.

Venham, L., Bengstron, D., and Cipes, M. (1978). Parent's presence and the child's response to dental stress. *Journal of Dentistry for Children*, 45, 213–217.

Volling, B.L. (2005). The transition to siblinghood: A developmental ecological systems perspective and directions for future research. *Journal of Family Psychology*, 19, 542–549.

Volling, B.L. (2012). Family transitions following the birth of a sibling: An empirical review of changes in the firstborn's adjustment. *Psychological Bulletin,* 138, 497–528.

Volling, B.L. and Elins, J.L. (1998). Family relationships and children's emotional adjustment as correlates of maternal and paternal differential treatment: A replication with toddler and preschool siblings. *Child Development*, 69, 1640–1656.

Volling, B.L., McElwain, N.L., and Miller, A.L. (2002). Emotion regulation in context: The jealousy complex between young siblings and its relations with child and family characteristics. *Child Development*, 73, 581–600.

Waldfogel, J., Craigie, T., and Brooks-Gunn, J. (2010). Fragile families and child wellbeing. The Future of Children; Princeton, 20, Issue 2.

Walker, L., Williams, S.E., Smith, C.A. et al. (2006). Parent attention versus distraction: Impact on symptom complaints by children with and without chronic functional abdominal pain. *Pain*, 122, 43–52.

Wildeman, C. and Western, B. (2010). Incarceration in fragile families. The Future of Children; Princeton, 20, Issue 2.

Wolfram, R.W. and Turner, E.D. (1996). Effects of parental presence during children's venipuncture. *Academic Emergency Medicine*, 3, 58–64.

Wright, G.Z. (1983). Parent-child separation. In: G.Z. Wright, P.E. Starkey, and D.E. Gardner (Eds.), Managing Children's Behavior in the Dental Office, 57–74. CV Mosby Co.

Wright, G.Z. and Stigers, J.I. (2011). Nonpharmacologic management of children's behaviors. In: J.A. Dean, D.R. Avery, and R.E. McDonald (Eds.), Dentistry for the Child and Adolescent, 9th ed., 27–40. Mosby.

Zeanah, C.H. and Fox, N.A. (2004). Temperament and attachment disorders. *Journal of Clinical Child and Adolescent Psychology*, 33, 32–41.

## Additional Reading

Arnup, K., Berggren, U., Broberg, A.G. et al. (2002). Attitudes to dental care among parents of uncooperative vs. cooperative child dental patients. *European Journal of Oral Science*, 110, 75–82.

Bowlby, J. (1969). Attachment and Loss. Volume 1: Attachment. Basic books.

Bowlby, J. (1972). Attachment and Loss. Volume 2: Separation. Basic books.

Eisenberg, N., Smith, C.L., and Spinrad, T.L. (2011). Effortful control. Relations with emotion regulation, adjustment, and socialization in childhood. In: K.D. Vohs and R.F. Baumeister (Eds.), Handbook of Self-Regulation: Research, Theory, and Applications, 2nd ed., 263–283. The Guildford Press.

Princeton University, Columbia University. *Fragile Families and Child Well-Being Study.* http://www.fragilefamilies.princeton.edu/.

Ganiban, J.M., Ulbricht, J., Saudino, K.J. et al. (2011). Understanding child-based effects on parenting: Temperament as a moderator of genetic and environmental contributions to parenting. *Developmental Psychology*, 47, 676–692.

Klingberg, G. and Berggren, R. (1992). Dental problem behaviors in children of parents with severe dental fear. *Swedish Dental Journal*, 16, 27–32.

Lucero, I. (2018). Written in the body? Healing the epigenetic molecular wounds of complex trauma through empathy and kindness. *Journal of Child & Adolescent Trauma*, 11, 443–455.

Martin, S.R., Chorney, J.M., Tan, E.T. et al. (2011). Changing healthcare provider's behavior during pediatric inductions with an empirically based intervention. *Anesthesiology*, 115, 18–27.

Powers, S.W. (1999). Empirically supported treatments in pediatric psychology: procedure-related pain. *Journal of Pediatric Psychology*, 24, 131–145.

Repetti, R.L., Taylor, S.E., and Saxbe, D. (2007). The influence of early socialization experiences on the development of biological systems. In: J. Grusec and P. Hastings (Eds.), Handbook of Socialization, 124–152. Guilford, New York, NY.

Rodriguez, D.M., Clough, V., Gowda, A.S. et al. (2012). Multimethod assessment of children's distress during noninvasive outpatient medical procedures: Child and parent attitudes and factors. *Journal of Pediatric Psychology*, 37, 557–566.

Rothbart, M.K. and Bates, J.E. (2006). Temperament. In: N. Eisenberg and W. Damon (Eds.), Handbook of Child Psychology: Vol. 3. Social, Emotional, and Personality Development, 6th ed., 99–166. Wiley.

Roustit, C., Chaix, B., and Chauvin, P. (2007). Family breakup and adolescents' psychosocial maladjustment: Public health implications of family disruptions. *Pediatrics*, 120, e984–e991.

Uman, L.S., Chambers, C.T., McGrath, P.J. et al. (2008). A systematic review of randomized controlled trials examining psychological interventions for needle-related procedural pain and distress in children and adolescents: An abbreviated Cochrane Review. *Journal of Pediatric Psychology*, 33, 842–854.

van der Gaad, C., Minderaa, R.B., and Keysers, C. (2007). Facial expressions: What the mirror neuron system can and cannot tell us. *Social Neuroscience*, 2, 179–222.

Versloot, J. and Craig, K.D. (2009). The communication of pain in paediatric dentistry. *European Archives of Paediatric Dentistry*, 10, 61–66.

5

# Societal Influences on the Contemporary Family

*Janice Townsend, Martha Wells, and Larry Dormois*

## Introduction

The dental practice of the not-too-distant past looks very different from today. Dentists are cognizant that the most meaningful changes are not in technology or materials but in the dramatically transformed patient population we now serve. Dental practices care for patients with different backgrounds, knowledge, priorities, expectations, and resources. The rapidly evolving societal influences on the contemporary family put pediatric dentistry at the fore-front of navigating these challenges.

Pediatric dentistry is no longer composed of a relatively homogenous patient base but reflects modern culture char-acterized by its diversity (Wells et al. 2018). Traditionally, diversity has been referred to as a "melting pot," welcoming people from many different countries, races, and religions, hoping to find ncw opportunities and a better way of life. Immigrants brought their heritage and traditions, which were passed down through generations. Today, the trend is toward multiculturalism, not assimilation. The "melting pot" is giving way to new metaphors such as "salad bowl," mixtures of various ingredients that keep their individual characteristics (Millet 2013). Immigrant populations are not being blended together in one "pot," but rather are trans-forming society into a multicultural mosaic.

The broader understanding of diversity refers to race eth-nicity, gender, sexual orientation, religion, and country of origin, among other factors (Goleman 2014). To extend the analogy, the "salad" is seasoned with generational differ-ences, regional/geographic influences, and a changing family structure where more women are working outside of the home adding significant income to family finances. Add in a dash of same sex parenting, religious and political divides, differing value systems, and unlimited access to information (and misinformation) via the Internet, and you begin to understand the challenges facing pediatric healthcare providers.

Not understanding the diversity of the patient base that one's practice serves can lead to misunderstandings, com-munication breakdowns, missed opportunities, loss of rep-utation, and frustration. The purpose of this chapter is to describe the influence of society on the contemporary fam-ily and to give dentists insight into why families behave the way they do today. It will offer some guidance on how to embrace the parent–professional relationship that has become increasingly complex and has moved away from the paternalistic model of "the doctor knows best." An understanding of these influences can help dentists com-municate with and guide parents so that dentists can best help their children. No two practitioners, practices, or com-munities are exactly the same. The observations in this chapter are generalizations, which will not fit everyone; however, commonalities help elucidate how parents might prcfcr to communicate and interact with healthcare profes-sionals. The topics covered in this chapter are meant as a starting place for dental providers to understand their unique practice environment and adjust to the unique expectations of their patient base.

## The Parents of Today

### Generational Influences

Modern parents are a conglomeration of individuals from different generational cohorts. All, or even most, parents do not share a common world purview. Generational cate-gories help practitioners understand how different world events, societal or economic shifts, and technological advances shape people's view of the world. In general, each cohort shares some over-arching attitudes and motivations that might be important to the healthcare professional (Table 5-1).

Baby Boomers have typically been over-protective, "heli-copter parents," hovering over their children, restricting

**Table 5-1**   Generational characteristics and shared tendencies among birth cohorts.

| Trait | Baby Boomers (1946–1964) | Generation Xers (1965–1980) | Millennials (1981–1996) | Generation Z-ers (1997–2012) |
|---|---|---|---|---|
| Core values | • Anything is possible<br>• Question everything | • Balance<br>• Diversity<br>• Independence<br>• Self-reliance<br>• Skepticism/cynicism | • Achievement<br>• Civic duty<br>• Diversity<br>• Extreme fun<br>• Like personal attention<br>• Self-confident | • Civic duty<br>• Community/collective good<br>• Authentic<br>• Ambitious<br>• Autonomous<br>• Success-oriented |
| Attributes | • Challenge authority<br>• Consumerism<br>• Most educated group<br>• Ethical<br>• Optimistic | • Adaptable<br>• Pampered by parents<br>• Highly educated<br>• Confident<br>• Competent<br>• Focused on family<br>• Results-oriented<br>• Pragmatic | • At ease in teams<br>• Highly educated<br>• Consumer mentality (even health care is a commodity to be consumed)<br>• Use Internet for health information<br>• Strong sense of entitlement<br>• Multi-taskers | • Most diverse<br>• Socially and technologically empowered<br>• Hard-working, value education<br>• Super multi-taskers<br>• Digital natives—Lifelong access to instant information<br>• Weaker people skills |
| As a consumer | • Brand-specific, loyal to a brand | • Discerning, information seeking, value convenience | • Value the "experience"<br>• Value ease and accessibility | • Value authenticity |
| Respect for authority | • Originally skeptical but time equals authority | • Skeptical of authority figures<br>• Will test authority repeatedly | • Will test authority but often seek out authority figures for guidance | • Less regard for hierarchy |
| Communication | • Diplomatic<br>• Like being called by first name | • Blunt/direct | • Polite | • Weaker social skills<br>• Texting over talking |
| Preferred method of communication | • Verbal<br>• Personal Interaction | • Voicemail<br>• Email | • Text message<br>• Instant messages<br>• Email | • Concise, visual<br>• Images, videos<br>• "Snack" media (short audio/video clips) |

*Source:* Adapted from Allen (2007); Fronstin and Dretzka (2018); Murphy (2007).

their exposure to challenging experiences, preventing failure, and solving their children's problems for them. This over-parenting has limited their children's ability to self-regulate emotions (see Chapter 2) and behaviors and independently manage difficult situations (Perry et al. 2018). These individuals are largely out of the parenthood arena since most of their children, the Millennials, are now becoming parents. However, millions of children are being raised by their grandparents who would fall into the Baby Boomer generation (Muthiah et al. 2019).

Parents of Generation X, sandwiched between the Baby Boomers and Millennials, represent the majority of parents of school-aged to high school children. Generation X waited longer to have children, which is a trend that continued into the next two generations as well (Livingston 2018). They have been called "stealth-fighters" as they are more hands-off until a concern reaches their threshold, then they forcefully and rapidly attack (Howe 2010; McBride 2017). They are adept in the digital world and will research information, practitioner credentials, and recommendations. Mothers and fathers spend significantly more time with their children than parents from the 1960s, while simultaneously working more, and have been credited with time-intensive parenting: playing with their children at home, facilitating their child's participation in extracurricular activities, and disciplining by explaining, discussing, negotiating, and reasoning (Ishizuka 2019).

Millennials represent the majority of new parents (Livingston 2018). Millennials have struggled more financially than previous generations and have been shaped by economic downturns as they were just beginning their careers. They prioritize experiences like traveling over home ownership (Halsall 2019). Even at a dental office, they desire a social-media-post-worthy "experience" (Radz 2018). They have waited even longer to have children, have changed jobs multiple times, and have different values compared to previous generations. These parents are less likely to be married, and both parents are likely to work, but they spend more time with their children than any previous generation, especially fathers (Pew Research Center 2015a). Like the "Gen Xers" before them, they believe parenting should be child-centered but are less likely to over-schedule their children. Millennial mothers are confident, and in surveys are likely to report that they are doing a very good job as a parent (Pew Research Center 2015b). They are technology savvy and grew up with information readily and immediately available. Unlike previous generations, these individuals seek information from the Internet and social media for help with parenting. They are the most informed generation regarding child development, though the information available online is overwhelming and can be wildly divergent (Hesselberth 2017).

Generation Z are digital natives with lifelong access to information and social media. While generational characteristics have been made of them in the workplace, there are too few of them in parenthood to draw inferences. Currently, they are expected to delay parenthood and value career success. However, parenthood can reshape the attributes of a generational cohort so the characteristics of Gen Z will change over time.

A commonality among the last three generations is that intensive parenting is the new cultural norm, in part because research has concluded that parenting behaviors predict a wide range of child outcomes (Ishizuka 2019; O'Connell et al. 2015). Parents of different social classes express remarkably similar support for child-centered and time-intensive parenting that is shared with mothers and fathers equally engaged, though their resources to provide that type of parenting may be vastly different. This extremely involved parenting style is not expected to change as "concerted cultivation" (fostering a child's talent by incorporating organized activities in their lives) is now the dominant cultural model for how children should be raised (Lareau 2003).

In dentistry, this is evident in that parents overwhelmingly prefer to be present with their children in the operatory; they feel they are expected to be present to help their child cope with an experience. However, all children eventually need to be responsible for and active in their own oral care. The clinician should promote autonomy, and this may need to be introduced to intensive parents slowly.

---

### Case 5.1

At the child's last examination visit, the dentist said: "Ms. Smith, Johnny will be 8 next time we see him, and we know that at home he has been brushing his teeth independently. We want him to have a chance to grow at the dentist's office too so that one day he will be in charge of his own oral health. Next time, we would like for Johnny to walk back by himself, let me look at his teeth, and answer a few one-on-one questions before you come back in the operatory with him." Mrs. Smith nods at the dentist.

---

***Case 5.1, Discussion:*** The dentist is setting the stage for the parent to allow Johnny to build some of his own coping skills for a dental appointment. Because Mrs. Smith nodding at the dentist is not necessarily a sign of agreement, the dentist says, "What are your thoughts about that?" While the dentist uses a consensus approach, she is also clearly outlining expectations for the parent (the parent will not be in the operatory at the beginning of the examination). Prior to Johnny's next visit, the receptionist reminds Mrs. Smith that Johnny is going to go back on his own for a few minutes. After a successful visit with Johnny, the dentist tells Ms. Smith: "Johnny was so fun today! He answered all of my questions and even told me about the new flavor of toothpaste he is using. Thank you for helping him grow into a great dental patient who is taking care of his teeth! We would like for Johnny to try even more on his own next time." Over time, this approach may allow many parents to give their child the opportunity for autonomy in the office. Even with parental resistance, this conversation sets goals for future behavior.

## Culture

The concept of culture is impacted by one's ethnic, racial, religious, and social affiliations (Donate-Bartfield et al. 2014; Marino et al. 2012; Scrimshaw 2003). Culture is not only a consideration for ethnic minorities but universally tied to identity (Mouradian et al. 2003). It is dynamic and constantly incorporating new elements; families may be members of several groups and their identification with these groups can change over time (Donate-Bartfield et al. 2014; Marino et al. 2012; Scrimshaw 2003). The impact of race and ethnicity is further impacted by acculturation or shifts in behaviors as a past and new culture merge (Crespo 2019; Tiwari and Albino 2017).

Societies worldwide are more diverse than ever before, and while diversity is inarguably beneficial, it brings challenges. Health disparities regarding oral health-care status are well documented in minority populations (Cote et al. 2004; Garcia et al. 2008; Ng 2003; Tiwari and Albino 2017). Barriers to care for children of ethnic minority background include insurance coverage and affordability, accessibility of providers, provider interest, language barriers, cultural barriers, and reduced trust (Cote et al. 2004; Garcia et al. 2008; Graham et al. 2005; Marino et al. 2012; Mofidi et al. 2002; Obeng 2007; Scrimshaw 2003; Sood et al. 2019; Tiwari and Albino 2017; Wong et al. 2005). Throughout the world, families, particularly those from disadvantaged and marginalized groups, receive care from providers who come from different backgrounds (Mouradian et al. 2003). Cultural dissonance between minority patients and their providers can result in inaccurate provider perceptions, inconsistent patient behaviors, attitudes, and compliance (Garcia et al. 2008). To treat diverse patients, practitioners must have sensitivity to subtle cues and skills to approach different groups. There is tension between understanding poignant aspects of different groups while avoiding stereotyping (declaring how all individuals within specific groups interact) (Goleman 2014; Marino et al. 2012). Knowledge of generalizations about certain groups can help identify when additional information is needed (Goleman 2014).

Culture significantly impacts oral health in various ways such as oral hygiene, diet, and care-seeking behaviors (Casamassimo 2003; Cote et al. 2004; Crespo 2019; Hilton et al. 2007; Ng 2003; Tiwari and Albino 2017). Susceptibility to caries varies by the country of origin, access to dental care, traditional diet, access to refined sugars, exposure to fluoride, and hygiene practices (Cote et al. 2004; Crespo 2019). Providers should not make assumptions about existing dental knowledge, especially with recent immigrants. In some countries, there may be no knowledge of "simple" prevention measures such as toothbrushing because access to toothbrushes and toothpaste are not available or affordable (Wong et al. 2005). These families will need detailed oral hygiene information and demonstrations. Even in populations who have established adequate oral hygiene habits, these may be insufficient to combat a new cariogenic diet (Hoeft et al. 2010; Tiwari and Albino 2017).

Race and ethnicity influence diet (Cote et al. 2004; Ng 2003). Specifically, prolonged bottle use is common in Mexican American, Native American, and Chinese families (Crespo 2019; Goleman 2014; Ng 2003; Wong et al. 2005). These families will need more detailed interviews to explore why the bottle is being used and specific strategies to address their circumstances. Race and ethnicity also impact health values such as importance of primary teeth (Goleman 2014; Ng 2003; Wong et al. 2005). Another prevailing view is that dental care is not necessary in the absence of pain (Cote et al. 2004; Crespo 2019; Goleman 2014; Hilton et al. 2007; Wong et al. 2005). For example, Chinese parents identified concerns that professional cleanings would loosen or scratch the teeth (Wong et al. 2005). One must seek to understand these potential misconceptions. Fatalism is a common barrier to preventive care and may have background in both cultural and socioeconomic background (Casamassimo 2003; Goleman 2014; Tiwari and Albino 2017). An example of fatalism in this regard is the belief that "my grandmother had dentures, my mom had dentures, and I'll have dentures too." It may be a result of a downward spiral of dental caries, tooth loss that cycles through generations who feel doomed to edentulism (Casamassimo 2003; Goleman 2014).

In health care, cultural competence is defined as "an understanding of the importance of social and cultural influences on patients' health beliefs and behaviors; considering how these factors interact at multiple levels of the healthcare delivery system; and, finally, devising interventions that take these issues into account to assure quality

**Table 5-2**  Four C's of Culture.

| Term | Suggested questions | Purpose |
|---|---|---|
| Call | • What do you call your problem?<br>• What do you think is wrong? | Symptoms may have different meanings in different cultures |
| Cause | • What do you think caused your problem? | Confusion may exist about the etiology of common dental disease |
| Cope | • How do you cope with your condition?<br>• What have you done to try to make it better?<br>• Who else have you been to for treatment? | Identify confusion about the cause of the disease and if nontraditional approaches have been attempted |
| Concerns | • What are your concerns regarding the condition?<br>• How do you feel about the recommended treatment? | Determine parents' perception of the course of illness and planned treatment |

*Source:* Based on Goleman (2014).

healthcare delivery to diverse patient populations" (Garcia et al. 2008). When interacting with families, one must be cognizant of the impact of culture on interpersonal interactions. For example, the Latino culture is known for formal but warm and friendly relationships with medical providers. The dentist would be expected to ask about family and school and work before beginning the appointment, and this formal friendly approach is called *personalismo* (Goleman 2014). Providers who do not show these characteristics may be perceived as cold or uninterested, but this same approach in other cultures may be interpreted as overly familiar and disrespectful. Another aspect of the appointment important for the provider is the uncertainty of physical contact (i.e., is a handshake expected or offensive?) If a dentist is unsure of desired or appropriate level of physical contact, she should wait and see how the family approaches and initiate a handshake if a hand is extended or smile and nod if not (Goleman 2014). If an averted gaze is noticed, it may be more comfortable to look at a shared handout to reduce direct eye contact (Goleman 2014).

Acceptability of behavior guidance techniques such as sedation, general anesthesia, and protective stabilization (passive immobilization) also varies according to race and ethnicity, and decision-making responsibilities are also influenced by culture (Chang et al. 2018; Goleman 2014; Hill et al. 2019; Wong et al. 2005). It is not uncommon for a mother to bring the child for a new exam and agree to treatment under general anesthesia only to fail to keep the appointment because the father does not understand or agree to the needed treatment. Childcare may be shared between generations (Crespo 2019; Hilton et al. 2007; Ng 2003). If elders do not share the same preventive goals or approve of treatment, then no progress can be made. Immigrants may also be pressured by family in their country of origin regarding the safety and financial aspects of recommended care (Obeng 2007; Wong et al. 2005).

Miscommunication can arise from lack of understanding about herbal medicines, home remedies, and regard for Western medicine (Crespo 2019; Goleman 2014; Tiwari and Albino 2017). Sometimes, medical or dental visits are in search of traditional care that is not offered in a new country. See Table 5-2 for the "Four C's of Culture" mnemonic which can facilitate communication (Goleman 2014).

When communicating with a diverse population, each piece of information should be short. If using a translator, the dental provider should make eye contact with the parent (not translator) and use common language, avoiding any dental jargon. Questions should be asked to learn more about the family's environment, resources, and beliefs. Recommendations should be tailored to fit the specific needs of that family. Tools such as "Ask-Tell-Ask" (Table 5-3) can

**Table 5-3**  Ask-Tell-Ask Technique.

| | |
|---|---|
| **ASK** | 1. Environment conducive to communication |
| | 2. Assess physical and emotional state |
| | 3. Assess informational needs |
| | 4. Assess patient's knowledge and understanding |
| | 5. Assess patient's attitude and motivation |
| **TELL** | 1. Keep information brief |
| | 2. Be systematic |
| | 3. Support prior successes |
| | 4. Personalize the information |
| | 5. Use simple language with no jargon |
| | 6. Do not unnecessarily alarm |
| | 7. Use visual aids and share supplemental resources |
| **ASK** | 1. Check for comprehension |
| | 2. Reassess physical and emotional state |
| | 3. Assess for barriers |

*Source:* Based on Goleman (2014).

ensure accurate understanding. Parents may be offered time to discuss treatment with family members not present before making decisions and given the opportunity to ask additional questions. Culturally competent care, knowledge of available resources, and accessibility of translators when needed can help reduce these disparities (Goleman 2014).

---

### Case 5.2

Maria brings her son, Jose, to the office and he has rampant caries. The family immigrated from Mexico a few years ago, and this is the first visit of the family to the dentist. The dentist gathers some information and asks Maria, "What do you think is wrong with Jose?" Maria replies the child is having pain and not eating normally. The dentist inquires, "what do you think is causing Jose to have pain and not eat?" Maria states that she is worried that Jose's teeth are not forming right because he isn't getting the vitamins he needs to make the teeth strong. The dentist says, "I see. What have you done to make Jose's teeth better?" Maria responds she has been giving him more milk once they noticed the teeth breaking down to try to fix the teeth but now the problem is getting worse.

---

*Case 5.2, Discussion*: At this point, the dentist should recognize that Maria is unfamiliar with dental caries and its causes. This is common with families immigrating from areas with high natural fluoride levels and a non-cariogenic diet. Brown discolored teeth from fluorosis are common, and caries may be unrecognized. The dentist should now counsel Maria about caries, its etiology, prevention, and needed treatment. This includes restorations, reducing milk consumption, and toothbrushing with fluoride. To ensure that Maria understands and to see if she has additional questions, the dentist says, "We have talked about a lot of things today. What are your concerns about the cavities and treating them?" Maria shares that she is still worried that other family members will still believe Jose's problem is due to malnutrition. The dentist educates Maria on other sources of calcium such as hard cheeses or supplements that will not cause cavities, and he encourages the family to see a pediatrician as well for a health assessment if they are concerned about malnutrition. He also provides Maria with a written brochure in Spanish about the caries process. Finally, he offers for other family members to attend future visits to discuss concerns with the dentist.

The dentist utilized the *Four C's of Culture* mnemonic. He was able to understand the underlying belief of what the parent thought caused the cavities and was able to educate the parent and allay concerns.

## Financial Status

Contemporary families have greater financial challenges than in recent decades, and most families have significant concerns about the cost of raising a child (Tucci et al. 2005). Families increasingly face financial insecurity with less employment stability and reduced savings. Living on the brink of insolvency is the new norm with two-thirds of households reporting that they fall into one of the following categories: have very little left over after meeting expenses, are only able to meet basic expenses, or fail to meet expenses (Pew Research Center 2015b).

Volatility from large-scale events such as rapid economic fluctuation, natural disaster, and conflict or family-level events such as unexpected illness can rapidly transform previously "middle class" families to poverty (Haley et al. 2010; Pascoe et al. 2016). Financial crisis alters dental care-seeking behavior for children and adolescents immediately and shifts care seeking from prevention to pain management (Sveinsdottir and Wang 2014). Families in financial decline are very good at masking poverty with previously purchased clothing or cars. "Difficult" behaviors such as questioning treatment may come from inability to pay. When the dentist suspects these circumstances, a discussion of the risks and benefits of deferred care is appropriate along with financial assistance resources.

Compassion is needed for families living in poverty, whether short-term or long-term. Poverty has profound effects on birthweight, infant mortality, brain development, language development, chronic illness, nutrition, and injury resulting in lifelong hardship (Council On Community Pediatrics 2016; Le-Scherban et al. 2016; Pascoe et al. 2016). Childhood poverty is strongly linked to adverse socioemotional outcomes, poor health, and disruption of adult socioeconomic advancement culminating in risk for intergenerational poverty (da Fonseca 2014; McEwenand McEwen 2017; Pascoe et al. 2016). Toxic stress, which is associated with child poverty, can cause heritable genomic changes (Council On Community Pediatrics 2016; McEwen and McEwen 2017; Pascoe et al. 2016).

Social determinants of health contribute to health disparities in childhood and include food and housing insecurity (Pascoe et al. 2016). Families with housing instability are not homeless but have difficulty paying rent, move frequently, are evicted, and may live in crowded or foreclosure conditions (da Fonseca 2014). Food security describes access to quality, variety, desirability, and quantity of diet (da Fonseca 2014). Robust programs that provide medical and social support can ameliorate the impact of poverty (Council On Community Pediatrics 2016; Pascoe et al. 2016), but even in countries with social safety net programs, socioeconomic disadvantage is associated with worsened oral health (Wamala et al. 2006). Obstacles to care include access to a provider that accepts government insurance, scheduling appointments when parents have no work leave, lack of convenient and reliable transportation, and wait time (Mofidi et al. 2002). Disadvantaged families have reported judgmental, disrespectful, and discriminatory behavior from staff and providers due to their public assistance status, which make future visits unlikely (Mofidi et al. 2002; Mouradian et al. 2003).

Financial insecurity and poverty affect parents' interaction with medical care professionals. These conditions activate the stress mechanisms of children and parents leading to depression, household conflict, impulsive behavior, and impaired interpersonal relationships (da Fonseca 2014; McEwen and McEwen 2017; Pascoe et al. 2016). Low-income families are significantly less trusting of physicians and are less satisfied with their own medical care than adults from higher-income families (Blendon et al. 2014). A child who is hungry, scared, abused, or overstressed can easily be mislabeled as "uncooperative"(da Fonseca 2014). Questions such as "Do you ever have problems making ends meet?" and "Is your housing ever a problem for you?" can help uncover the root of this behavior and connect families with needed resources (Klass 2016).

---

### Case 5.3

Linda presents to the office with her 18-month-old son Matthew. Matthew is obese, has ECC, and takes a bottle of milk to bed at night. When the dentist begins to counsel Linda about why she needs to stop the night-time, Linda becomes upset and says she has heard it all before with her older child. The dentist replies, "It seems like you are concerned about Matthew's health and know about the consequences of using the bottle at night. Is there anything else going on that is making it difficult to stop the bottle?"

---

***Case 5.3, Discussion***: By asking more about why the Linda is continuing to give Matthew the bottle at night, the dentist learns the family is staying with relatives in a cramped apartment because they have nowhere else to live. Linda is worried if the toddler cries at night, she will be asked to move out because the other family members work long shifts and need sleep. She gives Matthew the bottle because she is more worried about homelessness than teeth. The dentist thanks Linda for sharing this information, and the two strategize on behaviors that Linda could incorporate into her life such as brushing with fluoridated toothpaste after feedings, limiting snacks and sugared drinks in between feeding times, and returning for more frequent recare appointments on a three-month basis. These glimpses into the lives of our vulnerable families are heart-wrenching. Linda needs many things, but she does not need a lecture. Dentists can give advice about weaning and improved oral hygiene, but, most importantly, they should attempt to connect families with resources and support.

## Parenting Challenges

Parents perceive more pressure than ever to "succeed" at parenting. Both mothers and fathers agree parenting is very important to their identity and they care what their spouses, parents, friends, and neighbors think about how they are doing as a parent (Pew Research Center 2015b). Parents have always been held responsible for the behavior and development of their children, but in recent years, it has been reframed as a "job" requiring particular skills and expertise which can only be taught by a qualified professional (Gillies 2008). Parents are expected to provide security, stability, and safety and to act as educators for children (Gillies 2008). The majority of parents now feel both internal and community pressure to get parenting right and are concerned about their confidence as a parent (Tucci et al. 2005).

Parents today are in conflict about how best to parent. They have to choose between a style that is "helicopter" versus "free-range" or "nurturer" versus "Tiger"(Pew Research Center 2015b). Parents are bombarded with information and resolving conflicts and report feeling stressed, tired, and rushed (Figure 5-1) (Pew Research Center 2015b). Both men and women have significant conflict between their work and family obligations (Schor et al. 2003), and working moms are more likely to report that they spend too little time with children (Pew Research Center 2015b). Fathers have also received pressure to increase their involvement and influence on health and development (Yogman et al. 2016) and are less likely than mothers to say they are doing a very good job raising their children (Pew Research Center 2015b). Paternal involvement leads to more positive outcomes (Yogman et al. 2016), but the pressure for both parents to attend important events including dental visits can place an additional strain on family's time and finances and add more communication demands from the dentist.

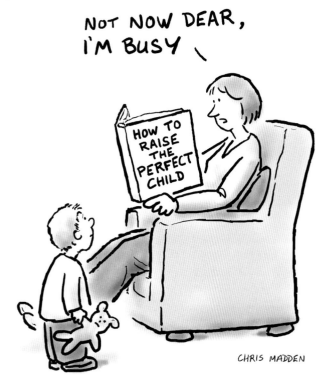

**Figure 5-1** Pressures on the contemporary parent. *Source:* Courtesy of Chris Madden.

Changes in family structure make meeting the increasing demands of parenting difficult. The share of children living in a two-parent household is at the lowest point in more than a century (Pew Research Center 2015b). Childbearing has been decoupled from marriage, and households often include a variety of family arrangements due to the prevalence of divorce, remarriage, and cohabitation (Pew Research Center 2015b). More mothers are working and are the primary bread winner in almost half of households (Pew Research Center 2015b). There is an increase in grandparenting, which further complicates family life.

This transition from parenting as a relationship to a job places stress on everyone, but the response to these pressures is significantly different between income groups. For higher-income families, income has trended up, and access to extracurricular activities and indulgences, such as electronics and travel, are unprecedented. There is a significant gap between these families and lower-income and nontraditional families without the financial means or time to comply with the demands of contemporary parenting (Gillies 2008; McEwen and McEwen 2017). Confidence in parenting is lower in families with fewer financial resources (Pew Research Center 2015b).

Changes in parenting are visible in the dental office with most pediatric dentists agreeing that they have seen changes over the course of their practice and that these changes were negative (Casamassimo et al. 2002). It is not surprising that the pressures parents feel boil over into the dental setting. Parents who are worried about the long-term impact of traumatic stress in children are unwilling to use behavior guidance techniques they perceive as aversive. Parents who take pride in their roles as parents and take part in "sharenting" (oversharing of information and images of their children on social media) are appalled at the idea of their child missing a tooth or having silver teeth. Fathers who feel guilty for spending inadequate time with their children intervene to "save" the child who is having a difficult time coping with a dental procedure. The driving impulse behind these misguided behaviors is the desire to be perceived as successful parents. The dentist has the ethical obligation to maintain the standard of care and to preserve a safe and respectful office environment for staff, but interpreting these actions through the lens of empathy can help give parents the reassurance they crave and open the door for a constructive conversation.

### The Trust Gap

Parents perceive more external threats to their children than ever before whether it be from catastrophe, the Internet, television, or bullying (Pew Research Center 2015b; Tucci et al. 2005). Sexual abuse scandals have shaken confidence in previously trusted figures including physicians (Pew Research Center 2015b). Insecurity encourages parents to desire more information (Tucci et al. 2005).

In some countries, there is rising distrust with medical leaders (Blendon et al. 2014). In the United States, public trust in the leaders of the U.S. medical profession fell from 73% having great confidence in 1966 to 34% in 2012 (Blendon et al. 2014). Distrust of health systems is rooted in unexpected costs that can result in bankruptcy, pharmaceutical and physician's complicity in the opioid epidemic, celebrity doctors challenging evidence-based treatment, and high profile lapses in accountability (Coulter 2002; Goldbach 2020). This distrust is most visible in the worldwide increase in vaccine refusal (Attwell et al. 2017).

Distrust of healthcare providers is more pervasive in certain demographic groups. Younger Americans are significantly less likely than Americans over 65 years of age to agree that US physicians can be trusted (Blendon et al. 2014). Asian and African American respondents are less trusting of their physician than Caucasian counterparts (Sood et al. 2019). Individuals with college degrees have been shown to be less trusting and more likely to seek a second opinion than those with less than a bachelor's degree (Sood et al. 2019). Previous studies have found an association between higher education and preference for more active involvement in decision-making (Say et al. 2006).

In guiding contemporary parents, having knowledge is no longer the essential value of the clinician as knowledge is readily and immediately available online. The majority of Millennials have sought information before receiving care: they have checked the quality of rating of the doctor, checked whether a health plan would cover a service, and found cost information. When surveyed, the majority of Millennials agree with the statement "I rely on myself, more than my primary doctor, to make decisions about my medical care" (Fronstin and Dretzka 2018). Clinicians are no longer the gatekeepers of knowledge, and the shift toward collaborative, consensus decision-making has arrived.

Parents increasingly turn to the Internet for information about child health. One study found that 97.8% of parents reported using the Internet to find health information for their children with almost half being frequent users who search for information a few times a month to every day (Pehora et al. 2015). Most searches start with generic search engines and may not access reliable sources of information (Sood et al. 2019). Conflicting online information significantly reduces trust in a pediatrician's diagnosis and increases the likelihood of seeking a second opinion (Sood et al. 2019).

The Internet may be a tool for patients who feel anxious about upsetting the patient–physician dynamic by questioning the physician (Pehora et al. 2015; Sood et al. 2019). Asymmetry of information and expertise between patient and provider is inherent to healthcare and can cause patients to feel vulnerable (Berry et al. 2017; Mouradian et al. 2003). This imbalance can lead to patients feeling confused but fearful of asking for clarification or desired treatment; patients may not want to risk alienating providers they are dependent upon (Berry et al. 2017). This turmoil has been called "white-coat silence" and can lead to perceived lack of interest, learned helplessness, and lack of compliance, degrading the therapeutic alliance (Berry et al. 2017). Patients and parents who feel disrespected by doctors are far less likely to trust doctors overall and are less likely to follow their advice (Wyman 2017). Families with past negative experiences may approach all health care with distrust or advocate for care in a way that may be perceived by providers as aggressive or dictatorial.

Trust must be earned over time, ideally within the framework of the dental home (American Academy of Pediatrics Ad Hoc Task Force on Definition of the Medical Home 1992). The dental home ( see Chapter 6) is based on the American Academy of Pediatrics (AAP_ policy on the medical home (American Academy of Pediatrics Section on Bioethics 2017, American Academy of Pediatrics Ad Hoc Task Force on Definition of the Medical Home, 1992). They stated, "The development of a trusting relationship between a pediatrician, parent, and child is at the center of the AAP concept of the medical home. Yet multiple barriers to the development of trusting therapeutic relationships exist. These include an increasingly mobile population, health insurance shifts, and situations in which a new relationship must be forged rapidly because of a medical crisis" (American Academy of Pediatrics Section on Bioethics et al. 2017).

The practitioner builds trust by showing her genuine concern for the patient and their family at every visit, by focusing on raising healthy children. The parent should feel their child's health is as important to the dental team as it is to them. Care must be taken by the whole dental team to communicate a "patient first" mentality.

The essential elements of trust are identified in the 2004 paper entitled "Trust in Healthcare"—they are: competence in knowledge; competence in social/communication skills; honesty; confidentiality and caring; and showing respect (Allinson and Chaar 2016).

## Practical Steps for Building a Patient-centered Practice

### Before the Patient Encounter

#### I. Understand Your Practice

*Begin with yourself.* What generational group are you in and how does it influence your approach to the practice of dentistry? What behavior guidance techniques are you comfortable with and what are you not willing to use? The doctor establishes the practice's values and influences its culture. This is often referred to as "branding your practice."

*Understand your team.* What are the strengths and weaknesses of each of your team members? In what generational groups are they? For what roles in the office are each suited and not suited?

*Finally, understand the patient base, your community, and the culture in which you practice.*

In what type of community is your practice? What ethnic, regional, education level, and socioeconomic backgrounds do the patients you treat come from?

#### II. Build a Diverse Team that Resembles the Patient Base of the Practice

A classic business book, *Good to Great* by Jim Collins, identifies principles for great businesses (Collins 2001). Two principles that have application are "get the right people on the bus," then "get the right people in the right seat." Effective teams, like society in general, will be multicultural. One must hire for personal skills as well as technical skills. A team member with excellent technical skills but weak communication skills would focus on clinical duties, whereas the more charismatic team member, who easily builds rapport with people, is trained to provide much of the pre- and post-operative communication with the parent. With the right people in the right positions, many of the challenges of caring for a diverse patient base can be successfully overcome.

### III. Learned Communication Skills for All Team Members

Poor communication and failure to acknowledge the patient's perspective are the source of most complaints and legal action (Coulter 2002). Communication skills and cultural competency are not natural skills. The foundation for all communication is the basic principles of self-awareness, respect for diversity, sensitivity in communication, and relationship building (Goleman 2014; Mouradian et al. 2003).

To prevent misunderstandings and errors, successful practices should have all team members use effective communication techniques: open-ended questioning, empathetic listening skills, exercising warmth and compassion during service delivery, and communicating clearly in layman terms (i.e., avoiding medical jargon, acronyms, and complex terms) (Ha et al. 2010). Providers who show empathy have improved patient outcomes with fewer complications from disease (Del Canale et al. 2012). Understanding these principles in theory is not the same as practicing them daily in the workplace. Improving communication skills is an ongoing process that is evaluated and monitored regularly.

## Principles and Practical Tips for the Patient Encounter

### I. Every Patient Encounter Matters

In the digital age where more interaction is online, it is increasingly important that all interpersonal interactions convey caring and respect. With the advent of online scheduling portals, the first personal interaction is often when the patient and parent enter the office. Their presence should be acknowledged with eye-contact and a smile, anticipating their arrival and greeting them by name whenever possible.

The décor of the office should reflect the diversity of the patient base (see Chapter 18). It is wise to consider if the office reflects the provider's personal tastes or is decorated for the comfort of the patients. A clean, up-to-date office communicates respect for patients as well as attention to quality. The look and feel of the office contribute to the "brand" of the practice and the "experience" of the parent, both of which resonate with contemporary parents.

### II. Enhance Understanding

With easy access to both information and misinformation via online searches, it will be common for patients to arrive with pre-conceived expectations. It is important to gain understanding of what information the parent is bringing into the visit. Lead with questions, not answers. Adopt the adage

"Listen first" even if a response seems readily apparent. Build upon the knowledge foundation the parent brings as the starting place to respectfully educate why the preconceived information does not best apply to their child in this case. Clarify with questions like, "Am I hearing that you would like . . ..?" Engage in dialog and debate, not coercion or condescension. The desired outcome is understanding. The Ask-Tell-Ask technique (Table 5-3) is described in detail later in this chapter and is an excellent tool for the dental team.

---

### Case 5.4

A mother brings James, her six-year-old son, with severely carious primary molars for an initial examination. The treatment plan includes crowns and pulpotomies.

Mother: "That seems like a lot of work, and money, for baby teeth that will fall out."

---

***Case 5.4, Discussion***: The dentist should use the principles of effective communication: building on the knowledge the parent already has, using words that the parent would understand, and asking open-ended questions at the end of the discussion to allow the parent to discuss any reservations or misunderstandings.

DENTIST: You are right; they are "baby teeth." And children do start losing baby teeth at James' age. However, these are his molars that are normally in the mouth for four to five more years. I am concerned that James will start hurting and possibly develop abscesses before then. If that occurs, our option will be to pull them which can cause other problems. These baby teeth hold space and will guide in his permanent teeth into their proper place.

MOTHER: Oh, I didn't realize that, but it is a lot of work. I don't know if I can afford it.

DENTIST: I understand. It is a lot of work and may feel overwhelming. I may be able slow the decay by placing fluoride medicine on the big cavities. It will turn the cavities dark black, but this could give us time to space James' dental work over several months. I will have Sofia in the business office work with you on the payment end. Would that be helpful? I know we both want James to have healthy teeth and a bright, big smile. We would love to work with you to reach that goal.

## Shared Responsibility

Informed consent is the hallmark of the doctor–patient relationship. The American Academy of Pediatric Dentistry Policy for Informed Consent states that dentists are required to provide relevant information concerning diagnosis and treatment needs to a patient so that the patient can make a voluntary, educated decision to accept or refuse treatment (American Academy of Pediatric Dentistry 2020a). Consent for advanced behavior management techniques such as sedation, general anesthesia, and protective stabilization (i.e., immobilization) should be obtained separately from consent for other procedures (American Academy of Pediatric Dentistry 2020b, 2020c). The obligation of the dentist is to diagnose and inform. In past paternalistic models, pediatric dentists may have been the last resort and felt obligated to provide care for every patient. In the era of shared-decision making, clinicians do not have to treat everyone. A parent or patient may be a poor fit for the provider and vice versa. Generally, consent concerns can revolve around radiographs, fluoride, "metal" restorations, bisphenol-A (BPA) in resins, and advanced behavior management techniques. If the den-

tist believes a parent's informed refusal violates proper standards of care, he should recommend seeking another opinion and/or dismissing the patient from the practice (American Academy of Pediatric Dentistry 2020c). If the parent has expectations that exceed the practitioner's training, skill, or comfort level, she should be referred to another practitioner who can better meet these expectations.

Medical models focus on shared decision-making processes that guide patients in the discussion from broad choices, to focused options, and finally decision-making (Elwyn et al. 2012). Decision aids are tools for shared decision-making that may be a combination of text, graphics, and flow charts, as shown in Figure 5-2. These aids that can provide information, including details of the decision, options, costs, and potential benefits, encourage patients to recognize their own values and share values

**Your dentist has advised your child has a larger cavity on their primary tooth that needs treatment. You have three options. Each option has different benefits, risks, costs, and probable outcomes.**

**Silver Diamine Fluoride**
- No additional visits
- The cost is $75
- The cavity will appear dark brown or black
- Cavity may become bigger and cause pain or infection
- Tooth may need extraction later ($210) and space maintainer ($360)

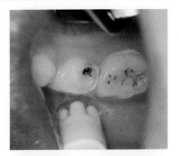

**Stainless Steel Crown**
- One visit will be needed
- The cost is $310
- This tooth will appear to be silver
- The crown will be in the mouth until it falls out at around age 9–11
- This is the most durable option

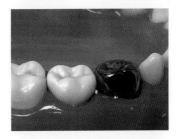

**White Zirconium Crown**
- One visit will be needed
- The cost is $410
- The tooth will look white but may be a different shade from the surrounding teeth
- More tooth is taken away with these crowns which may result in the nerve being exposed and a nerve treatment ($225) may be needed

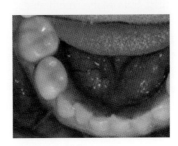

- These crowns don't fit all tooth sizes and a stainless steel crown may be needed
- There is little long-term data on this type of crown but they are probably more likely to fall off or break compared to silver crowns

**Figure 5-2** Example of Shared Decision Aid. *Source:* Photos provided by Drs. William Waggoner and Dustin Janssen.

with a healthcare provider (Hulin et al. 2017; Parker et al. 2017). Shared decision-making has been linked to improved decision-making, outcomes, and patient satisfaction (Say et al. 2006).

## Parent Guidance Techniques

Having "expertise," the specialized knowledge that is the outcome of years of training and experience, is the science of dentistry. However, having expertise does not automatically entail the ability to effectively use this knowledge in discourse. There is no "one way" for communication to be effective, but the soft skills that result in a clinician's "bedside manner" are the art of pediatric dentistry. They are the heart of the dentist–parent relationship.

### Ask-Tell-Ask

While Ask-Tell-Ask can be used for children, it is an excellent tool for parents. It is a collaborative communication method that includes asking open-ended questions and assessing a parent's existing knowledge before sharing information (Table 5-3). This technique involves inquiring about the patient's visit and feelings about any planned procedures (ask); explaining the procedures through demonstrations using causal language (tell); and again, inquiring if the parent understands and how he feels about the impending treatment (ask) (American Academy of Pediatric Dentistry 2020b).

---

**Case 5.5**

Mary is the third child of a single mom. She is three years and six months old and arrives at the office with a smile on her face and teddy bear in hand. She hops in the chair and shows the dentist "Beary" who has a pacifier attached to him. Upon examination, the dentist notices an open bite consistent with a non-nutritive sucking habit. The dentist tells Mary's mom that the pacifier is changing her bite and that she needs to take it away. He acknowledges that taking away a pacifier is hard for the parent and child. He goes on to tell her several ideas for stopping the habit and that if she can stop giving Mary a pacifier, the change in her bite might correct itself. He says that Mary has nice teeth otherwise, and he will check her again in six months.

---

*Case 5.5, Discussion*: This type of communication style is common: Tell-Tell-Tell, and it does little to change patient behavior. Usually, unhealthy habits are not occurring

because the parent lacks knowledge but because of other barriers. The dentist could have used the Ask-Tell-Ask approach for Mary's mother. *Ask*: "When I show you Mary's bite, what concerns do you have about it?" "What do you think is causing it?"

> *TELL*: "Yes, you are right, most times the top teeth come over the bottom teeth when you bite down. Using the pacifier is probably causing this. The good news is that if we stop the habit, her bite might correct itself over time. I understand, though, it is hard on a parent and child to stop a pacifier habit. Could I share with you some ideas that parents have given me over the years and some that I used with my own children?"
>
> *ASK*: "We talked about several ideas. What will make it difficult for you to take away the pacifier? Yes, I understand that it will be hard for her to fall asleep without it. How do you think you will manage that? As you are trying some of these ideas, if you need our advice, please call us. We're always here to help parents through these changes. What other questions or concerns do you have?"

The Ask-Tell-Ask technique is also especially helpful in ensuring that a parent understands a complex treatment plan and alternatives to that plan.

---

**Case 5.6**

Mr. Wang brings his three-years-old son in for his first dental visit. He has rampant caries. The dentist asks Mr. Wang, "What concerns do you have about Daniel's teeth?" Mr. Wang replies that he knows Daniel has cavities, that he really wants Daniel to have his teeth fixed, and that he has heard about crowns for baby teeth. The dentist says, "My assistant, Susan, will go over several different options that we have for taking care of Daniel. After you've had a chance to talk with Susan, I will talk with you again." Susan talks over several options with Mr. Wang including active surveillance, treatment with silver diamine fluoride, and restorative treatment with general anesthesia. The dentist returns and asks Mr. Wang, What questions do you have?

---

*Case 5.6, Discussion:* The Ask-Tell-Ask style of communication is more time-consuming than presenting a single treatment plan. The dentist in a busy practice may not always have the time to effectively engage this way, but a well-trained auxiliary can offer a parent this type of conversation. Susan should also show Mr. Wang pictures of stainless-steel crowns and silver diamine fluoride staining to ensure understanding of esthetic constraints, and she should avoid asking a question about understanding that can have a "yes" or "no" response.

Once the dentist returns, he may say: "This is a complicated decision. What questions do you have?"

> Mr. Wang: "I would like you to crown Daniel's teeth."
>
> Dentist: "I always like to check in with my parents to make sure my staff and I have explained everything clearly. Could you tell me what you're expecting Daniel's teeth to look like after they have been crowned and how we're going to get Daniel to be able to cooperate to receive these crowns?"
>
> Mr. Wang: "Daniel needs crowns on all of his back teeth, and they will look silver. Daniel will be asleep in the surgery center for the treatment."
>
> Dentist: "Yes, you are right on track. This is a big decision, and I am sure you might like to discuss it with other family members. If you have any additional questions later on, please call us. What other questions might you have now?"

Alternatively, the dentist could offer to talk with the parent another time, especially if the patient presents with a complex medical history and/or dental needs (i.e., "Mr. Wang, there are several options that we could offer Daniel, and I really would like the chance to spend some time thinking about his dental needs and the best course of action. Could I schedule another time to speak with you either in person or on the phone so that I can have some dedicated time to go over the options with you?") If the treatment options are ambiguous or complicated, the dentist should offer the parent a recommendation based on his/her expertise and knowledge.

## Motivational Interviewing

Motivational interviewing (MI) is a patient-centered, collaborative counseling approach designed to strengthen an individual's intrinsic motivation toward a positive behavior change, and when used with parents, it has been shown to improve pediatric behaviors (Borrelli et al. 2015). The key components of MI are: asking **o**pen-ended questions to assess a parent's readiness for change, **a**ffirming and empathizing with the parent, **r**eflecting on what factors motivate or worry the patient, and **s**ummarizing what the patient has expressed (OARS). Many times, a visual "menu" of potential goals that the individual may select is utilized.

---

**Case 5.7**

Charlie is an 18-months-old, healthy boy, and Mrs. Martin's only child. Mrs. Martin is a 38-year-old lawyer who calls Charlie her special gift because she thought she would not have children. Dr. Devi says "Hi, Mrs. Martin. It's so nice to meet Charlie; we're so glad you're sharing him with us today. Tell me a little about him. What is it like to be his mother? ... It sounds like he's a fun toddler to raise. What concerns do you have for his teeth? ... So, it sounds like you want him to have less cavities than you had as a child and that you didn't like your smile for a long time but that brushing is stressful because he fights you. On one hand, you're worried that Charlie may get cavities in his teeth because he doesn't get his teeth brushed every day, but on the other hand you really don't like to make him cry when you brush them."

---

*Case 5.7, Discussion:* Dentists are often faced with challenging "at-home" behaviors. Utilizing the OARS approach, the dentist may say, "I understand. It is hard for a parent to see their child upset. Many of my other parents feel a lot like you. May I share with you some of the ideas that other parents have used? I have a 'menu' of some options we could try. Let's take a look and see what you might feel most comfortable with. . . I agree that brushing every night could really help Charlie's teeth stay healthy. Many of my parents have found that wrapping their toddler in a towel with his arms by his sides after a bath and laying him on the floor to brush his teeth is the easiest way to handle brushing a toddler who fights having his teeth brushed. They also would tell you that if you had a crystal ball and could look into the future, you'd be really surprised that when Charlie is older, like 4, he'll hop right up on the bathroom stool and look forward to getting his teeth brushed! But right now, it is hard when he cries. What do you think might be hard for you with this plan? Is there anyone who can help?". . . "It sounds like you would like to try brushing every night. That's a great plan! Would it be ok with you if my assistant, Jennifer, calls you in 2 weeks to see how it is going with Charlie and to see if you have any additional concerns?" During the conversation, when a parent uses "change talk" such as "I can probably brush his teeth at least at night," the clinician recognizes that language and builds on it with reflection and open-ended questioning. The dentist provides education when the parent expresses some readiness for change and helps the parent select an appropriate goal (i.e., a goal that moves in the direction of a healthy behavior but may not fully encompass the behavior). This type of interviewing has been shown to build rapport with the parent and elicit change behaviors (Weinstein et al. 2006).

## Managing the Rise of Paternal Involvement

Although mothers continue to provide the majority of primary care for the child, dentists are likely to see more fathers as the parent accompanying children to appointments. A father may be a biological, foster, or adoptive father; a stepfather; or a grandfather. He may or may not be living with the family and/or have legal custody. Although parenthood status is usually straightforward, circumstances in which parental rights are unclear may involve complex legal issues, including implications in terms of parental access to the child's protected health information and ability to consent to care (Yogman et al. 2016). Little research is available for how fathers interact with dental providers compared to mothers; however, in medicine, research has shown that fathers ask fewer questions than mothers, appreciate direct, straightforward communication, and are satisfied with physicians who communicate in a family-centered way (Cousino et al. 2011). Practitioners may ask more open-ended questions to fathers to engage them in the appointment. Some practitioners have offered to use video conferencing for the parent who was unable to accompany the child so that both parents can understand the treatment plan and have the opportunity to ask questions. Advice for pediatric healthcare providers includes (1) welcome fathers and express appreciation for their attendance; (2) explore the family composition, cultural beliefs about men's roles in families, and the division of childcare tasks within the family; (3) emphasize how children look to their fathers as role models of behavior including oral hygiene practices; and (4) offer written material that the father can share with the other parent if treatment plans are complex or require advanced techniques (Yogman et al. 2016).

## Use of Digital Technology for Parent Education, Engagement, and Guidance

Contemporary parents expect to be engaged digitally, and they demand convenience as consumers. eCommerce has radically changed how goods and services are delivered, primarily because of its superior convenience and cost-effectiveness (Levy 2019). As healthcare consumers, Millennials (and the generations to follow) expect digital access, expect to be able to complete healthcare forms, pay their bills, and schedule an appointment online without ever speaking to a person. They value convenience, are dissatisfied with having to wait on a doctor at an appointment, and are likely to use telehealth if it is offered; they are more likely to self-diagnose, use home remedies or alternative therapies, and seek cost information prior to receiving care (PatientPop 2019). In recent years, mobile healthcare applications (mHealth apps) have exploded, with the number of downloads for mHealth apps doubling from 2015 to 2017 (Terry 2016). As Millennials display entirely new patterns of social and purchasing behavior, teledentistry and mHealth may play roles in implementing strategies to meet the new model of healthcare consumer.

Dentists treating children will need an online presence with a well-designed, mobile-friendly website. The vast majority of patients have searched online to find a healthcare provider and prefer to schedule and pay their bills online. These parents also spend a lot of time on social media; a practitioner can become a resource for contemporary parents by sharing his/her expertise on one of the social media platforms and by encouraging followers to schedule preventive visits at appropriate intervals. mHealth and/or teledentistry can be utilized as part of the motivational process with encouragement notifications or follow-up video conferences and has been successfully used in medicine this way (Shingleton and Palfai 2016). While there is much research that can be done to determine "best practices" for these technologies, successful clinicians will embrace how consumer demand is reshaping healthcare delivery.

Given that today's parents are connected to social media, many may wish to videotape their child at the dentist's office. While a child laughing when getting her teeth "tickled" may make a heartwarming video, it is a bit disconcerting to have a parent take out a phone during the middle of a difficult procedure and starting filming. Several factors must be considered: health information privacy violations, especially of other patients, privacy rights of staff, and malpractice risk management for photos or videos taken out of context (Litch 2015). While a designated area or photo booth could be utilized, one must be cautious to not inadvertently photograph or record any other individual, part of a patient's record, or another patient's voice. The simplest approach is to have a "no video or photo" policy such as: "We respect the privacy rights of all our patients and our staff. Therefore, we do not allow photography (video or otherwise) on the premises" (Litch 2015). Additionally, if a dentist wishes to use a patient's image, such as for a "no cavities" bulletin board or website page, an authorization and consent from the parent is required (Litch 2015).

## Managing Negative Online Reviews

With an Internet presence comes the risk of a negative online review. An estimated 80–90% of consumers read online reviews before selecting a business including health care, and positive reviews make consumers more likely to use a business (Murphy 2019). Important factors in reviews are their recency, the number of total reviews, the overall rating of the business, and the legitimacy of the review. The vast majority of review readers do read a business' response to a review. The recommendations for managing a negative review range from no response to a standard statement such as: "Our office strives to provide the best service and we do our best to succeed with this goal. I would like to learn more about what happened and hope you will contact us as soon as possible" (American Dental Association 2017). Any response must protect the patient's privacy. A practical suggestion is to ask the many satisfied parents in your practice to leave a positive review and "bury" the negative review as most review readers do not read past the first page of search results (Erskine 2017).

## Managing the Angry Parent

Despite a dentist's best efforts to offer a supportive, communicative dental environment, clinicians will inevitably encounter parents with complaints about the quality of their child's care. The NURSE technique (Name, Understand, Respect, Support, Explore) can be utilized to help the clinician be more effective at conflict resolution with a displeased parent (Back et al. 2005).

---

### Case 5.8

Joe Hernandez brings his daughter, Lily, to a recall visit. The upper right first primary molar has a failing resin restoration, and the recurrent caries is large. The dentist explains the extent of decay and recommends treatment with a pulpotomy and stainless-steel crown. The father's consent is obtained and documented in the patient record. Mr. Hernandez returns with Lily who receives treatment with ease. The staff reviews the post-operative instructions and Lily is smiling leaving the appointment. Two months later, Lily and her mother present for an emergency visit because her "gum has a bump on it." After the examination, the dentist explains that Lily's tooth is infected and will need to be extracted. Lily's mother is not smiling and is visibly upset.

---

*Case 5.8, Discussion:* Dentists are often presented with one parent bringing the child for one type of visit and the other parent accompanying the child for a subsequent visit. Documenting which parent accompanied the patient is critical to avoid miscommunication. For a treatment visit with a different parent than the one who presented for the planning visit, a dentist or staff should review which parent gave consent, summarize the planned treatment, and ask if the accompanying parent has any additional questions. For an upset parent, the dentist should use the tenets of effective communication: empathy, compassion, listening, and reflection.

The dentists says, "I was worried about this. Mr. Hernandez and I discussed this as a possibility. Some parents in this situation would be frustrated." Mrs. Hernandez remarks that she's squeezed in this appointment over lunch and has to return to work and that she's not sure how she will manage to take off time from work again. The dentist says, "I understand why you'd be upset by this." Mrs. Hernandez states that she doesn't want her daughter to have to go through another appointment and the dentist says "I appreciate that you've brought Lily to see me even though it is hard to take off work. I'm sorry the tooth didn't respond the way we had hoped." Mrs. Hernandez tells the dentist, "Well you did tell Joe that it was a large cavity and that we may not have caught it in time." The dentist responds, "I know this is inconvenient for you. Luckily, Lily is not in pain so we can do this another time so that you can return to work today. We will try to work with your schedule and find a time that works for you." In naming the emotion, the dentist did not say "I can see you are angry" because people do not like being told what they are feeling (Back et al. 2005). Additionally, the dentist conveyed that he believed in the veracity of the parent's concerns and validity of her emotions; this is important even when dentists do not consider those complaints to be reasonable or appropriate (Steinman 2013). While the parent in this scenario was effectively satisfied, some upset parents may not be easily appeased. Complaints often arise from unmet expectations (Steinman 2013). *Active listening* gives the parent the opportunity to describe, explain, and criticize and conveys a sincere interest in hearing the parent without interrupting to clarify or solve. It is beneficial to summarize unmet expectations, especially when they may be unreasonable (i.e., "What I hear you saying is that you are frustrated that the cavity was very large and that the tooth wasn't able to heal with the nerve treatment we tried."). The dentist may offer an apology for the emotions the patient is experiencing without accepting responsibility. This apology is often an avenue for providing an explanation without appearing defensive (i.e., "I am sorry that you are upset that Lily's tooth became infected. I always want to save teeth if possible, but pulpal treatment doesn't work for every tooth with a large cavity, and some teeth abscess despite our best efforts save them."). Apologizing may seem counterintuitive and imprudent, especially for complaints that are unjustified. Apologies, however, can decrease blame, anger, and antagonistic responses and restore trust and strengthen relationships (Robbennolt 2009). The dentist then strives to satisfy the patient: "What would you like me to do to help Lily?" Finally, the dentist proposes a plan: "Thank you for telling me how you feel. Here's what I would like us to do next."

Many clinicians are not comfortable, confident, or adept at working with unhappy parents and may experience anxiety, avoidance, fear, anger, and frustration. Utilizing a technique like NURSE can serve as a framework to help clinicians remain calm during a confrontational encounter and give them an effective plan of action.

## Conclusion

For decades, the AAP has advanced the need for family-centered care for children, with the medical home as the standard for pediatric medical care. Its policy statement "Patient and Family-Centered Care and the Pediatrician's Role" states "the perspectives and information provided by families, children, and young adults are essential components of high-quality clinical decision-making" and "patients and families are integral partners with the health care team" (Committee on Hospital Care and Institute for Patient- and Family-Centered Care 2012). This principle is a core AAP strategic priority. As dental healthcare providers, patients come to our practices with this expectation.

Implementing true family-centered care is difficult, requiring study, effort, and commitment, but its rewards are improved patient care and less stress for the dental provider. Trust is a fragile concept; once interpersonal trust is lost, it can be difficult to rebuild (Hupcey and Miller 2006).

Just as the patients and parents that walk into the dental practice are diverse, so are the readers of this chapter. This chapter is meant as an introduction to the societal and cultural trends at the time of its writing. The information presented may not apply to the culture of every reader; however, the principles presented can be crafted to equip all readers to better create a truly patient-centered practice. Society constantly changes. While clinical competency is an important part of doctor–patient trust, it is no longer the only requirement to be a successful healthcare practitioner. Healthcare providers must possess cultural competency and effective communication skills as well. Those who master both will thrive no matter where the future leads.

## References

Allen, R. (2007). Generational Differences Chart, West Midland Family Center [Online]. Available at: http://www.wmfc.org/uploads/GenerationalDifferencesChart.pdf. Accessed 26 May 2020.

Allinson, M. and Chaar, B. (2016). How to build and maintain trust with patients [Online]. Available at: https://www.pharmaceutical-journal.com/eye-care/how-to-build-and-maintain-trust-with-patients/20201862. article?firstPass=false#fn_15. Accessed 21 May 2020.

American Academy of Pediatric Dentistry. (2020a). *Informed Consent.* Reference Manual of Pediatric Dentistry, 439–442. Chicago IL: American Academy of Pediatric Dentistry.

American Academy of Pediatric Dentistry. (2020b). *Behavior Guidance for the Pediatric Dental Patient.* Reference Manual of Pediatric Dentistry (pp. 266–279). Chicago, IL: American Academy of Pediatric Dentistry.

American Academy of Pediatric Dentistry. (2020c). *Protective Stabilization for Pediatric Dental Patients.* Reference Manual of Pediatric Dentistry (pp. 280–285). Chicago, IL: American Academy of Pediatric Dentistry.

American Academy of Pediatrics Section on Bioethics, Leuthner, S.R., Vizcarrondo, F.E. (Eds.) (2017). American Academy of Pediatrics bioethics resident curriculum: Case-based teaching guides. [Online]. Available at: http://www.aap.org/sections/bioethics/default.cfm. Accessed 22 May 2020.

American Academy of Pediatrics Ad Hoc Task Force on Definition of the Medical Home: The Medical Home. (1992). *Pediatrics, 90,* 774.

American Dental Association. (2017). How to handle online negative reviews. [Online]. Available at: https://www.ada.org/en/publications/ada-news/2017-archive/september/how-to-handle-online-negative-reviews. Accessed 22 May 2020.

Attwell, K., Leask, J., Meyer, S.B. et al. (2017). Vaccine rejecting parents' engagement with expert systems that inform vaccination programs. *Journal of Bioethical Inquiry,* 14(1), 65–76.

Back, A.L., Arnold, R.M., Baile, W.F.et al. (2005). Approaching difficult communication tasks in oncology. *CA: A Cancer Journal for Clinicians,* 55, 164–177.

Berry, L.L., Danaher, T.S., Beckham, D. et al. (2017). When patients and their families feel like hostages to health care. *Mayo Clinic Proceedings,* 92, 1373–1381.

Blendon, R.J., Benson, J.M., and Hero, J.O. (2014). Public trust in physicians–U.S. medicine in international perspective. *New England Journal Medicine,* 371(17), 1570–1572.

Borrelli, B., Tooley, E.M., and Scott-Sheldon, L.A. (2015). Motivational interviewing for parent-child health interventions: A systematic review and meta-analysis. *Pediatric Dentistry,* 37, 254–265.

Casamassimo, P.S. (2003). Dental disease prevalence, prevention, and health promotion: The implications on pediatric oral health of a more diverse population. *Pediatric Dentistry,* 25, 16–18.

Casamassimo, P.S., Wilson, S., and Gross, L. (2002). Effects of changing U.S. parenting styles on dental practice: Perceptions of diplomates of the American Board of Pediatric Dentistry presented to the College of Diplomates of the American Board of Pediatric Dentistry 16th Annual Session, Atlanta, GA, Saturday, May 26, 2001. *Pediatric Dentistry,* 24, 18–22.

Chang, C.T., Badger, G.R., Acharya, B. et al. (2018). Influence of ethnicity on parental preference for pediatric dental behavioral management techniques. *Pediatric Dentistry,* 40, 265–272.

Collins, J. (2001). Good to Great. New York City, New York. Harper Collins Publishers.

Committee on Hospital Care and Institute for Patient- and Family-Centered Care. (2012). Patient- and family-centered care and the pediatrician's role. *Pediatrics,* 129, 394–404.

Cote, S., Geltman, P., Nunn, M. et al. (2004). Dental caries of refugee children compared with US children. *Pediatrics,* 114, e733–740.

Coulter, A. (2002). After Bristol: Putting patients at the centre. *British Medical Journal,* 324, 648–651.

Council on Community Pediatrics. (2016). Poverty and Child Health in the United States. *Pediatrics,* 137, e20160339

Cousino, M., Hazen, R., Yamokoski, A. et al. Multi-site Intervention Study to Improve Consent Research, T. (2011). Parent participation and physician-parent communication during informed consent in child leukemia. *Pediatrics,* 128, e1544–1551.

Crespo. (2019). The importance of oral health in immigrant and refugee children. *Children,* 6, 102.

da Fonseca, M.A. (2014). Eat or heat? The effects of poverty on children's behavior. *Pediatric Dentistry,* 36, 132–137.

Del Canale, S., Louis, D.Z., Maio, V. et al. (2012). The relationship between physician empathy and disease complications: An empirical study of primary care physicians and their diabetic patients in Parma, Italy. *Academic Medicine,* 87, 1243–1249.

Donate-Bartfield, E., Lobb, W.K., and Roucka, T.M. (2014). Teaching culturally sensitive care to dental students: A multidisciplinary approach. *Journal of Dental Education,* 78, 454–464.

Elwyn, G., Frosch, D., Thomson, R. et al. (2012). Shared decision making: A model for clinical practice. *Journal General Internal Medicine,* 27, 1361–1367.

Erskine, R. (2017). 20 Online reputation statistics that every business owner needs to know [Online]. Available at: https://www.forbes.com/sites/ryanerskine/2017/09/19/20-online-reputation-statistics-that-every-business-owner-needs-to-know/#581b7a38cc5c. Accessed 22 May 2020.

Fronstin, P. and Dretzka, E. (2018). Consumer engagement in health care among Millennials, baby boomers, and Generation X: Findings from the 2017 consumer engagement in health care survey [Online]. Available at: https://www.ebri.org/docs/default-source/ebri-issue-brief/ebri_ib_444_millennialhealthcare-5mar18.pdf?sfvrsn=3f35342f_4. Accessed 30 March 2020.

Garcia, R.I., Cadoret, C.A., and Henshaw, M. (2008). Multicultural issues in oral health. *Dental Clinics of North America,* 52, 319–332.

Gillies, V. (2008). Perspectives on parenting responsibility: Contextualizing values and practices. *Journal of Law and Society,* 35(1), 95–112.

Goldbach, P. (2020). The erosion of trust in healthcare: How did we get here? [Online] Available at: https://www.healthdialog.com/blog/erosion-trust-healthcare how-did-we-get-here. Accessed 28 May 2020.

Goleman, J. (2014). Cultural factors affecting behavior guidance and family compliance. *Pediatric Dentistry,* 36, 121–127.

Graham, M.A., Tomar, S.L., and Logan, H.L. (2005). Perceived social status, language and identified dental home among Hispanics in Florida. *Journal of the American Dental Association,* 136, 1572–1582.

Ha, J.F. and Longnecker, N. (2010). Doctor-patient communication: A review. *Ochsner Journal,* 10, 38–43.

Haley, J.M., McMorrow, S., and Kenney, G.M. (2010). Despite recent improvement, one in six children lived in a family with problems paying medical bills in 2017. [Online]. Available at: https://www.urban.org/sites/default/files/publication/100909/children_in_families_with_problems_paying_medical_bills.pdf. Accessed 28 May 2020.

Halsall, A. (2019). Millennials may be history's most competent parents. *Here's why [Online].* Available at: https://winnie.com/blog/why-millennials-are-historys-most-competent-parents. Accessed 03 April 2020.

Hesselberth, J. (2017). App time for nap time: The parennials are here [Online] Available at: https://www.nytimes.com/2017/11/04/style/millennial-parents-parennials.html?_r=0#nws=mcnewsletter. Accessed 03 April 2020.

Hill, B., Fadavi, S., LeHew, C. et al. (2019). Effect of caregiver's race and ethnicity on acceptance of passive immobilization for their child's dental treatment. *Journal of Dentistry for Children,* 86, 3–9.

Hilton, I.V., Stephen, S., Barker, J.C. et al. (2007). Cultural factors and children's oral health care: A qualitative study of carers of young children. *Community Dental and Oral Epidemiology,* 35, 429–438.

Hoeft, K.S., Barker, J.C., and Masterson, E.E. (2010). Urban Mexican–American mothers' beliefs about caries etiology in children. *Community Dentistry and Oral Epidemiol,* 38, 244–255.

Howe, N. (2010). Meet Mr. and Mrs. Gen X: A new parent generation [Online]. Available at: https://www.aasa.org/SchoolAdministratorArticle.aspx?id=11122. Accessed 03 April 2020.

Hulin, J., Baker, S.R., Marshman, Z. et al. (2017). Development of a decision aid for children faced with the decision to undergo dental treatment with sedation or general anaesthesia. *International Journal of Paediatric Dentistry,* 27, 344–355.

Hupcey, J.E. and Miller, J. (2006). Community dwelling adults' perception of interpersonal trust vs. trust in health care providers. *Journal of Clinical Nursing,* 15, 1132–1139.

Ishizuka, P. (2019). Social class, gender, and contemporary parenting standards in the United States: Evidence from a National Survey Experiment. *Social Forces,* 98, 31–58.

Klass, P. (2016). Saving Tiny Tim–Pediatrics and childhood poverty in the United States. *New England Journal of Medicine,* 374(23), 2201–2205.

Lareau, A. (2003). Unequal Childhoods: Class, Race, and Family Life. University of California Press, Berkeley.

Le-Scherban, F., Brenner, A.B., and Schoeni, R.F. (2016). Childhood family wealth and mental health in a national cohort of young adults. *SSM Popul Health,* 2, 798–806.

Levy, M. (2019). Marketing medicine to millennials: Preparing institutions and regulations for direct-to-consumer healthcare. *California Western Law Review,* 55(2), Article 9.

Litch, S. (2015). Litch's law log: Best practices for in-office photos and videos that parents wish to take [Online]. Available at: http://www.pediatricdentistrytoday.org/2015/September/L/5/news/article/414/. Accessed 26 May 2020.

Livingston, G. (2018). More than a million Millennials are becoming moms each year [Online]. Available at: https://www.pewresearch.org/fact-tank/2018/05/04/more-than-a-million-millennials-are-becoming-moms-each-year/. Accessed 04 April 2020.

Marino, R., Morgan, M., and Hopcraft, M. (2012). Transcultural dental training: Addressing the oral health care needs of people from culturally diverse backgrounds. *Community Dentistry and Oral Epidemiology,* 40(Suppl 2), 134–140.

McBride, T. (2017). The Mindset List® of Generation X [Online]. Available at: https://themindsetlist.com/2017/05mindset-list-generation-x/. Accessed 03 April 2020.

McEwen, C.A. and McEwen, B.S. (2017). Social structure, adversity, toxic stress, and intergenerational poverty: An early childhood model. *Annual Review of Sociology,* 43, 445–472.

Millet, J. (2013). From melting pot to salad bowl [Online]. Available at: https://www.culturalsavvy.com/ understanding_american_culture.htm. Accessed 20 May 2020.

Mofidi, M., Rozier, R.G., and King, R.S. (2002). Problems with access to dental care for Medicaid-insured children: What caregivers think. *American Journal of Public Health,* 92, 53–58.

Mouradian, W.E., Berg, J.H., and Somerman, M.J. (2003). Addressing disparities through dental-medical collaborations, part 1. *The role of cultural competency in health disparities: training of primary care medical practitioners in children's oral health. Journal of Dental Education,* 67, 860–868.

Murphy, R. (2019). Local consumer review survey [Online]. Available at: https://www.brightlocal.com/research/local-consumer-review-survey/. Accessed 22 May 2020.

Murphy, S. (2007). American association of retired persons, leading a multigenerational workforce [Online]. Available at: https://assets.aarp.org/www.aarp.org_/articles/money/employers/leading_multigenerational_workforce.pdf. Accessed 26 May 2020.

Muthiah, N., Adesman, A., and Keim, S. (2019). Grandparents raising grandchildren: Are they up to the job? *Pediatrics*, 144 (2 Meeting Abstract), 77.

Ng, M.W. (2003). Multicultural influences on child-rearing practices: Implications for today's pediatric dentist. *Pediatric Dentistry,* 25, 19–22. https://www.ncbi.nlm.nih.gov/pubmed/12627696

O'Connell, L.K., Davis, M.M., and Bauer, N.S. (2015). Assessing parenting behaviors to improve child outcomes. *Pediatrics,* 135, e286–288.

Obeng, C.S. (2007). Culture and dental health among African immigrant school-aged children in the United States. *Health Education,* 107, 343–350.

Parker, K., Cunningham, S.J., Petrie, A. et al. (2017). Randomized controlled trial of a patient decision-making aid for orthodontics. *American Journal of Orthodontics and Dentofacial Orthopedics,* 152, 154–160.

Pascoe, J.M., Wood, D.L., Duffee, J.H. et al. (2016). *Mediators and adverse effects of child poverty in the United States. Pediatrics,* 137. doi: 10.1542/peds.2016-0340

PatientPop. (2019). 7 ways Millennials are changing healthcare—and how your practice must adapt [Online]. Available at: https://info1.patientpop.com/rs/677-NCQ-300/images/WP%2020190621%20-%207%20Ways%20Millennials%20Changing%20Healthcare.pdf. Accessed 23 May 2020.

Pehora, C., Gajaria, N., Stoute, M. et al. (2015). Are parents getting it right? A survey of parents' Internet use for children's health care information. *Interactive Journal of Medical Research,* 4, e12. doi:10.2196/ijmr.3790

Perry, N.B., Dollar, J.M., Calkins, S.D. et al. (2018). Childhood self-regulation as a mechanism through which early overcontrolling parenting is associated with adjustment in preadolescence. *Developmental Psychology,* 54, 1542–1554.

Pew Research Center. (2015a). Raising kids and running a household: How working parents share the load [Online]. Available at: https://www.pewsocialtrends.org/2015/11/04/raising-kids-and-running-a-household-how-working-parents-share-the-load/. Accessed 04 April 2020.

Pew Research Center. (2015b). Parenting in America. Retrieved from https://www.pewresearch.org/wp-content/uploads/sites/3/2015/12/2015-12-17_parenting-in-america_FINAL.pdf

Radz, G. (2018). Will millennials kill private practice dentistry? [Online]. Available at: https://www.dentaleconomics.com/practice/marketing/article/16384950/will-millennials-kill-private-practice-dentistry. Accessed 03 April 2020.

Robbennolt, J.K. (2009). Apologies and medical error. *Clinical Orthopaedics and Related Research,* 467, 376–382.

Say, R., Murtagh, M., and Thomson, R. (2006). Patients' preference for involvement in medical decision making: a narrative review. *Patient Education and Counseling,* 60(2), 102–114.

Schor, E.L. and American Academy of Pediatrics Task Force on the Family. (2003). Family pediatrics: Report of the task force on the family. *Pediatrics,* 111(6 Pt 2), 1541–1571.

Scrimshaw, S.C. (2003). Our multicultural society: Implications for pediatric dental practice. Keynote speaker, 17th annual symposium, Denver, Colorado, Saturday, May 25, 2002. *Pediatric Dentistry,* 25, 11–15.

Shingleton, R.M. and Palfai, T.P. (2016). Technology-delivered adaptations of motivational interviewing for health-related behaviors: A systematic review of the current research. *Patient Education and Counseling,* 99, 17–35.

Sood, N., Jimenez, D.E., Pham, T.B. et al. (2019). Paging Dr. *Google: The effect of online health information on trust in pediatricians' diagnoses. Clinical Pediatrics,* 58, 889–896.

Steinman, H.K. (2013). A method for working with displeased patients-blast. *Journal of Clinical and Aesthetic Dermatology,* 6(3), 25–28. Retrieved from https://www.ncbi.nlm.nih.gov/pubmed/23556033

Sveinsdottir, E.G. and Wang, N.J. (2014). Dentists' views on the effects of changing economic conditions on dental services provided for children and adolescents in Iceland. *Community Dent Health Journal,* 31, 219–223.

Terry, N. (2016). Will the Internet of things disrupt healthcare? [Online]. Available at: https://papers.ssrn.com/sol3/papers.cfm?abstract_id=2760447. Accessed 22 May 2020.

Tiwari, T. and Albino, J. (2017). Acculturation and pediatric minority oral health interventions. *Dental Clinics of North America,* 61, 549–563.

Tucci, J., Mitchell, J., and Goddard, C. (2005). The changing face of parenting: Exploring the attitudes of parents in contemporary Australia. Australian Childhood Foundation, Ringwood, Vic.

Wamala, S., Merlo, J., and Bostrom, G. (2006). Inequity in access to dental care services explains current socioeconomic disparities in oral health: The Swedish National Surveys of Public Health 2004–2005. *Journal of Epidemiology and Community Health,* 60, 1027–1033.

Weinstein, P., Harrison, R., and Benton, T. (2006). Motivating mothers to prevent caries: Confirming the beneficial effect of counseling. *Journal of the American Dental Association,* 137, 789–793.

Wells, M.H., Dormois, L.D., and Townsend, J.A. (2018). Behavior guidance: That was then but this is now. *General Dentistry,* 66, 39–45.

Wong, D., Perez-Spiess, S., and Julliard, K. (2005). Attitudes of Chinese parents toward the oral health of their children with caries: A qualitative study. *Pediatric Dentistry,* 27, 505–512.

Wyman, O. (2017). Right place, right time: Improving access to health care information for vulnerable patients. [Online]. Available at: https://www.oliverwyman.com/content/dam/oliver-wyman/v2/publications/2017/jan/right-place-right-time/RPRT_Altarum.pdf. Accessed 22 May 2020.

Yogman, M., Garfield, C.F., and Committee on Psychosocial Aspects of Child and Family Health. (2016). Fathers' roles in the care and development of their children: The role of pediatricians. *Pediatrics,* 138. doi:10.1542/peds.2016-1128

## 6

## Establishing a Dental Home
*Ari Kupietzky and Anna B. Fuks*

### Introduction

The recognition of and treatment for early childhood caries (ECC) has been a major concern for the dental profession. Indeed, concerns about the dental treatment directed toward infants were reported at the beginning of the twentieth century (Cunha et al. 2004). Although dental caries in children declined from the early 1970s until the mid-1990s, the National Institute of Dental and Craniofacial Research (NIDCR) reported that this trend has reversed: the reversal being more severe in younger children (Dye et al. 2007; NIDCR 2018). To combat this form of early dental caries, pediatric dentists in the 1980s began recommending that dental examinations for children should commence at one year of age or earlier.

Education, a less costly alternative, also has been a focus in solving the ECC problem. One of the earliest centers for delivering an educational program was the Baby Clinic, established in 1986 at the Londrina State University in Brazil. The aim of the Baby Clinic was to provide education to parents and to maintain or re-establish a good oral health status, creating a positive attitude in parents and children toward dentistry (Cunha et al. 2000). Education for improving oral health starts very early, and lectures on prevention of oral diseases are included in prenatal delivery preparation courses for parents (Casamassimo 2001). A model for the delivery of preventive education to the parent and very early oral examination of the infant has been termed the *Dental Home*. Reports describing new programs indicate the profession's acceptance of this approach, and indeed, an entire book has been published recently on infant dentistry (Berg and Slayton 2015).

This chapter approaches the dental home from a different viewpoint—the patient management perspective. How can the dental home have an impact on future child dental behavior and the relationship between the pediatric dentist and parent? The chapter also presents the technical aspects of examining and managing a one-year-old child, the recommended age to establish a dental home. The management of a one-year-old presents the clinician with entirely different circumstances as compared to older children. Although there is only a year separating a one-year-old from a two-year-old child, there are great cognitive, physical, and dental differences (see Chapter 2).

### Rationale

All of the patient management techniques discussed in the preceding and following chapters have in common the need for effective communicative management. This leads to the conclusion that there is a need for a congenial relationship. Proper patient management and treatment can be achieved in a friendly, familiar environment. This concept has been labeled the "medical home" by our pediatric medical colleagues. The medical home concept was introduced by the American Academy of Pediatrics (AAP) in 1967. At the time, it was envisioned as a central source for all the medical information about a child. It focused primarily on those with special needs and in low socioeconomic groups, as underprivileged children were seeking basic medical treatment in hospital emergency rooms. In 1992, the concept was expanded, and the medical home was defined as a strategy for delivering family-centered, comprehensive, continuous, and coordinated care for all infants and children. In 2002, the organization further extended and operationalized the definition, including the requirement that each patient have an ongoing relationship with a personal physician trained to provide first contact and continuous, comprehensive care. The medical home is now applied to all children and suggests that a strategy be developed that ensures a familiar healthcare provider for each family. This concept argues for a place that does not change each year with the vagaries of the third-party payment system, governmental support, or practitioner market. The strategy worked: studies show that the medical home public health model allows appropriate care to be initiated more often in the primary care center than in the emergency room. Furthermore, it is associated with better preventive health, higher levels of disease management, and lower resource utilization and costs (Devries et al. 2012; Hearld and Alexander 2012).

The guideline on infant oral care was adopted by the American Academy of Pediatric Dentistry (AAPD) in 2001. In 2010, the AAPD reaffirmed its "Policy on the Dental Home," and defined the term *Dental Home* as "the ongoing relationship between the dentist and the patient, inclusive of all aspects of oral health care delivered in a comprehensive, continuously accessible, coordinated, and family-centered way. Establishment of a dental home begins by twelve months of age and includes referral to dental specialists when appropriate" (AAPD reference manual 2020). This concept supports a place where all families feel they will be welcomed for regular, comprehensive care and where they are understood and valued. Empirical evidence suggests great value to a long relationship with child patients as it allows additional learning and reframing of experiences after difficult procedures. This can only occur if the family has a comfortable relationship with the dental home. The present alternative is a system that leads to episodic and emergency care (Feigal 2001).

In a familiar and welcoming environment, relationships can be made that ease the stress of health care for children. A dental home enhances the likelihood of establishing parental compliance with early and regular care. It is a cornerstone of prevention in dentistry, and it is much more likely to lead to better child acceptance of dental procedures.

A major goal of the dental home concept is the prevention of ECC. Although not yet substantiated by extensive research, researchers and clinicians state that the benefits of the dental home are substantial and intuitive with an increasing emphasis on disease prevention and management, advancements in tailoring care to meet individual needs, and better health outcomes (Nowak and Casamassimo 2008). The benefits of the dental home include early dental attendance and preventive services, resulting in lower future treatment costs, and a decrease in more invasive, complex dental treatments (Doykos 1997; Nowak et al. 2014; Savage et al. 2004). The establishment of a dental home, especially among high-risk, low-income populations, is not limited to decreasing the prevalence of ECC but also reduces the practice of cariogenic feeding behaviors (Kierce et al. 2016). Untreated dental problems may lead to hospitalization and expose children to additional health risks associated with conscious sedation and general anesthesia (Newacheck et al. 2000). However, among the non-tangible advantages of this approach to dental care is the fact that a dental home established early in life may also

reduce children's anxiety or fear of dental care. This is the reason for including this chapter in a book devoted to patient management. Again, the emphasis is on the prevention of disease and its consequences.

## The Dental Home and the Pediatric Dentistry Treatment Triangle

With introspect, one may conclude that establishing a dental home is simply the early foundation of a healthy, balanced, stable, and harmonious pediatric dentistry triangle (see Figure 6-1). The first-year visit provides ideal conditions for development of the dentist–parent–child relationship. The child is free of pain, and the accompanying parent is free of stress and anxiety. The healthy triangle has at its base the dentist and parent acting as a foundation for the apex of the triangle: the child. The dental team and parent are team members, on the same side of the triangle supporting the child through the dental experience. Conversely, when a two-year-old child appears at the dentist for the first time with ECC and possibly pain, the pediatric dentistry triangle is far from ideal (see Figure 6-2). Many parents are filled with feelings of guilt when their child is diagnosed with ECC, often with anxiety and stress. As the dentist explains the cause of the disease and discusses the treatment options, many parents take on the role of child protector. The dental team is then situated on one side of the triangle opposite the child and parent. The dental team, bearing the weight and balancing force of the unstable and fragile triangle, is at a disadvantage. The early establishment of the dental home allows the avoidance of such an unfavorable start.

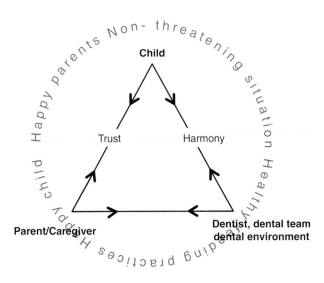

**Figure 6-1**  The pediatric dentistry triangle founded under ideal circumstances: during the establishment of a dental home at age one year. *Source:* Courtesy of Dr. Ari Kupietzky.

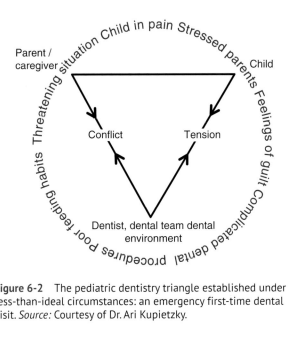

**Figure 6-2** The pediatric dentistry triangle established under less-than-ideal circumstances: an emergency first-time dental visit. *Source:* Courtesy of Dr. Ari Kupietzky.

---

### Case 6.1

Mrs. G. telephoned a pediatric dentist's office to make a first-time appointment for her 13-month-old daughter. The receptionist sensed much hesitation in the mother's voice. "My friend told me that I should bring Kayla in for an appointment. But when I asked my dentist at what age to start with my daughter's dental appointments, he told me not before four or five years old! I was wondering how the dentist would get Kayla to open her mouth. She gives us trouble when taking a bath and even I, as her mom, can't brush her teeth."

The receptionist reassured her that Dr. Ann and the entire staff have much experience dealing with young children, even younger than Kayla. She told Mrs. G. that a pediatric dentist is similar to a pediatrician and will be able to help Mrs. G and Kayla through the visit. Mrs. G made the appointment.

---

***Case 6.1, Discussion:*** The receptionist is the first contact with the dental office, and in this case needed to reassure the mother that bringing in her child for the one-year visit was the right thing to do. It is clear how important it is for Kayla to establish a dental home. Her mother mentioned on the phone that Kayla is not getting proper preventive dental care at home. She will need to be instructed on proper feeding habits, fluoride usage, and how to brush a young child's teeth. Her predicament and uncertainty about this visit are typical, especially if Kayla is her first child. Contradicting

information regarding the proper timing for the first dental visit is widespread in the dental profession. Referral from a pediatrician or family doctor lends more credibility to the concept. Many general dentists give parents misinformation either out of ignorance or perhaps because they themselves cannot manage a very young child and therefore do not comprehend the validity of such an early dental visit. Having a website explaining much of the above helps alleviate parents' initial anxieties.

Although the dental home concept was introduced more than 10 years ago, a 2011 survey of parent leaders confirmed that the majority of parents are not aware of it (Kagihara et al. 2011). The majority of respondents (84.8%) said parents do not know about the recommendation to establish a dental home for their child by 12 months of age. They elaborated on their answers with comments including the following:

- "I just learned this (age-1 dental visit concept) myself within the last week—and I'm supposedly in the loop."
- "Some families need to be informed. Other families tell us that they have attempted to get that oral health screening from their dentist at age one and have been turned away because the dentist did not follow this as the standard of care."
- "Many believe they can wait until either the child starts school or they lose their baby teeth."
- "No way! Age three is what we always heard!"
- "Yes, but if the child is chronically ill, other health issues often come first and many children who do not feed by mouth are often taken to the dentist later because of other health complications."
- "Not at all, as oral health care is not considered a priority in light of other medical diagnoses a child might have, and because most families don't think baby teeth are important."

Despite the AAPD's recommendation that all children have a dental visit following the eruption of the first tooth or no later than 12 months of age, changes within the dental profession were initially slow. In 1997, approximately 73% of AAPD members surveyed agreed with the policy, but only 47% reported performing evaluations on children 12 months old or younger (Erickson and Thomas 1997). Many pediatric dentists had not accepted the AAPD Policy on the Dental Home, nor did they perform infant oral evaluations a decade after the initial policy statement.

However, over the last decade, AAPD members' attitudes and practices have improved significantly. A survey of the AAPD membership on infant oral healthcare beliefs revealed that 91% agreed with the policy, and 90% performed infant oral evaluations in their practice (Bubna et al. 2012). And recently, respondents of the 2017 AAPD membership survey reported, on average, that 75% of their patients had established a dental home. But there still seems to be a lingering doubt about the value of the dental home and early care. When the question was posed to Academy members in a different way, a large discrepancy was revealed in practitioners' beliefs in the AAPD policy. When asked at what age asymptomatic children should have their first oral health evaluation, only 47% of respondents said by 12 months. When practitioners were asked why they did not perform infant oral evaluations in their office, several reasons were noted. Surprisingly, the most common reason was that practitioners felt the "parents do not see the value of the infant oral evaluations." The second most commonly cited answer was that "existing conditions should dictate evaluation time."

Thus, it seems that one of the major difficulties in establishing early prevention is getting support within the profession. Most caregivers have not been counseled on proper infant oral health care and the various factors that contribute to dental disease. Many parents are unaware that the inappropriate use of a baby bottle could result in harm to their child's developing dentition. How, then, is early education to be dispensed to parents? One suggestion made by AAPD members is to educate pediatricians and primary care physicians about the value of early dental evaluations. The AAP has a policy which recommends that pediatric health-care professionals perform oral health risk assessments on all patients beginning at six months, and that patients who are at risk for developing dental caries enter an "aggressive anticipatory guidance and intervention program provided by a dentist between six and twelve months of age" (Hale 2003).

Another equally important suggestion made by AAPD members was to educate and train general dentists, as well as dental students and residents, about infant oral health care and the establishment of a dental home. Surveys in Iowa and Ohio have revealed that fewer than 15% of dentists believe in or perform infant oral examinations (Siegal and Marx 2002; Wolfe et al. 2006), and few general dentists examine children younger than three years old (Seale and Casamassimo 2003). Currently, undergraduate education in infant dentistry is lacking. The report of McWhorter et al. (2001) on infant oral health education in US dental school curricula found that the average didactic curricular time devoted to the topic of infant oral health is 2 hours and 20 minutes, and over half of the pre-doctoral programs provided no hands-on experience in infant oral health examinations. A recent survey (Marcelle et al. 2016) emphasized the importance of ensuring that predoctoral curriculums promote a greater awareness among students about the importance of risk assessment and management of oral diseases. Since general dentists far outnumber pediatric dentists and ultimately examine the majority of children, the recommendation has great importance.

### Case 6.2

Dr. Sue brought 18-month-old Joey and his mother into the operatory for the child's first dental examination. She seated the mother in the dental chair with the child lying backward on her. Dr. Sue was handed a mirror to examine the child's mouth and teeth, and the assistant adjusted the dental light. Joey refused to open his mouth. When the dentist forcibly opened his mouth, Joey started crying. The mother became very upset and interrupted the procedure. She accused Dr. Sue of not being patient and not knowing how to deal with her child. "If you would have just explained to Joey why he needs to get his teeth checked, he would not have cried. Joey understands everything. We never do anything to him without an explanation and his consent."

***Case 6.2, Discussion***: The child was placed in "mommy wrap" position (in which the guardian lies on the chair and wraps her arms around the infant or toddler). While this position is commonly used with children by general practitioners, it is not the recommended position for examining toddlers. The mother lying back in the "mommy wrap" position may feel vulnerable and not in control. She cannot observe what is being done on her very young child and may assume the worst. In contrast, in the "knee to knee" position (see below), the child is able to see the mother's face while she controls the child's movement. This is reassuring for both child and parent. In the former position, the child only sees the dentist and assistant and, of course, the overhead bright light.

The dentist did not start with initial counseling, anticipatory guidance, and preparation of the mother for realistic expectations for an 18-month-old child (see Table 6-1 for development milestones of a toddler). Comprehending the importance of a dental examination is usually beyond an 18-month-old's capacity. A first-time modern parent may have false expectations.

Toddlers should ideally be scheduled early in the day, avoiding nap time. A favorite toy or blanket may accompany the child. If possible, either through a written letter or on a website, parents should be advised not to communicate any of their fears to the child. They also could be informed on the procedure that generally takes place.

There are various positions to facilitate the toddler's examination. For example, the dental chair is raised and adjusted to simulate a physician's examination table. The infant lies at the foot of the dental chair that is covered with a fresh towel or sheet. This position allows the dentist to peer directly into the child's mouth.

**Table 6-1** A child's developmental milestones – 12–18 months.*

| Cognitive Milestones | Language Milestones | Social/Emotional Milestones | Physical Milestones |
|---|---|---|---|
| • Identifies family members in photographs <br> • Enjoys cause-and-effect relationship <br> • Is able to make choices between clear alternatives <br> • Begins to solve problems <br> • Remembers more | • Has expressive vocabulary of 4–10 words (by 13–15 months) <br> • Has expressive vocabulary of 10–20 words (by 18 months) <br> • Can listen and respond to simple directions | • Prefers to keep caregiver in sight while exploring environment <br> • Demands personal attention <br> • May reveal stubbornness <br> • Unable to share <br> • Responds to simple requests | • Picks up small objects with pointer finger and thumb <br> • Can build a tower of cubes <br> • Can throw a ball <br> • Walks well <br> • Turns pages in a book <br> • Can walk while holding an object |

*Source:* *Based on ACT: Quality Professional Development for Childhood Care and Education Professionals, Department of Human Resources, http://www.acetonline.org/ child_dev_milestone.pdf.

## The Knee to Knee Examination

The most effective and comfortable position for the patient, parent, and dentist is the "knee to knee" position. Position the child in the seated adult caregiver's lap (Figures 6-3–6-6). Interact warmly with both the child and the caregiver. The dentist and parent sit opposite one another with knees touching. With the child facing the dentist, touch the child's hand. Tickle the arm. Speak gently and smile. During this "warming up" time, brief counseling may occur. Ask the parent to turn the child 180 degrees so that the child is now facing them. The child is placed on the parent's lap, facing the parent, with the child's legs wrapping around the parent's waist. While the parent is holding the child's hands, the child is laid back, resting the head in the dentist's lap. This position enables the child to see and feel the parent while the dentist performs the examination with minimal restraint. The position allows for excellent visualization of the oral cavity by both the parent and dentist.

Another option for the knee-to-knee exam is using a cushion device (Figure 6-7). A lap cushion device flexes with the baby, allowing the tilt-back to feel more secure. Some parents may prefer it over the infant lying directly on the dentist's lap. On the other hand, it might startle the child, introducing a new device which may make the exam more formal and threatening.

When approaching the very young patient (or any other patient, for that matter), begin with a digital examination. Because the young child often does not comprehend the procedures, the clinician starts slowly with an extraoral examination, gently rubbing the child's face and talking calmly. Vocal quality is important with all youngsters and may be one of the dentist's greatest assets in managing behavior, especially when dealing with very young children. Even if the child does not comprehend the language, a soothing voice helps relax the patient. Before performing an intraoral examination, the dentist explains to the parent that the procedure does not hurt the child and that even

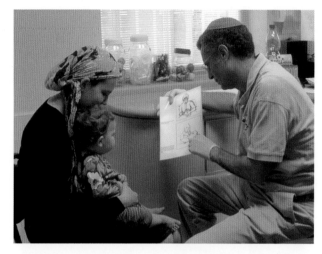

**Figure 6-3** Infant exam: Initial counseling and anticipatory guidance. Even if the child does not comprehend the language, a soothing voice helps to relax the patient.

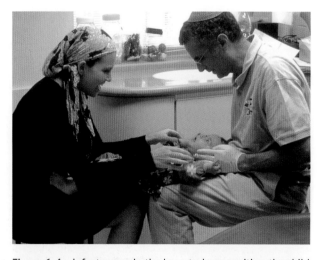

**Figure 6-4** Infant exam: In the knee-to-knee position, the child is able to see the mother's face while she controls the child's movement. The mother is able to observe and communicate with the child and dentist.

(a)

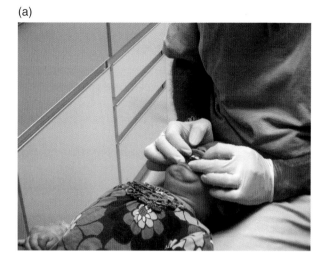

(b)

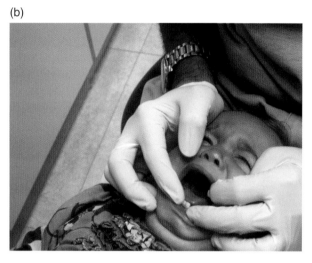

**Figure 6-5** Infant exam: Begin with a digital examination and without instruments (a). Crying may facilitate the exam. As the child cries, the mouth remains open (b).

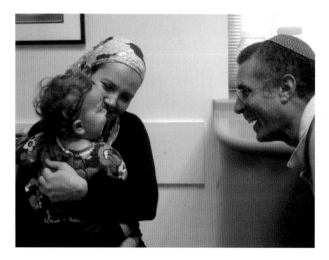

**Figure 6-6** Infant exam: Most children will regain composure immediately, as they sit up and receive a hug from the parent.

(a)

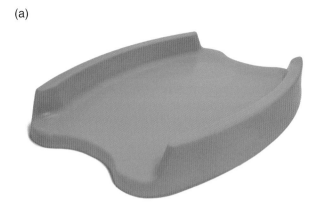

(b)

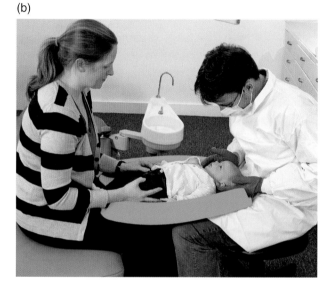

**Figure 6-7** A lap cushion device flexes with the baby, allowing the tilt-back to feel more secure (a). Some parents may prefer it over the infant lying directly on the dentist's lap (b). On the other hand, introducing a new device which may make the exam more formal and threatening might startle the child. *Source:* Courtesy of Specialized Care Co, Inc. Hampton, NH. specializedcare.com

though the young patient appears cooperative, many children begin to cry during an oral examination. Most parents appreciate the forewarning. It may also be necessary to explain this to other children in the office to avoid upsetting them. Since the child is in the parent's arms, the dentist has to attempt to communicate with the child and parent simultaneously. It is not unusual for a young patient's mouth to remain closed since the child does not understand what is expected. The mouth is easily opened by sliding an index finger between the teeth or gum pads and cheek, and pressing lightly against the ramus of the mandible. However, a gentler approach, which often achieves the same end, is to have the dental assistant rub the child's tummy. This relaxes many infants and toddlers, and their mouths often open spontaneously. Once access to the oral cavity is gained, every attempt is made to complete the oral examination before withdrawing from the child's mouth.

In summary, several points are important when examining infants and very young children:

1) Begin with a digital examination and without instruments, and perform as much of the examination as possible. Instruments can be cumbersome in a small mouth and potentially harmful if the child makes sudden, unexpected movements.

2) Avoid using the operatory light if possible. If it is used, care should be taken to keep the light out of the infant's eyes.

3) Place a finger near the tine of the explorer when entering or leaving the mouth or moving the instrument from tooth to tooth. The finger in this position helps to prevent harm in the event of a quick turn of the child's head.

4) Use a mouth prop for young children who do not keep their mouths open. A small Molt mouth prop can be of great advantage when a child fails to keep the mouth open. A less threatening type of prop, which can be prepared beforehand, consists of four or five tongue blades wrapped in adhesive tape, or can be purchased ready-made (see Figure 6-8).

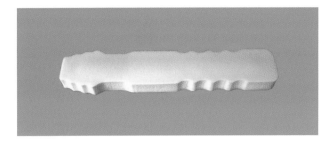

**Figure 6-8** Mouth prop. *Source:* Courtesy of Specialized Care Co, Inc. Hampton, NH.

---

### Case 6.3

Two four-year-olds arrived at the pediatric dentist's office following a collision of heads at nursery school. Both children had bleeding from the mouth and were accompanied by their parents. Sue had been at the dentist initially at age two and had since returned for a checkup the previous year. Jack had never been to any dentist, and this emergency visit was the first for both himself and his mother. Jack was crying and very frightened, and his mom was visibly upset and tense. Conversely, Sue was a little nervous but was familiar with the office, staff, and dentist. She was looking forward to receiving the prize to be given later. Her mom remembered being told by the dentist that such incidents might occur and are indeed expected. "Kids will be kids. Maybe that is why they grow up with baby teeth." On the other hand, Jack's mom reacted aggressively toward the dentist when she was told that her son's lip was indeed lacerated but that his teeth were not fractured due to the fall; rather they were severely decayed and only appeared broken. The mother had given Jack a baby bottle of apple juice to calm him. She was shocked when told that Jack needed extensive dental work not only on his front teeth but also his molars, as they showed advanced signs of ECC.

Sue was discharged after an X-ray. Jack refused to take an X-ray and was to return for restorative treatment under general anesthesia, his parent's preference.

---

***Case 6.3, Discussion***: Obviously Jack's mother was at a disadvantage. Her first encounter with her child's dentist was emergent and under duress. This could have been avoided if she had the opportunity to establish her child's dental home earlier. The dental home should not only be analyzed on its effects on the child's oral health and anxiety but also on how it might change the dental anxiety of parents. This is not a trivial point.

Chapter 1 described the cycle of dental fear. Maternal anxiety and its impact on a child's dental health, anxiety, and behavior has been extensively studied (see Figure 6-9). This anxiety can affect the child's oral health and have long-term rippling effects on the child's future adult dental health (Shearer et al. 2011). As parents bear the responsibility for their preschool children's oral health, anxiety may influence parental attitudes and habits regarding the child's oral health care. Mothers with severe dental anxiety may be reluctant to expose their young child to the expected "terrifying" dental experience. Although there are clear, common ECC etiological pathways involving bacteria and diet, these can be modulated by the relative contribution of other factors, including socioeconomic, cultural, and ethnic backgrounds and paternal dental anxiety (Seow et al. 2009). Thus, research suggests that preventive strategies for children's oral health should pay closer attention not only to the child's characteristics and those of his family, but also to maternal dental anxiety-related behaviors (Goettems et al. 2012).

The dentist had alerted Sue's mother to the possibility that trauma might occur, especially during the growing period of two to four years of age, when toddlers seek independence and learn to walk. She was told what to expect and how to act in the event of a traumatic episode involving her child's teeth. Anticipatory guidance should not be limited to explanations about caries, but also include emergency situations. Other topics include oral development (pattern of eruption and teething facts), fluoride, oral hygiene at home, breastfeeding's effects on the mouth, pacifier use versus thumb-sucking effects, and nutrition and diet.

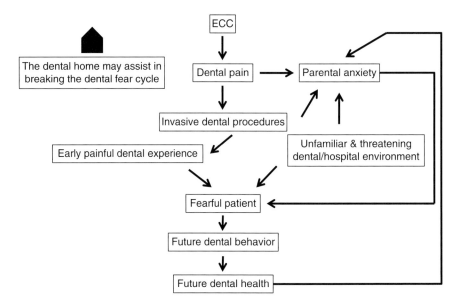

**Figure 6-9** The dental fear cycle may be broken or avoided by establishing a dental home early. *Source:* Courtesy of Dr. Ari Kupietzky.

## Summary

This chapter has provided some of the background for the dental home, a relatively new concept. It was included in this book because children who are indoctrinated into a dental home generally have fewer major dental problems and, importantly, they and their parents have better attitudes toward oral health care. Cases were provided to elucidate these points. For those inexperienced with examination procedures for the infant patient, a detailed description was provided.

## References

American Academy of Pediatric Dentistry Policy on the Dental Home. (2020). *The Reference Manual of Pediatric Dentistry* 2019–2020, p. 15.

American Academy of Pediatric Dentistry. (2018). The 2017 Survey of Pediatric Dental Practice. Available at: https://www.aapd.org/globalassets/media/aapd_chws_survey_pediatric_dentistry_final_2017.pdf. Accessed on March 2, 2020

Berg, J. and Slayton, R. (2015). Early Childhood Oral Health, 2nd ed. Wiley-Blackwell, Ames, Iowa.

Bubna, S., Perez-Spiess, S., Cernigliaro, J. et al. (2012). Infant oral health care: Beliefs and practices of American Academy of Pediatric Dentistry members. *Pediatric Dentistry*, 34, 203–209.

Casamassimo, P. (2001). Maternal oral health. *Dental Clinics of North America*, 45, 469–478.

Cunha, R.F., Delbem, A.C., Percinoto, C. et al. (2000). Dentistry for babies: A preventive protocol. *ASDC Journal of Dentistry for Children*, 67, 89–92.

Cunha, R.F., Matos, J.X., and Marfinati, S.M. (2004). Dentistry for babies: Why do parents seek dental care?. *Journal of Clinical Pediatric Dentistry*, 28, 19–34.

Devries, A., Li, C.H., Sridhar, G. et al. (2012). Impact of medical homes on quality, healthcare utilization, and costs. *The American Journal of Managed Care*, 18, 534–544.

Doykos, J.D. III. (1997). Comparative cost and time analysis over a two-year period for children whose initial dental experience occurred between ages 4 and 8 years. *Pediatric Dentistry*, 19, 61–62.

Dye, B.A., Tan, S., Smith, V. et al. (2007). Trends in oral health status: United States, 1988–1994 and 1999–2004. National Center for Health Statistics. *Vital and Health Statistics*, 11, 1–92.

Erickson, P.R. and Thomas, H.F. (1997). A survey of the American Academy of Pediatric Dentistry membership: Infant oral healthcare. *Pediatric Dentistry*, 19, 17–21.

Feigal, R.J. (2001). Guiding and managing the child dental patient: A fresh look at old pedagogy. *Journal of Dental Education*, 65, 1369–1377.

Goettems, M.L., Ardenghi, T.M., Romano, A.R. et al. (2012). Influence of maternal dental anxiety on the child's dental caries experience. *Caries Research*, 46, 3–8.

Hale, K.J. (2003). Oral health risk assessment timing and establishment of the dental home. *American Academy of*

*Pediatrics Section on Pediatric Dentistry. Pediatrics*, 111, 1113–1116.

Hearld, L.R. and Alexander, J.A. (2012). Patient-centered care and emergency department utilization: A path analysis of the mediating effects of care coordination and delays in care. *Medical Care Research and Review*, 69, 560–580.

Kagihara, L.E., Huebner, C.E., Mouradian, W.E. et al. (2011). Parents' perspectives on a dental home for children with special health care needs. *Special Care Dentistry*, 31, 170–177.

Kierce, E.A., Boyd, L.D., Rainchuso L. et al. (2016). Association between early childhood caries, feeding practices and an established dental home. *Journal of Dental Hygiene*, 90, 18–27.

Marcelle, M., Mugayar, L., Tomar, S.L. et al. (2016). The impact of an Infant Oral Health Program on Dental Students' Knowledge and Attitudes. *Journal of Dental Education,* 80, 1328–1336.

McWhorter, A.G., Seale, N.S., and King, S.A. (2001). Infant oral health education in U.S. dental school curricula. *Pediatric Dentistry*, 23, 407–409.

National Institute of Dental and Craniofacial Research (NIDCR). (2018). Dental caries (tooth decay) in children (Age 2 to 11). Available at: https://www.nidcr.nih.gov/research/data-statistics/dental-caries/children

Newacheck, P.W., McManus, M., Fox, H.B. et al. (2000). Access to health care for children with special health care needs. *Pediatrics*, 105, 760–766.

Nowak, A.J. and Casamassimo, P.S. (2009). The Dental Home in Early Childhood Oral Health (Eds. J. Berg and R. Slayton), 154–169. Wiley-Blackwell, Ames, Iowa.

Nowak, A.J., Casamassimo, P.S., Scott J. et al. (2014). Do early dental visits reduce treatment and treatment costs for children? *Pediatric Dentistry*, 36, 489–493.

Savage, M.F., Lee, J., Kotch, J. et al. (2004). Early preventive dental visits: Effects on subsequent utilization and costs. *Pediatrics*, 114, 418–423.

Seow, W.K., Clifford, H., Battistutta, D. et al. (2009). Case-control study of early childhood caries in Australia. *Caries Research*, 43, 25–35.

Seale, N.S. and Casamassimo, P.S. (2003). Access to dental care for children in the United States: A survey of general practitioners. *Journal of the American Dental Association*, 134, 1630–1640.

Shearer, D.M., W.M. Thomson, J.M. Broadbent et al. (2011, July 7). Does maternal oral health predict child oral health-related quality of life in adulthood? *Health and Quality of Life Outcomes.* 9, 50.

Siegal, M. and Marx, M. (2002). Ohio dental care providers' treatment of young children. *Journal of the American Dental Association*, 136, 1583–1591.

Wolfe, J.D., Weber-Gasparoni, K., Kanellis, M.J. et al. (2006). Survey of Iowa general dentists regarding the age 1 dental visit. *Pediatric Dentistry*, 28, 325–331.

# 7

# Non-Pharmacologic Approaches in Behavior Management

*Ari Kupietzky and Gerald Z. Wright*

*Eyal Simchi and Debra A. Cohen (contributed to section on Magic in Pediatric Dentistry)*

## Introduction

The previous chapters of this volume have focused on the child patient and the family. The remaining chapters deal specifically with techniques or strategies of behavior management which are used in the practice of dentistry for children.

The present chapter is devoted to non-pharmacologic approaches that are commonly used by dentists today. Most of these methods have evolved from generations of dental practitioners. Consequently, some of the references may seem historic, but they are still valid today. The methods in this chapter are extremely important because they are the basis for behavior management. If a child's behavior cannot be managed, then it is difficult, if not impossible, to carry out any dental treatment. Behavior management is therefore one of the cornerstones of pediatric dentistry (Roberts et al. 2010).

Many of the psychological terms used in this chapter are derived from learning theory. Learning theory is an all-embracing term for a body of psychological research that describes how people modify their behavior patterns as a result of personal experience or the experiences of a role model. In the language of learning theory, learning is the establishment of a connection or association between a stimulus and a response. It is often referred to as *S-R theory*.

In the original edition of this book, this chapter contained a section on learning theory. However, little has changed in this area in the past 40 years, and that section is omitted in the present edition. Instead, to be more relevant and practical, the chapter will interweave dentistry and psychology.

The importance of behavior management and its relationship to psychology has resulted in considerable coverage of the topic in the literature. Some are anecdotal writings. Some are based on psychological principles. Some are controlled studies. Some survey professional practices. Together, they provide a wealth of information. To organize and present the chapter in a meaningful way, and include the pertinent non-pharmacologic literature, it is divided into seven parts: getting to know your patient, pre-appointment behavior modification, effective communication, non-pharmacologic clinical strategies, retraining, hypnosis, and the use of magic in behavior management.

## Getting to Know Your Patient

This section deals with getting to know new child patients. With all of these procedures, the primary goals are to (1) learn about patient and parent concerns and (2) gather information which enables a reasonably reliable estimate of the child's cooperative ability.

Knowing as much as possible about the new patient prepares the dentist to deal with new patient situations in a meaningful way. Information collection begins at the first contact. Assuming that a parent telephones the dental office for a child's appointment, the receptionist begins to create a record. The important demographic information is usually recorded onto the digital patient record or chart. However, an astute receptionist will determine who referred the child patient, why the child has been referred to the office, and whether or not this is the child's first dental visit. The responses to these questions can be very enlightening.

Once a new patient arrives in an office, dental teams conduct inquiries in two ways: (1) using a questionnaire completed by a parent or caregiver and (2) by directly interviewing the child and parent. In some offices, one method may predominate, while in others, a combination of techniques is used.

### Questionnaires

Questionnaires can be important tools for gaining information because probing questions can uncover critical facts about a family's child-rearing practices, a child's school experiences, or a child's developmental status. Rather than including lengthy lists of questions that can be found in other sources, those items that have been found to be most helpful in clinical situations are shown in Table 7-1. Questions such as these provide some clue or insight into a child's background.

The first question pertains to the intellectual capacity of the child. If "slow learner" is checked, then it is necessary to explore the matter further with the parent. The other four questions have direct clinical relevance (Wright and Stigers 2011). The question related to the child's medical experience is from the investigation of Martin et al. (1977), and it relates to the child's history with physicians. Much has been written about the relationship between past medical history and a child's cooperative behavior in the dental environment. It seems the influential feature is the *quality* of medical contacts. That is, if a child relates positively to a physician and is well-behaved, there is a relatively good chance for cooperation at the dentist.

**Table 7-1** These are clinically relevant questions that can be copied into the health history form.

| How do you consider your child is learning? | ☐ Advanced in learning |
| | ☐ Progressing normally |
| | ☐ A slow learner |
| How do you think your child has reacted to past medical experiences? | ☐ Very well ☐ Moderately well ☐ Moderately poorly ☐ Very poorly |
| How would you rate your own anxiety (nervousness, fear) at this moment? | ☐ High ☐ Moderately high ☐ Moderately low |
| Does your child think there is anything wrong with his/her teeth such as a chipped or decayed tooth, gumboil? | ☐ Yes ☐ No |
| How do you expect your child to react in the dental chair? | ☐ Very well ☐ Moderately well ☐ Moderately poorly ☐ Very poorly |

With respect to the response to the medical question, there is another factor worthy of consideration. To the very young child, the term "doctor" means a physician, and an appointment at the doctor's office, whether physician or dentist, is all the same. The child generalizes the past experience. When the basis for generalization involves a language label, it is called "mediated generalization." To the child approaching school age, language labels form the basis for many generalizations, hence the importance of word selection.

The next question asks parents to rate their own anxiety. Studies have documented a significant relationship between mothers' anxieties and their children's cooperative behaviors in the dental office. Many of these studies were conducted at a time when mothers primarily accompanied their children to the dental office. At the present time, many fathers or both parents now bring children for dental appointments. Since the paternal role has yet to be entirely established, the clinician can only speculate at this time that fathers' responses, like mothers' responses, will be similarly correlated. Some contemporary findings support the role of the father in transferring dental fear from parent to child (Lara et al. 2014). Evidence is mounting that the person closest to the child (mother, father, or guardian) is usually the one with whom the child is most likely to identify and the person most likely to transfer dental fear (Majstorovic et al. 2014).

The fourth question asks whether the child believes that there is anything wrong with their dentition. An affirmative response indicates that something has been identified by the child and, consequently, apprehension is likely to be greater (Wright and Alpern 1971). The final question emphasizes the role of parents as legitimate members of the pediatric dental treatment triangle in that they can predict their children's cooperativeness with a high degree of accuracy. This question was found to be highly significant in studies by Martin et al. (1977), Johnson and Baldwin (1968), and, in a more recent study, by Sharma et al. (2017).

After reviewing the questionnaire responses, it is possible that the clinician may be concerned that the child will be uncooperative. Forehand and Long (1999) have referred to some uncooperative children as strong-willed. They are often described as being independent, persistent, and confident. While qualities such as these are quite positive, most strong-willed children can also be stubborn, argumentative, and defiant, leading to non-compliance. In an effort to learn more about these children, the questionnaire in Table 7-2 was developed based on the work of Forehand and Long. This questionnaire can be provided as a supplementary set of questions after examining the initial responses.

**Table 7-2** Situations in which uncooperative children may display problems.

| Situations in which strong-willed children often display problems |
| --- |
| **Situations:** |
| • Going to bed |
| • Getting up in the morning |
| • Mealtime |
| • Bathtime |
| • When you are on the phone |
| • When you have visitors at home |
| • When you visit others |
| • Riding in the car |
| • Grocery shopping |
| • Eating in restaurants |
| **In the above situations:** |
| • Is there a problem? |
| • How often? |
| • What do you do? |
| • What does your child do? |

*Source:* Adapted from Forehand and Long (1999).

Many of the foregoing questions came from behavioral science research that is now more than 40 years old. Limited research of this type is conducted in pediatric dentistry these days, so there is little new material to call upon. Nonetheless, the clinician should give serious consideration to incorporating such questions into a behavioral or health questionnaire. The list of questions is potentially endless, but that would be impractical. These questions have proven to be worthwhile. Careful scrutiny of the responses can tip off the astute clinician to a potential behavior problem.

## The Functional Inquiry

In medical practice, a functional inquiry is a series of symptom-related questions posed in a personal interview that elicit new information and obtain further details about a presenting problem. In pediatric dentistry, it is used to learn about dental problems, explore the behavior of the new child patient, understand the parent's attitude, and assess the potential for patient and parent compliance. A questionnaire offers a starting point. It provides general information and clues, and it guides the functional inquiry. To begin, consider the first question related to learning efficiency. If a parent has indicated that the child is a "slow learner," more factual information is necessary. A leading question might be, "Is your child in a special class or special

school?" Knowing that the child attends a special education class or school can offer a clue about the functioning level of the patient. If the child is behind in school or in a special program, then slow learning is an important part of the patient's profile. The child may have to be guided through dental experiences more slowly, with clear, concrete, and repeated explanations and visual aids. Conversely, a parent may indicate that a child is "advanced in learning." The child may attend a school for the gifted. An important part of managing bright children often involves giving detailed explanations, catering to their curious natures.

For very young patients, two interesting questions are "What time does your child go to bed?" and "Is your child toilet trained?" If a child goes to bed at a regular hour, such as 7:00 p.m. or 8:00 p.m. and is toilet trained by the age of 24–36 months, the implication is that child-rearing practices in the home are structured. On the other hand, a three- to four-year-old child who does not go to bed as scheduled or who is not toilet trained arouses the experienced clinician's suspicion about the home environment. Is the parent overly permissive? Is the child's behavior generally non-compliant? More information can be obtained through the questionnaire in Table 7-2.

There is no limit to the depth of the functional inquiry, but if it is to be productive, questioning must be thoughtful. The information on the questionnaire helps to make this efficient. Other avenues to be explored include rewards and reinforcement in the home environment. These may provide some insight into the type of behavior management techniques that would be acceptable to the parent. Learning in advance that a parent does not believe in physical punishment can prevent a future confrontation if aversive techniques are employed.

## Recall Patients

The discussion so far has been directed toward the new child patient. However, consider the case of this recall patient.

### Case 7.1

Susan, 11 years of age, came to the dental office with her father for a recall appointment. After a few minutes, Susan was summoned into the treatment room by the dental hygienist and, without hesitation, the youngster followed the hygienist. At the conclusion of the appointment, the dentist reported to her father that Susan's teeth were excellent and that she was a good patient. Susan's father replied, "I'm surprised. She stayed up most of the night worrying about this visit." "Oh," said the dentist, "I didn't know!"

***Case 7.1, Discussion***: This case points out that functional inquiries are not limited only to new patients. When children have been patients for a long time, situations change and a periodic history review is in order. Based upon her father's remarks, the child was quite anxious. If the dentist had known about Susan's emotional state, she might have managed her differently or spoken to her about the problem. How was the dentist to know?

A recall history review is not as detailed as a new patient inquiry. It is generally conducted with a written questionnaire that provides an update on administrative information and health history. However, there are other questions to be asked, as shown in Table 7-3. The first question asks about oral hygiene. If a parent notes that the home care is adequate and, on examination, the child's oral hygiene appears neglected, something is wrong. It may be that the parent's expectations differ from those of the dentist. In this instance, consultation is necessary to re-establish hygiene goals. Or it may be that the child attends to the oral hygiene but requires further instruction.

The second question is a behavioral one. If a child really approaches the office with fear, after being a patient in the office for several years, the dental team must make every effort to reduce the fearfulness over future appointments. A good way to begin is by asking "Were you nervous coming here today?" Children are usually truthful and will confirm or deny the suspicion. "Tell me why." Sometimes, the answer is simple: "I don't like the taste of that (fluoride gel)." Many dentists keep several fluoride flavors in the office and can reply, "We have several kinds here. Today, you choose one. We will find one that you like." The point is—as in Susan's case—important information may be missed or problems undiscovered. The pediatric dentistry treatment triangle variables are constantly changing, and the astute clinician keeps patient information up-to-date.

**Table 7-3** Responses to these questions can be helpful when updating the health history. They can alert the dental team to a potential problem.

---

How do you think your child has maintained his/her oral hygiene?

☐ Good ☐ Fairly good

☐ Not very well ☐ Poor

Does your child have concerns about coming for this dental appointment?

☐ No anxiety ☐ A little anxiety

☐ Anxious

---

## Pre-appointment Behavior Modification

Psychologists have developed many techniques for modifying patients' behaviors by using the principles of learning theory. Behavior modification, sometimes called *behavior therapy*, may be defined as the attempt to alter human behavior and emotion in a beneficial manner and in accordance with the laws of learning theory (Eysenck 1964). These laws state that rewarded behavior tends to occur more often in presence, and unrewarded or punished behavior tends to be extinguished or disappear. Behavior therapists use various conditioning techniques to effect behavior changes. In this section, pre-appointment behavior modification refers to anything that is said or done to positively influence a child's behavior before entering the dental operatory. In recent years, some of the methods employed include pre-appointment e-mail messages, audiovisual modeling, and patient modeling.

Why use pre-appointment behavior modification? Dental anxiety represents a general state in which the individual is apprehensive and is prepared for something negative to happen (Klingberg 2008). It persists in our society. In a survey of 583 9–12-year-old children, only 64% reported liking their last dental visit, while 11% didn't like their visit and 12% were afraid to go to the dentist (AlSarheed 2011). With data like this, it is apparent that dental anxiety remains a common problem. It appears to develop mostly in childhood and adolescence (Locker et al. 2001). Consider the following scenario and what can be done to prevent it.

---

### Case 7.2

Sally, a four-year-old, had not visited any dentist previously. It was now time for her first dental visit, and her crying could be heard as she and her parent approached the office. As they came nearer, Sally's crying had a crescendo effect, alerting the entire dental office team to the presence of the new, anxious patient. Entering the office, the parent said, "Quiet! I told you that you would not get a shot today."

---

***Case 7.2, Discussion***: There are many possible reasons for Sally's behavior. Her apprehension may have originated in the family unit. It may be caused by (1) behavior contagion, (2) threatening the child with the dentist as a punishment, (3) well-intentioned but improper preparation, (4) discussing dentistry problems within earshot of the child, or (5) sibling attitudes. The question is, what can be done to ease the child's introduction to dentistry?

## Pre-appointment contact

Many parent and child concerns can be alleviated. Pre-appointment contact can provide directions for preparing the child patient for an initial dental visit and, therefore, increase the likelihood of a successful first appointment. It also can diminish a parent's apprehension. The sequence of events in many dental offices is (1) the parent phones to make an appointment, (2) the appointment is made for some time in the future, and (3) the parent is contacted as a reminder the day before the dental appointment. Years ago, Tuma (1954) suggested sending a pre-appointment letter explaining what is to be done at the first visit. He hinted that this could modify the behavior of some children. In addition to serving as an appointment reminder, it established good public relations. He explained that child management in dentistry was based on sound principles of psychology, and he suggested rewards for good behavior or as tokens of affection—not as bribery. He implied that rewards for negative behavior only reinforced it and established bad habits. Thus, Tuma explained basic pediatric dentistry management techniques in psychological terms to parents.

Following up on Tuma's suggestion, Wright et al. (1973) conducted a randomized, controlled study that demonstrated the beneficial effect of the pre-appointment letter. They mailed these letters to mothers of children three to six years of age who had appointments for first dental visits. The behavior of these children was compared with that of another group who had not received letters. As a result of the contact, children were better prepared by their mothers for their dental visits and were more cooperative. This was especially true for three- to four-year-old children.

A simple letter can do much to relax a mother and help her prepare her child for the dental visit. In the study of Wright et al. (1973), mothers acknowledged their appreciation of the dentist's thoughtfulness. They welcomed the concern for their children. The demonstrated effect is of great importance to the clinician. It reduced maternal anxiety and favorably affected the patient's dental office behavior. Box 7-1 is a sample letter.

Nowadays, parental anxiety still needs to be considered, and new technology offers different options for pre-appointment contact. Many pediatric dentists have websites, and a pre-appointment letter can be put on the site. Many patients provide their e-mail addresses to the

---

**Box 7-1   The pre-appointment letter**

Your Child's First Dental Visit

Dear (Name),

I am writing to you because I am pleased with the interest you are showing in your child's dental health by making an appointment for a dental examination. Children who have their first dental visit when they are very young are likely to have a favorable outlook toward dental care throughout life.

At the first appointment we will examine your child's teeth and gums, and take any necessary x-rays. For most children, this proves to be an interesting and even happy occasion. All of the people on our staff enjoy children and know how to work with them.

You parents play a most important role in getting children started with a good attitude toward dental care, and your cooperation is most appreciated. One of the useful things that you can do is to be completely natural and easy-going when you tell your child about the dental appointment. This approach will enable your child to view the appointment primarily as an opportunity to meet some new people interested in maintaining good oral health.

Good general health depends in large part upon the development of good habits, such as sensible eating and sleeping routines, exercise, recreation, and the like. Dental health also depends on good habits, including proper tooth brushing, regular dental visits and avoidance of excessive sweets. We will have a chance to discuss these points further during your child's appointment.

Best wishes, and I look forward to meeting you.

Sincerely,

(Name)

*Source:* Wright et al. (1973).

dental office, and letters can be sent directly to them. Other technology software programs enable practices to send pre-appointment reminders and instructions to ensure parents remember and are well-prepared for appointments with their dentist. These programs can leave the information in various languages.

The work of Bailey et al. (1973) has also supported pre-appointment contact. By comparing maternal and child anxiety levels, they observed that a youngster exposed to a parent's positive attitude toward a dental visit reacted more positively. Behavior was better for children prepared properly by parental discussion. It appears, then, that if the elements of surprise and lack of information are removed by parent preparation, children are more likely to cooperate.

Recommendations for many types of pre-appointment mailings have been made. Correspondence has run the gamut from the simplest welcoming letter to bombarding the mailbox with all manner of mailings. These have included pre-appointment questionnaires, dental society information flyers, commercial booklets, complicated statements of office policy, and even dental comic books. Numerous mailings can make too much of the first dental visit. Over-preparation can confuse the parents or provoke anxiety. Thus, the final effect of some of these approaches may be opposite the intention. The uncomplicated pre-appointment letter welcomes the patient; spells out the basic, first-appointment procedure avoiding dental terminology; and generally states the philosophy of good dental health care. This is sufficient.

## Audiovisual Modeling

This strategy can be applied before the appointment and in the clinic. The social learning theory proposed by Bandura (1977) has become perhaps the most influential theory of learning and development. While rooted in many of the basic concepts of learning theory, Bandura believed that direct reinforcement could not account for all types of learning. His theory added a social element, arguing that people could learn new information and behaviors by watching others. Factors involving both the model and the child patient can play a role in the success of observational learning (modeling). The child has to pay attention, remember what was observed, reproduce the behavior, and have good reason (motivation) to want to adopt the behavior. Without these factors, observational learning becomes ineffective.

Since the child must pay attention, anything that detracts attention will have a negative effect on observational learning. If modeling by audiovisual means in the dental office, a staff member should be present to direct the child's attention to the model.

The ability to store information is also an important part of the learning process. Retention can be affected by a number of factors, so it is helpful if the staff member points out key parts of the presentation. The staff may question the child to reinforce the learning. Later, it is vital for the child to recall information and act on the observational learning. Once the child has paid attention to the model and retained the information, he should be led to the operatory with the parent. The procedure in the operatory should follow the model as closely as possible so that the child can actually reproduce the behavior.

Finally, for observational learning to be successful, the child has to be motivated to imitate the behavior that was modeled. Reinforcement plays an important role in motivation. For example, if a child sees a departing patient praised for their good behavior and given a prize, that motivates the new patient.

During the 1970s, there were at least eight investigations into the merit of using video modeling. Most of these studies used different procedures. For example, some had an assistant working with a child, while others left the child alone. The video presentations differed. As a consequence, results from these studies were mixed. A most supportive study was that of Malemed et al. (1975). They divided children between 5 and 11 years of age into two groups. One group viewed an unrelated film, and the other watched a modeling film. Their results, which are summarized graphically in Figure 7-1, demonstrate the benefit of modeling.

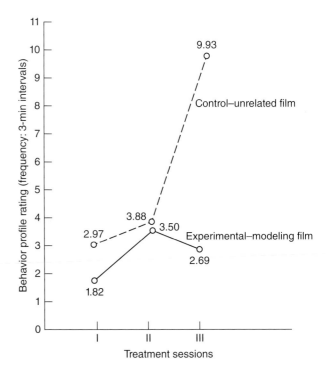

**Figure 7-1** The graph shows mean behavioral differences. The higher behavior profile rating indicates less cooperation. Note the wide difference in behavioral profile ratings between the two groups. *Source:* Adapted from Melamed et al. (1975).

Greenbaum and Melamed (1988) contended that research on modeling indicates that this technique offers dentists a means of reducing fear in child patients of all ages. They recommend it for children who have had no prior exposure to dental treatment. They further suggested that with video technology, the practitioner has the means to incorporate patient viewing of pre-recorded modeling tapes as part of the usual waiting period. Such a procedure creates a prepared patient, and the dentist will spend less time in behavioral management tasks.

However, an audiovisual presentation has two obvious disadvantages: (1) there is expense, as it requires special equipment and space, and (2) unless the presentation is developed by the dentist, it can be impersonal change to However, an audiovisual presentation has an obvious disadvantage, unless the presentation is developed by the dentist, it can be impersonal. For this reason some practitioners prefer live models.

## Live Models

There are three types of live models in a general practice: siblings, other children, and parents. Research by Ghose et al. (1969) evaluated the benefit of sibling models. The study concentrated on the effect of siblings on three- to five-year-old children without previous dental experiences. Sibling pairs entered the clinical area together, and the older child was examined first. Next, the younger child was examined while the older child observed. Similarly, dental prophylaxes and radiographs were performed for the children. At a second visit, a local anesthetic was administered and a restoration was completed. Sibling pairs serving as a control group were examined and treated separately. The study concluded that the presence of the older sibling had a favorable effect on the behavior of younger child at the first visit (Figure 7-2). The presence of

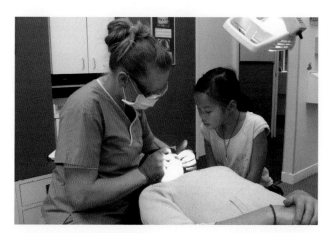

**Figure 7-2** The older sibling models for the younger one. Both children learn when an explanation is provided by the dentist.

a big brother or sister also seemed to maintain or even improve the younger child's behavior during subsequent visits. Recall appointments in particular provide an excellent modeling opportunity for children (similar to parent recall appointments).

Farhat-McHayleh N. et al. (2009) compared mothers versus fathers as live models for their children in the dental setting and concluded that mothers were more effective than fathers. However, in older children, the effect of live modeling with the father increased. They suggested that a child's relationship with his or her father evolves with age, such that use of the father for modeling is favored at older ages, when the father has become more integrated in the child's life.

Using non-related children as models is also beneficial. Investigating this strategy, White (1974) employed an eight-year-old model for four- to eight-year-old children. They divided subjects into three groups and compared the beneficial effects from either a modeling or a desensitization approach, with a control group having no preparation. They observed less avoidance behavior with both experimental groups and found that those children with the model seldom asked for a parent to be present. Similar results in the clinical setting were described by Adelson and Godfried (1970). They emphasized that the model was given a high status and rewarded for good behavior in the presence of the observing child.

A third type of modeling utilizes a plush doll, stuffed animal, or puppet. The counting of teeth and use of an intraoral mirror are demonstrated on the "model," who of course is a model patient! The need to keep the mouth open and not move is explained to the child (Figures 7-3 and 7-4).

The merits of modeling procedures using audiovisual, live models or toys are recognized generally by psychologists. The merits are as follows: (1) stimulation of new and positive behaviors, (2) facilitation of behavior in a more appropriate time, (3) decrease of fear-related, inappropriate behavior, and (4) extinction of fears. These procedures offer the clinician some interesting ways to modify children's behaviors before they are seated in the dental chair. Unfortunately, in the years since the 1970s, there has been little behavioral science research on this subject. Hopefully, this area will be visited again in the near future.

## Effective Communication

Although communication can occur in different ways, most non-pharmacological strategies are highly dependent upon verbal communication. There are many facets to good verbal communication.

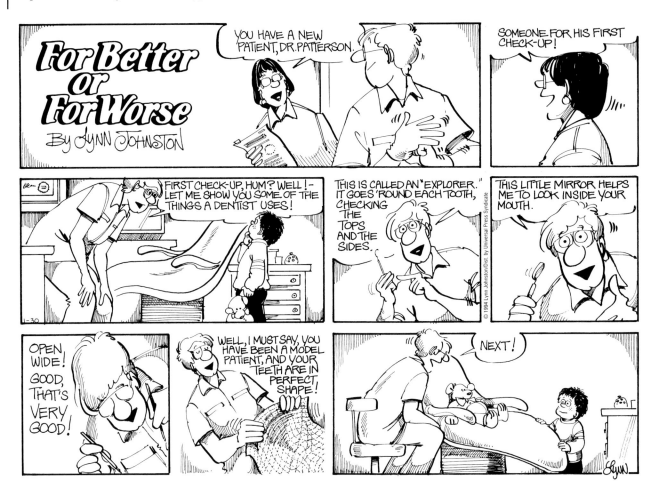

**Figure 7-3** For better or for worse. *Source:* © (1995). Lynn Johnston Prod. Used courtesy of the creator and Universal Uclick. All rights reserved.

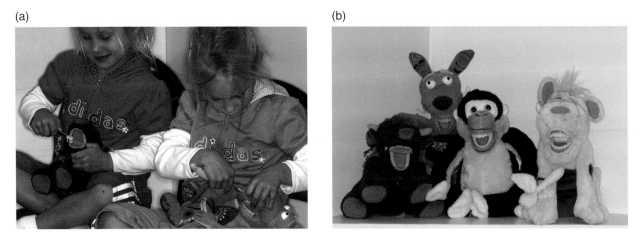

**Figure 7-4** Allowing children to "teach" their favorite stuffed toy or a puppet can make the setting more memorable and more personally relevant for pediatric patients (a). Demonstration dolls are available for this purpose (b). *Source:* Courtesy of Dr. Ari Kupietzky.

## Establishing Communication

It is widely agreed that the first objective in the successful management of a young child is to establish communication. By involving a child in conversation, a dentist not only learns about the patient, but also relaxes the youngster. There are many ways to initiate verbal communication.

---

### Case 7.3

Dr. A.: Do you go to school?

Jimmy: Yes.

Dr. A.: Do you like school?

Jimmy: Yes.

Dr. A.: Well, let's see your teeth.

---

*Case 7.3, Discussion*: Jimmy responded to Dr. A.'s questions but was not actively involved in communicating. Dr. A. was in a hurry "to get to the mouth." Welbury et al. (2005) refer to this type of communication as a *preliminary chat*. They suggest initiating conversation with non-dental topics. Many young children are very proud of their new clothing, and they like to be asked about it. Older children often wear team sweaters, school crests, or group uniforms (e.g., Brownies, Cubs, Beavers), and they like to be questioned about their activities. Whatever the ploy for initiating a conversation, questions should be phrased so that a child cannot offer a simple "yes" or "no" reply. Next, ask an open-ended question such as "What are those badges for?" This tends to establish communication. The process of drawing a child out and into communication with others around them is referred to as *externalization*. If other children in the family have attended the office previously, there should be information such as siblings' names, pets, schools, or hobbies to call upon. This makes the initial questioning much more personal.

Children are often shy and reluctant to talk when they are first exposed to a new experience and to new people. When they have gained confidence and are comfortable in the unfamiliar environment, they will usually speak more freely. During the first dental visit, they may speak more readily to a dental assistant. This enables the dentist to listen and make an evaluation of the comprehension and emotional maturity of the child.

## Message Clarity

A common theme throughout the literature in pediatric dentistry is that effective communication is essential to the development of a trusting relationship with the child patient. It is a critical requisite for the pediatric dentist in gaining cooperation (Nash 2006). To be effective, the message has to be clear. To ensure clarity, be certain that the child is addressed at the appropriate level of comprehension. This can be easily overlooked. Consider this example.

---

### Case 7.4

Dr. B. is preparing a tooth for a restoration. Access is difficult, and the child's head must be still. The child moves her legs, causing her entire body to shift slightly, and Dr. B. says in a calm voice, "Jenny, you must sit still. This will only take a minute. Do you understand?" Jenny nods her head affirmatively, but again changes her leg position, causing her head to move. So, Dr. B. repeats the instructions in a firm voice. Jenny does not move for about 20 seconds, during which time half of the preparation is complete. She then moves again. This time, Dr. B. repeats instructions in a firm, displeased tone. "Jenny, sit still. Don't move." The cavity preparation was completed without further difficulty, and the child is complimented for her behavior.

---

*Case 7.4, Discussion*: Two aspects of this case are noteworthy. First, the patient was four years old, and the message may not have been understood. Dentists sometimes fail to communicate effectively (Chambers 1976). That may have been the problem in this case. If we say to a child "Open your mouth" or "Climb up into the chair," the child likely will understand the instruction. But when the dentist said, "Sit perfectly still. This will only take a minute." Dr. B. probably thought that the instructions to Jenny were clear and that good communication was established. That assumption may be incorrect. It is possible that the child did not truly understand what was meant by "sit still," and it is probable that she had no concept of what constitutes a minute because she began moving after 20 seconds. Second, when the instructions were given on the first two occasions, they were delivered in a calm voice. On the third occasion, a firm displeased tone seemed to gain the result, and the child was still. This is known as voice control.

There are other ways to deal with this situation. Dr. B. could have been more explicit and explained the problem to the child. "Jenny, the tooth that I am going to fix is way back here," he could have said, pointing to the tooth. "I need you to help me. This is very important. If your head moves, even a little, then your tooth moves too. If you move your legs, it moves your head and your head moves the tooth. Try not to move your head, your arms or your legs while I am working on the tooth. I am going to count out loud and when I finish counting, we will be done."

By stressing the importance, the child's awareness of the situation may be enhanced. By asking her to help, she is a member of the team.

Clarity only occurs when the message is understood in the same way by the sender and the receiver. There has to be a "fit" between the intended and understood messages. For children with limited vocabularies, more detailed verbal communication is often needed, and sometimes it has to be supplemented in other ways. Consider a common experience in the home environment. A three-year-old approaches the hot stove. Her mother says, "Go away, its hot." If the child does not understand the meaning of "hot," she may try again. On the other hand, if the mother clarifies the verbal command and supplements it by picking up the child, placing the hand near the hot plate, and explaining that "hot hurts," the message becomes clearer. An analogy in pediatric dentistry is the three-year-old who lifts a hand to the mouth while the dentist is using an explorer. Saying "put your hands down" gives a command, but the child may not pay much attention to it. In effect, it scolds the child. Demonstrating the sharpness of the instrument and telling the child to keep his hands down in order not to get hurt is more effective communication.

To improve message clarity with young children, pediatric dentists and their office personnel have to use euphemisms sometimes. These are non-offensive word substitutes. For most pediatric dentists, euphemisms are like a second language. The following is a small glossary of word substitutes that can be used to explain procedures to children.

| Dental Terminology | Word Substitute |
|---|---|
| Air blast | Wind |
| Alginate material | Pudding |
| Burr | Brush |
| High speed suction | Vacuum cleaner |
| Explorer | Tooth feeler/counter |
| Rubber dam | Rubber raincoat |
| Stainless steel crown | Tooth hat |
| Study models | Statues of teeth |
| X-ray film | Tooth picture |
| X-ray equipment | Tooth camera |
| Pit-fissure sealant | Tooth (nail) polish |

## Multisensory Communication

The spoken word is not the only means of communication. Nonverbal communication, such as stroking the hand of a young child, communicates the feeling of warmth. A dental assistant's smile conveys approval and acceptance. Similarly, these feelings can be transmitted through the eyes. Since communication is a reciprocal process, children who avoid eye contact are telling the dentist that they are not yet ready to cooperate fully. Hence, effective communication occurs through a multisensory approach.

Whenever communication occurs there is a transmitter, a medium, and a receiver. The dentist or dental health team is the transmitter, the office environment provides an array of media, and the child is the receiver. It is widely recognized that certain characteristics are typical of all three for good behavior management (Moss 1972).

The transmitter may be one or all of the members of the dental health team during a child's dental visit. However, one fundamental rule must be recognized. Verbal transmission may come from only one direction at any given time. Children cannot divide their attention between two adults simultaneously or be distracted (Figure 7-5). If the dentist has entered into a discussion with the child, then the assistant must refrain from commenting. Typically, the error of two adults speaking to the child at one time occurs under stress. If a child resists an injection, the dentist may be trying to control her, and often a well-meaning dental assistant chimes in with words for the child. The communication then comes from two directions, and the message becomes unclear.

The attitude of the transmitter is often conveyed through the voice. Voice intonation, tone, and modulation can express empathy and firmness. Often, it is not what is said but rather how it is said that creates an impact. Young children do not always hear or understand words and sentences, and thus repetition is almost always required. The transmission must be constant. A kind pattern can give a young child a feeling of security and promote behavior management.

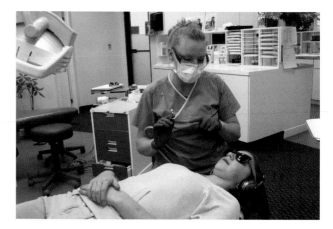

**Figure 7-5** The dentist explains the procedure to the child patient. Note that the child has earphones in place. Effective communication can only come from one source at a time. Avoid earphones and other distractors when communicating.

Since communication is multisensory, posture, movements, and position of the dental health team are extremely important nonverbal communication signs. Generally, movements should be slow and smooth, designed to convey a positive attitude, and instill a feeling of security in the patient. Rough or gentle application of instruments also conveys an operator's attitude. When speaking to a child, approximate the child's level in the dental chair rather than tower above him.

The medium in the dentist-patient communication system is complex. While it obviously involves the projections of the office personnel, it also encompasses the dental office environment. Office design, pictorial displays, and background music all are media of communication. They convey messages and should therefore be considered. When we deal with the school-age group, the latest music group may be preferable. Quiet background music, however, would be more likely to promote a settling effect for the very young child. The importance of the dental office environment is discussed in greater detail in Chapter 18.

The visual channel must always be considered in multisensory communication. Sometimes, those things which may seem natural to the dentist may be unsettling to a patient. A case in point is cited by one of the authors:

---

### Case 7.5

One week, two children were referred to Dr. C. as behavior problems. After chatting with both of these children, Dr. C. did not understand why they were considered behavior problems. Trying to comprehend the reasons for their misbehaviors, Dr. C. asked them what frightened them during their previous dental experiences. Both children (from the same office) referred to the "ugly" posters in the dentist's office. When checking with the dentist, Dr. C. learned that the office had new charts on the operatory walls, which were produced by a commercial company to demonstrate the progress of periodontal disease. It was a family practice, but the office medium catered to adults.

---

*Case 7.5, Discussion*: A friendly atmosphere sets the mood when a child patient and parent enter the reception room (see Chapter 16). The welcoming smile of the receptionist, the décor of the room, and a homey atmosphere can all play an important role in establishing communication. The dentist treating children in general practice has to seriously consider how children react to the office environment.

Children in their roles as receivers also have characteristics that need to be recognized by the dental team for effective behavior management. Their focus of attention is narrow and indivisible. The messages being communicated must be continuous to hold their attention. If the dentist has to leave the operatory, someone else must transmit; otherwise, the receiver builds up concerns. This oversight commonly occurs when the dentist leaves the operatory and the dental assistant focuses on chores (such as cleaning instruments) without communicating with the child. When left alone, fear can develop in these children.

Other senses of the receiver can be used to advantage. In school, children are encouraged to touch. Let them touch the rubber dam, prophylaxis cup, cotton roll, and other non-harmful objects. Children should also be allowed to use their sense of smell and be made to feel comfortable. The positioning of the patient in the chair is important, and so is the positioning of light. Light shining in a child's eyes can upset her potential as the receiver. Most children are good receivers. The message to be communicated is that the child can relax and need not be afraid.

Previous research has shown that the ability to assess non-verbal communication in children is closely related to the ability to observe. Using videos, Brockhouse and Pinkham (1980) studied the observational abilities of 141 participants and found that significant patterns evolved. One pattern was that pediatric dentists were more accurate in their abilities to predict behavior as compared to other experience levels. Dental assistants were significantly less accurate than others, including student groups. This finding was somewhat surprising, as many dental assistants had spent more chair time with children in the clinic than any other group. Another pattern revealed that freshman students had poorer predictive abilities than other dentist or student groups. They lacked clinical or didactic experience. The investigators concluded that experience appears to be the best means of developing the ability to assess non-verbal communication in children, but formal education is also important, perhaps because of the complexity of the communication process.

### Confident Communication

Speaking confidently to a child can lead to cooperative behavior. Many former dental students can relate to the following case.

---

### Case 7.6

Ms. N., a senior dental student, attempts a cavity preparation for seven-year-old Tyler. Each time she begins cutting the tooth, the child frets. The behavior baffles Ms. N., who is unsure of the depth of anesthesia, and she summons an instructor.

The instructor greets the child and runs the handpiece slightly above the tooth. When Tyler frets again, the instructor stops, explains the noise, solicits the child's cooperation, and completes the procedure without incident.

---

*Case 7.6, Discussion*: To support the point that confidence is an important ingredient in communicating with the pediatric patient, a study of communication patterns was reported by Wurster et al. (1979). They examined communication patterns among sixteen randomly selected senior dental students and their child dental patients. Interactions were videoed during regular treatment appointments. The data showed that the probability of a child's behavior following a practitioner's behavior was related. Patterns of behavior employed by clinicians will lead to a certain type of behavior on the part of the child. If the communication pattern is appropriate, the desired behavior likely will be achieved. In this same study, the operator's confidence level was considered, and the results showed that less confident operators were responsible for 95% of coercive behavior, 86% of permissive behavior, and 87% of uncooperative behavior.

### Voice Control

Gaining a child's attention is the ultimate aim of voice control. Without the attention of the child, there is no means of communication, and without communication, the child will never learn to be a good dental patient. The patient will miss the cues, lack motivation, respond improperly, and miss the rewards of approbation by his parents and the dental staff. As well as being a method of communication, voice control is thought of as a management technique; therefore, it will be described more fully with the non-invasive techniques in this chapter.

### Active Listening

Listening is important in the treatment of all children. Active listening (Wepman and Sonnenberg 1979) or reflective listening (Nash 2006) has the positive effect of reassuring children that what they are going through is a normal part of the human experience. Ways in which children's feelings can be acknowledged include (1) listening quietly, (2) acknowledging the feeling with a word such as "I see," or (3) giving the feeling a name: "Are you really nervous about coming to see me today?" In dealing with older children, listening to the spoken words may be more important than it is with younger children when attention to non-verbal behavior is often more crucial. An example of good listening follows:

---

**Case 7.7**

Dr. S. was preparing to place a rubber dam on nine-year-old Mary. She said, "I don't want that in my mouth."
  Dr. S. replied, "You don't like the tooth raincoat?"
  Mary said, "No. I can't breathe when you put that in my mouth."

---

*Case 7.7, Discussion*: By listening, Dr. S. learned what bothered Mary. The dentist then acknowledged her concern and told her that a big hole will be cut in the raincoat so that she will be comfortable. Dr. S. didn't add new information. She merely listened. The dentist communicated with the youngster, showed an interest in her feelings, and recognized the issue.

### Problem Ownership

If a dentist treats an adult and the marginal ridge fractures on the new restoration, the fault is mainly that of the dentist. Similarly, if a child reacts negatively, the problem belongs with the dentist. Often, the first attempt to resolve such a problem involves giving orders to the child, such as "You must stop crying!" and "You must sit still!" These messages tell children that they have no control over the situation, no matter what they are feeling. This is not an unusual scenario:

---

**Case 7.8**

Dr. F. is fitting a band on five-year-old Harry's maxillary second primary molar. The saliva-covered band is slippery. The child, who has a small mouth, whimpers and fidgets in the dental chair. Dr. F. is afraid of dropping the band in Harry's mouth and says, "You must sit still and stop crying!"

---

*Case 7.8, Discussion*: Most people (including children) do not like to be told what to do, and this approach often increases their resistance. These are "you" messages such as "You are too old to behave like that!" or "You know better than that!" These are negative messages that undermine the rapport that a child could develop with the dentist.

An alternative is to send "I" messages. Effectively communicated, "I" messages establish the focus of the problem where it belongs. They are not negative evaluations of the child, but they identify a problem and establish ownership of it. For example, "I can't fix your teeth if your mouth is not open wide" and "It will take me a lot longer to fix your teeth if you don't open your mouth wide!" The "I" statements are more than just a change in phrasing from "you" statements, which carry an evaluative statement about the child—the "I" statements disclose how the dentist is feeling. They describe a situation that needs to be altered if the dentist is to be able to solve the problem.

Wepman and Sonnenberg (1979) discussed a set of techniques that seemed well-suited to increase the flow of information between the dentist and child patient. Owning the problem and active listening are the first two steps. Both encourage genuine communication. The patient is stimulated to express feelings, and the dentist does the same—a necessary process in communication. If the child behaves in a way that causes an emotion in the dentist, the dentist can and should express, within reason, not only the quality of emotion, but also its strength. Consider the following straightforward approach with a whining child: "Please don't cry. It makes me feel bad. I don't like to feel bad. I like to feel good! You like to feel good too. So, why are you crying?" This brings the problem right to the surface, and the dentist is prepared to listen.

## Non-Pharmacologic Clinical Strategies

Management techniques should be part of an integrated patient approach (Forehand and Long 1999). They contend that it is not a matter of choosing among techniques but a matter of incorporating the best techniques into a plan. A flow chart or plan for behavior management is shown in Figure 7-6. The flow chart begins with learning about child development, children's behavior, and family environments. These are the topics of earlier chapters in this book. Gaining knowledge about families and children is important to behavior management. It is comparable to dentists learning dental material science before performing operative dentistry.

Getting to know your patient is the next stage of the continuum. This was discussed earlier in this chapter. Probing for information and responses from parenting can direct the future management technique.

A review of the literature reveals that there are many sources of uncooperative behavior. Most of these behaviors, however, can be attributed to manifestations of

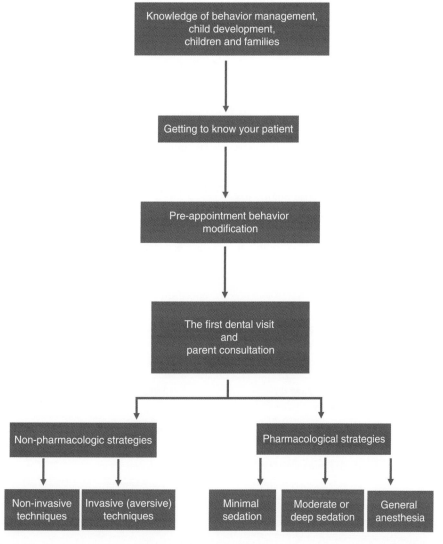

**Figure 7-6** This behavioral management plan or flow chart illustrates that the treatment of a child is complex. It involves knowledge of child development, family environments, and behavior management combined with a variety of potential strategies.

anxiety. Thus, pre-appointment behavior modification, discussed earlier in this chapter, is an important part of the behavioral plan.

The plan escalates in intensity as the dentist (or dental hygienist)–child patient interaction occurs during the first visit. Usually, this involves the oral examination, and taking any necessary radiographs and perhaps includes a dental prophylaxis and oral hygiene instructions. At this time, if the child requires treatment, the dentist has to determine what management technique will be recommended. Discussion with a parent ensues, and the examination findings, course of treatment, and management strategies are discussed.

The American Academy of Pediatric Dentistry (2019) lists numerous management techniques in their guidelines. Some of these are more acceptable to parents than others. In an attempt to explore their acceptability, a group of studies have been conducted over three decades. These studies showed videos of management techniques to parents while treatment was performed. Parents rated their acceptability of management techniques using a visual analogue scale. The findings are presented in Table 7-4.

Comparison of the four studies shown in Table 7-4 reveals that parental attitudes changed over the three decades with increasing approval of pharmacological management and decreasing approval of physical management. While tell-show-do (TSD) is rated consistently as the most acceptable technique, the rankings show that sedation and general anesthesia have increased in acceptability over the past three decades. Passive restraint (papoose board) has been in the lower range of acceptability in all studies. Hand-over-mouth (HOM) acceptability progressively decreased over the years, making it the least acceptable in the Eaton study (2005). Current AAPD guidelines have removed HOM as a behavior management technique, and it was not included in the most recent study.

Data from these studies helps the clinician to select management techniques, but this data has limitations. Parental attitudes change over time. Thus, it is important to keep abreast of new surveys and studies. The children's past dental experiences, which could have influenced the findings, were not explored. Techniques that are acceptable in public university/hospital setting may not be suitable for use in private practice. Social and cultural variables could influence parental attitudes. Nonetheless, before making any management recommendation, dentists should be aware of the acceptability of techniques regionally.

Non-pharmacologic techniques may be classified in different ways. There are those that are non-threatening, which Roberts et al. (2010) refer to as universally accepted techniques. Another group of techniques—those that are used with uncooperative children—limit the movements of child patients. They have been referred to as *controversial techniques*, and they are not universally accepted. Another way of classifying the two groups of techniques is to refer to them as "non-invasive" or "invasive."

The remainder of this chapter will describe non-pharmacological techniques that are used in pediatric dentistry. Those that are non-invasive include TSD, behavior shaping, reinforcement, operant conditioning, modeling, voice control, desensitization, visual imagery, humor, distraction and contingency distraction, and parent presence/absence. The invasive techniques are HOM and physical restraint.

## Tell-Show-Do (TSD)

This technique was formalized and developed into a training technique by Addelston (1959). Specifically, the TSD procedure is as follows. The dentist explains to the child what is going to be done in language that the child can understand. This is done as slowly and with as much repetition as necessary until the child is aware of what the procedure will be.

**Table 7-4** Behavior management techniques ranked by parental acceptance in four similar studies.

| Murphy et al. 1984 | Lawrence et al. 1991 | Eaton et al. 2005 | Patel et al. 2016 |
|---|---|---|---|
| 1) Tell-show-do | 1) Tell-show-do | 1) Tell-show-do | 1) Sedation |
| 2) Positive reinforcement | 2) N2O | 2) N2O | 2) General anesthesia |
| 3) Mouth prop | 3) Voice control | 3) General anesthesia | 3) Active restraint |
| 4) Voice control | 4) Active restraint | 4) Active restraint | 4) Passive restraint |
| 5) Active restraint | 5) Hand-over-mouth | 5) Sedation | |
| 6) Hand-over-mouth | 6) Passive restraint | 6) Voice control | |
| 7) Sedation | 7) Sedation | 7) Passive restraint | |
| 8) General anesthesia | 8) General anesthesia | 8) Hand-over-mouth | |
| 9) Passive restraint | | | |

*Source:* Adapted from Patel et al. (2016). Highlights showing change in ranking added.

Lengthy, complicated procedures are broken down into steps for easier communication. Armed with the knowledge of language development at various ages, the dentist and all office personnel can use the "tell" portion of the technique advantageously by phrasing instructions with words that are at the child's language level. Second, the dentist shows the child what will be used, how it works (e.g., high-speed drill), and how the procedure will be carried out, demonstrating on an inanimate object to be sure that understanding is complete. Third, without deviating from the explanation or demonstration, the practitioner proceeds directly to perform the previewed operation.

When demonstrating to the child, all team members must be fully aware of their transmitting roles. Sudden movements or unexpected noises should be avoided, as these changes can disrupt rapport. An X-ray machine, for example, is large and potentially frightening. After talking about it and demonstrating its use on yourself or an assistant (with the current off), introduce the machine by bringing the X-ray head slowly to the child. Noisy instruments should be demonstrated to children at a distance to avoid startling them. Gradually bring the instrument closer for demonstration and inspection. Operating a hand-piece without touching the child, or letting the patient feel the vibration without cutting the tooth, allows the child to extinguish any learned association between noise and vibration and pain and undesirable behavior. This is a desensitizing technique or, as it is sometimes called, "approach by successive approximations."

The TSD method can be used on a young child who lacks dental preconditioning at a first visit. It can be used for a child who is fearful because of a prior painful experience in another dental office, or for one who is apprehensive because of information received from parents or peers. The method permits the child to learn a stimulus-response association. It allows the dentist to complete procedures properly and provides a satisfying experience for both individuals. The child visiting the dentist for the first time learns by successive approximations. The dentist or dental team member leads the child step by step. The initiation of TSD may begin not in the treatment room but rather in the bridging or education room (see Chapter 18). In lieu of a bridging room, bridging chairs may be used in the treatment room (see Figure 18-12).

Nothing evokes fear or anxiety more than the unknown. In the TSD technique, attempts are made to remove the unknown. However, one simple piece of armamentarium is important to the technique and often overlooked: a mirror (Figure 7-7). If a mirror is not used, how can a child see a rubber dam on the tooth? Although the mirror may sometimes interfere with the working area, it is a small inconvenience when the end result is considered.

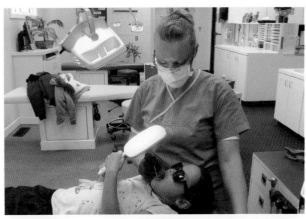
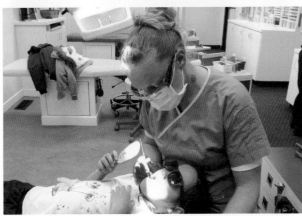

**Figure 7-7** The child patient holds a mirror during treatment. If the patient is unable to see what is happening, then tell-show-do is not really occurring. Note that the large mirror blocks the light (top). Use of a small mirror is recommended so that the light is not blocked (bottom).

The TSD technique works because it avoids the fear of the unknown, but another factor that really makes it effective is consistency in not hurting the child. Over the years, the TSD technique has not been used as a preface to local anesthesia. Some clinicians are of the opinion that showing the child the needle and syringe, more often than not, leads to a breakdown in dentist–patient rapport. Because the administration of local anesthesia plays a significant role in a daily pediatric dentistry practice, two conflicting views should be considered.

Some are of the opinion that the sight of the needle can be frightening and suggest that the child need not see the syringe if it is carried properly to the mouth (see Chapter 9). On the other hand, Addelston (1959) used TSD during local anesthesia administration with great success. He advocated letting the child observe the injection with a mirror. Since this is the only procedure omitted in the TSD technique, he has contended that its omission builds fears in children. He has suggested that many clinicians perhaps do not allow children to observe injection procedures due to their personal concerns and apprehensions. Thus, there are two opposing attitudes toward using TSD and the injection technique. Again, clinicians are charged with the responsibility of determining which method works best for them and their patients.

## Behavior Shaping

By definition, behavior shaping is that procedure which very slowly develops behavior by reinforcing successive approximations of the desired conduct until it comes to be. Thus, this technique is a simple method of teaching the child step-by-step what is expected in the dental operatory. At the same time, it is a procedure which obviates apprehension. Behavior shaping can be looked upon as a form of behavior modification because it is used to alter conduct according to established principles. The method is used with children who demonstrate sufficient cooperation to establish communication. With those who demonstrate negative behavior, a reasonable level of cooperation must first be established.

For both behavior shaping and TSD, an office's dental team members should follow an established office protocol for introducing new procedures or instruments to children. That protocol might be:

1. State the goal at the outset. "Today we are going to check your teeth."
2. Divide the explanations. "First, we have to count your teeth. We will count the upstairs teeth first. Now, we need to count your downstairs teeth. Next, we have to feel your teeth to make sure they are strong. Let me show you my tooth feeler. This is how I use it (placing explorer on fingernail)."
3. Use age-appropriate language. For young children, use euphemisms.

Behavior shaping is a learning model. It is well-recognized that programs which most closely follow the learning theory model will be the most efficient. Those which deviate from the model will be less efficient, with the loss of efficiency directly related to the amount of deviation from the model. Thus, by developing an understanding of psychological principles and by modifying familiar techniques to better fit the model, improved results in the practice of behavior management can be obtained.

Although TSD and behavior shaping are similar, there are some subtle differences. They are:

1. Behavior shaping requires positive behavior throughout the procedure. TSD makes no mention of the reactive behavior.
2. Behavior shaping allows retracing of steps. If you have completed telling the child about the procedure and the child looks away when showing an instrument, the clinician has to return to the telling stage. To get the child's attention, it may be necessary at this point to speak firmly to the child.
3. Behavior shaping includes positive reinforcement throughout. TSD makes no mention of reinforcement.

### Positive Reinforcement

An integral part of behavior shaping is reinforcement. In the process of establishing desirable patient behavior, it is essential to give appropriate feedback. Positive reinforcement is an effective technique to reward desired behaviors and strengthen their recurrence.

Reinforcement is an important concept of learning theory. If a response results in obtaining a goal, this response is rewarded or reinforced. A stimulus such as a painful tooth is the motivation for a child to visit the dental office. The visit is the response. The elimination of pain is the goal. A pleasant appointment resulting in oral comfort satisfactorily attains the goal, and therefore rewards or reinforces the child's behavior. Similarly, if a child is afraid of injections, and the dentist convinces the child that there will be no pain, delivering a painless injection reinforces the positive cooperative behavior that has been attained.

There are different types of reinforcements. Consider a child who is receiving instructions. During this conversation and any subsequent explanations or demonstrations, when there is a positive response to a suggestion, the child is reinforced by a smile and a variety of sounds of approbation (verbal social reinforcers)—"right" or "great" or "that's good." Most reinforcements of everyday life are social in nature. A smile reinforces behavior because the person who is smiling is more likely to supply subsequent reinforcements than one who is not (Ferster 1964). Even a small child has learned this fact. Consider this scenario in which the child is having a tooth restored.

---

**Case 7.9**

Dr. A.: "We are almost finished with the job. You are being a good helper!"

A LITTLE WHILE LATER:

Dr. A.: "Can you open your mouth a little wider? Oh, you are a good helper!"

A LITTLE WHILE LATER:

Dr. A.: "Jimmy, can you open your mouth a little more? What a good helper!"

*Case 7.9, Discussion*: Three times the dentist congratulated Jimmy by telling him that he is a good helper. There is nothing wrong saying that, but it is not an effective reinforcement. "You are a good helper!" is a general statement. For the compliment to be truly effective, the reinforcement has to be specific. When children are rewarded specifically, such as "you are really helping me by opening your mouth wide," the reinforcing statement unsurprisingly causes the child to open wider.

Clinical research in psychology has confirmed that immediate reinforcement is more effective than delayed rewards in enforcing behavior shaping and modification. Skinner (1953) demonstrated the existence of a temporal gradient. Accordingly, reactions followed by immediate reinforcement are better learned than those more removed from the reinforcement. The more immediately reinforcement follows the response, the stronger the association between the cue (good behavior) and the response (verbal approval). The desired behavior will be learned more readily.

The value of immediate social rewards cannot be overstated. Complimenting a child immediately on any aspect of their behavior which we would like to reinforce should be an integral part of the conversation in the dental office. Praise should concern the child's efforts and achievements, not his personality attributes. This is what immediate social rewards should sound like: "Wow, you're really helping today. I didn't know you could open this wide," or "You are the best patient we've had all day." These comments should come not only from the dentist but from all the members of the staff. The reinforcements, of course, are used only for acceptable behavior.

Any excuse can be used for a compliment. If a child is whimpering or fidgeting, try to ignore it. Consider it minor inappropriate misbehavior. When the patient stops for a while, that is the point to reward the correct response. "Now you're doing great. You are sitting really still. I hope you can keep it up." If the inappropriate response occurs and is not reinforced, the strength of the response progressively decreases, and it is eventually eliminated. Consider the following strategy for five-year-old Ralph, who is scheduled for a one-hour restorative appointment. After 15 minutes, this conversation occurred.

---

**Case 7.10**

RALPH:   "When can I go home?"
DENTIST:   "Soon you can go, Ralph."

FIVE MINUTES LATER:
RALPH:   "When can I go home?"
DENTIST:   "It will be a little longer."

---

*Case 7.10, Discussion*: Ralph continued to ask similar questions, slowing the progress of the appointment and irritating the dental team. Note that the dentist did not give Ralph an exact estimate of the time. Saying 45 minutes would likely mean little to him. However, this was not the problem. By replying to Ralph's questions, the dentist gave the child attention, thereby reinforcing the undesirable attention. A better approach might have been not to reply to the first question and in reply to the second question, simply say "This will take quite a bit longer. When you ask me that, I have to stop working, and it makes it slower. So, I can't stop to answer your questions anymore." When a response occurs but is not reinforced, it can eventually be eliminated. This is an example of response extinction. However, when inappropriate behavior—such as raising the hand, clutching at the operator's arm, or moving the head from the headrest—interferes with the treatment, social aversive conditioning by means of voice control will suppress the response. This is especially effective if an alternative response is available for obtaining positive reinforcement. One could say, "No, don't do that," in a loud, firm tone. Then, in a warm, friendly tone, say, "That is better, good." Children will work for rewards and try to be deserving of them.

Overt demonstrations of affection, such as holding and kissing the small, young child, are also a type of immediate social reinforcement useful in maintaining a behavior pattern. However, if the dentist is not customarily overtly affectionate or demonstrative, it may be awkward, and both the dentist and the child may be uncomfortable. It is better to be natural. Touching a young child or holding his hand is fine, or an affectionate arm around the shoulder may suffice. These demonstrations of affection, however, have their limitations. Children over 9 or 10 years of age have reached a more independent stage and can be very aloof. They may feel uncomfortable in this kind of close situation and may take offense when affection is demonstrated. Parents, too, may object to this type of reinforcement, especially with older children. Even children who have been with a practitioner from the age of two or three years may be offended by the "touching" display of affection that is used for reinforcement or rapport maintenance.

Finally, reinforcements or rewards also can be described as *intangible* or *tangible*. Verbal compliments are intangible rewards. Prizes or tokens are tangible and particularly effective with some patients. However, in some offices, they are given indiscriminately at the end of an appointment. Rather than serving as a reward, they are given automatically and have little meaning.

## Operant Conditioning

One method of behavior modification that has been effective in beneficially altering children's behaviors is operant conditioning. It involves verbal reinforcements followed by tangible rewards. Children are praised verbally, and approval of their behavior is acknowledged. Token systems are used as a tangible reinforcement. Tokens may be many different things: stars, points, poker chips, check marks on a chart, or stamps. When the child has accumulated a sufficient number of tokens, they can be exchanged for back-up reinforcements such as toys, badges, a favorite activity, or food (with a parent's approval). The initial token may not elicit much of a response from a child, but the back-up reinforcements acquire important reinforcing properties. Operant conditioning usually occurs over several appointments. Therefore, unless a child has a lengthy series of appointments, such as for orthodontic treatment, it likely is not the best strategy to use.

It is clear that positive reinforcement is an important part of TSD, behavior shaping, and operant conditioning. It is more than simply saying "You are a good helper." Rosenberg (1974) points out that "one should learn and then practice to praise effectively." A learned response does not always remain strong, so reinforcement should occur whenever possible. In S-R theory, consistency is critical when reinforcing behavior or ignoring behavior. Otherwise, learning does not happen.

## Modeling

A description of the modeling procedure in conjunction with pre-appointment behavior modification was provided earlier in this chapter. Modeling, however, can also serve as a management technique. It can be useful in many ways, but it is particularly helpful in dealing with the adolescent needle phobic patient. As practicing pediatric dentists are aware, these children present some of the most challenging management problems. Wright et al. (1983) described a plan, incorporating psychologically valid principles, to deal with these problem cases. Part of the plan involves the use of nitrous oxide analgesia. However, the nitrous oxide sedation alone is likely to fail in these difficult cases. Wright suggests augmenting the procedure with modeling and reinforcement. The modeling can be done with a videoed procedure or a live model. The advantage of live models is that they can answer questions and explain to the needle-phobic patient that they, too, used to be afraid of needles. It is advantageous if the model is of the same sex and close to a similar age. This procedure is an example of expanding behavior management technology that has been urged by behavioral scientists (Kuhn and Allen 1994).

## Voice Control

This technique was mentioned briefly in the communication section, as it is a communication technique. It is also a management technique. There can be a fine distinction between communication and patient management. The general goal of communication is to impart understanding, whereas that of patient management is to encourage cooperative behavior.

When using voice control for management, sudden and firm commands are used to get the child's attention or to stop her from whatever she is doing. Once the dentist has the child's attention, conversation should revert to a quieter tone. Monotonous, soothing conversation is supposed to function like relaxing music to set the mood.

Chambers (1976) theorized that voice control is most effective when used in conjunction with other communication, such as tapping a child on the chest or clapping the hands loudly. In these cases, it is what is heard that is important because the dentist is attempting to influence behavior directly and not through understanding. A sudden command to "stop crying and listen to me" may be a necessary preliminary measure, preparing the way for future communication. The same message shouted in a foreign language would probably be equally effective in stopping disruptive patient behavior that is preventing proper communication.

Greenbaum et al. (1990) conducted one of the few studies to determine the effectiveness of voice control. Study subjects—three to seven years old—were assessed as potential management problems and were assigned randomly to an experimental group (voice control group) or a control group (no voice control). Restorative treatment was performed, and treatment sessions were videoed. Whenever behavior interfered with treatment, the dentist used firm voice tones. In the group with no voice control, if the children misbehaved, the dentist asked them to desist in a normal, conversational voice. The investigators found that children in the voice control group showed less disruptive behavior immediately after the use of a firm voice than the no-voice counterparts. This is one of the few studies to provide empirical data on this technique.

The American Academy of Pediatric Dentistry (2020) succinctly states that voice control guidelines are (1) to gain the patient's attention and compliance, (2) to avert negative or avoidance behavior, and (3) to establish adult-child roles. The latter refers to establishing authority in dealing with the uncooperative and inattentive but communicative child patient. The dentist, however, must realize that this technique is not acceptable to all parents. In Eaton's study (2005), voice control was in the lower range of acceptability; therefore, if a parent is present, they should be informed about the technique beforehand.

## Desensitization

Another method of behavior modification used in dentistry is desensitization. Systematic desensitization, or reciprocal inhibition as described by Wolpe (1969), is the elimination of anxiety response habits by first presenting a stimulus that evokes a mild response. When it no longer causes anxiety, progressively stronger stimuli are introduced until direct control is exerted over the strongest anxiety-producing stimulus. Desensitization involves patient training in progressive deep muscle relaxation. The bond between the stimulus and the anxiety is gradually weakened in the presence of relaxation. Anxiety and deep muscle relaxation are incompatible and do not occur together.

Unless the clinician is very keen to use this technique, desensitization may be impractical for use in the dental office. It is time-consuming. The clinician also requires special training for it to be effective. It has been included, however, for the clinician to gain an understanding of the technique and to realize that some psychologists can help dental patients by using this approach.

## Contingency and Distraction Techniques

Distracting a child from a potentially difficult or painful procedure is a well-established technique in pediatric dentistry (Allen et al. 1990; Ingersoll et al. 1984; Venham et al. 1981). Many types of audio-visual distractors have been used in either a contingent or non-contingent format, some of which are described in Chapter 18. Verbal distraction also is used effectively during local administration.

Overall, contingency studies have yielded mixed results. Nonetheless, they offer some interesting approaches to behavior management and may be the way of the future. They are also practical as the clinician does not have to invest in special training or equipment. The two contingency techniques that have received attention from behavioral scientists are contingent distraction and contingent escape (Kuhn and Allen 1994). Both are designed for the child who is not cooperating in the dental clinic.

Ingersoll and colleagues (1984) suggested that children's disruptive behavior can be reduced by using a distractor such as an audio tape, which is dependent (contingent) on cooperative behavior, as opposed to providing unlimited access to audio tapes. In the experimental group, three- to nine-year-old children were informed that they could listen to taped material through headphones as long as they were cooperative. If the child became disruptive or uncooperative, the dentist immediately terminated the audio presentation and did not reinstate it until the child exhibited cooperative behavior. The children in the contingent group decreased levels of disruptive behavior, whereas the non-contingent control group had no behavioral change.

Contingent escape takes advantage of the powerful motivation to escape and uses it to promote more cooperative behaviors. It is based on "raising the hand" to stop treatment, which is a non-verbal management technique that allows a child some control over the dental routine. In contingent escape, brief periods of escape from ongoing dental treatment are provided contingent upon cooperative behavior. Instead of raising a hand, the child can receive praise and brief escape from dental treatment by simply being very still and quiet. Any disruptive behavior by the child delays escape until cooperation is regained.

Contingent escape is based on well-established learning principles and is designed to not only diminish undesirable behavior, but to increase desirable behaviors (Kuhn and Allen 1994). Delayed consequences not tied to specific behaviors fail to teach children how to behave. Contingent escape provides immediate feedback to teach children more adaptive coping behaviors.

## Visual Imagery

Another technique which may be considered by some as being hypnosis-based is visual imagery. It is a technique that can be helpful in certain situations. The visual imagery technique is believed to work with children because they have good ability to imagine and fantasize. The approach may be effective for the elimination of phobic behavior without the disadvantage of the time required to train the patient in relaxation techniques.

Ayer (1973) describes visual imagery where children were asked to imagine that they were playing with their dogs and that the dogs were yelping louder and louder. The children were asked to open their mouths and sit as still as possible. The clinician talked constantly throughout the visits, distracting the children with the imagined setting.

Ayer reported on the successful treatment of three 10-year-old patients who were identified as needle phobic. All of the children cooperated fully and displayed only moderate anxieties during the injections. Each child had three appointments during which extractions were completed. Subsequent contact with the parents of these children, as well as the children's own comments, indicated that the youngsters were no longer fearful of injections and they were now model patients.

Ayer emphasizes an important ingredient for effecting behavior change, indicating that a necessary variable in the successful application of behavioral change techniques—and one that is seldom noted—is time. Behavior change requires both time and patience on the part of the clinician. The time factor, he theorizes, may be one of the main reasons that the recommendations of behavioral scientists are so slow to be implemented in the dental office.

Ayer's writing seems to have gotten lost in the historical literature. Those interested in using visual imagery will find it well worth their time to read Ayer's original paper. The technique has application in the dental office— particularly with needle phobic adolescents. If the Ayer technique is combined with nitrous oxide analgesia, it can be extremely effective in solving needle phobic cases (Wright 1979).

### The Use of Humor

Planned humor assessment and interventions are relatively recent in medical and dental care. However, in recent years, there has been a general acceptance of the role of humor in building and maintaining relationships, emotional health, and cognitive function. This part of the chapter will discuss the development of humor and how it can be used to improve conventional management techniques. An understanding of this development will assist pediatric dentists in anticipating the various types of humor unique to each stage of childhood and develop individualized humor interventions (Dowling 2002).

A full discourse on humor theory is beyond the scope of this text, but certain basic definitions are essential. From a psychological perspective, humor involves cognitive, emotional, behavioral, psycho-physiological, and social aspects (Mora-Ripoll 2010). In general, the term "humor" can refer to a stimulus (such as a video), which is intended to produce a humorous reaction—a mental process (perception of amusing incongruities) or a response (laughter and exhilaration). Humor and laughter are typically associated with a pleasant emotional state. For the purpose of this discussion, humor is defined as a stimulus that helps people laugh and feel happy. Laughter is a psychophysiological response to humor that involves both characteristic physiological reactions and positive psychological shifts. Sense of humor is a psychological trait that varies considerably and allows a person to respond to different types of humorous stimuli.

Two main theories explain the functions of humor: the relief theory and the incongruity theory. According to the relief theory, which focuses on the relief of tension, people experience humor and engage in laughter because they sense that stress is reduced in doing so (Kuiper et al. 1993). The incongruity theory focuses on contradictions between expectations and experiences. It purports that people laugh at things that surprise them or that violate an accepted

**Table 7-5** Stages of Children's Humor as described by McGhee (2002).

| Stages | Example | Dental Application |
|---|---|---|
| Stage 0: First 6 months. Laughter without humor (the pre-humor stage). | Tickling | Smiling and making funny noises |
| Stage 1: 6 to 12–15 months. Laughter at the attachment figure. | Peek-a-boo | Counting fingers and continuing to tickle the arm |
| Stage 2: 12–15 months to 3–5 years. Treating an object as a different object. | Using a bowl as a hat | Finger as a toothbrush |
| Stage 3: 2–4 years. Misnaming objects or actions. | Calling a cat a dog | Misnaming colors; calling a mirror blue or a chair red |
| Stage 4: 3–5 years. Playing with word sounds (not meanings). | "Daddy, Faddy, paddy" | While using the nasal mask, tell patient to breathe through their *nose* and not through their *toes* |
| Stage 5: 6–7 years to 10–11 years. Riddles and jokes. | Why did the boy tiptoe past the medicine chest? He did not want to wake the sleeping pills. | Q. What flowers are the kissing flowers? A. Tulips. Q. Why did the tree come to the dentist? A. To get a root canal. |

*Source:* McGhee (2002). © 2002. Reproduced with permission of Paul McGhee.

pattern—with a difference close enough to the norm to be non-threatening, but different enough to be remarkable. The incongruity theory emphasizes cognition (Wilkins and Eisenbraun 2009).

Using a cognitive approach to humor, McGhee (2002) developed a theory which traces the development and appreciation of humor in children through defined stages and continues to form the framework for research in this area. It contains six stages, each based on the children's cognitive abilities that enable them to recognize and produce cognitive incongruities (Cunningham 2005). A summary and description of these stages is presented in Table 7-5. The first two stages of child development (Stages 0 and 1) are interesting, but Stage 2 (12–15 months to 3–5 years) and later stages have more clinical relevance. Understanding the developmental stages can be of practical benefit to dentists who are interested in using humor effectively in the dental setting.

## Treating an Object as a Different Object

At Stage 2, children begin producing "jokes" nonverbally by performing incongruous actions such as putting a bowl on their head as a hat or pretending to talk into their shoe. These jokes are any incongruous actions with an object. Another form of typical humor is using the correct object, but applying it to the wrong object; for example, the child may ask: "Brush ear?" In these cases, the same behavior may be just as funny if it is the mother, father, or another sibling who initiates it (McGhee 2002). This stage is significant since it presents the earliest self-created humor. It is the parallel of incongruous actions toward objects from the initial McGhee system of humor development.

In Stage 3, children from two–three or four years of age begin to misname objects or actions. Once the child's vocabulary increases, the young child can extend incongruity humor to misnaming objects or actions: calling a cat a dog, calling a shoe a sock. After age two years, parents are asked by their child to name people and things. Toddlers are very excited by the realization that everything has a name, and they begin playing with those names. Many parents first see this new form of humor in the "Show me your nose" game. Even if the parent has always played the game straight, the day always arrives when the child is prompted to "Show me your nose" and exhibits a mischievous grin and points to his or her ear. The child may or may not laugh, but there's no doubt that this is pretty funny to them.

At Stage 4, children aged three–five years start to play with word sounds, if not their meanings. As children's verbal competence grows, they are less dependent on objects as the source of humor. The preschooler may experiment with rhyming words, made-up silly words, and other humorous play that does not directly link to concrete objects within their reach. Many children are especially fond of the verbal expression of humor found in stories and poems like Dr. Seuss' *The Cat in the Hat*. Humor includes playing with word sounds—not meanings—altering funny words or creating nonsense words. Children become attuned to the way words sound and begin playing with the sounds themselves. This often takes the form of repeating variations of a familiar word over and over, such as: "daddy, faddy, paddy" or "silly, dilly, willy, squilly" (McGhee 2002). In the latter part of this stage, previously labeled "Conceptual incongruity," there is a dramatic change in the form of humor which emerges due to the fact that children begin to develop conceptual thought (Loizou 2006). Humor is centered on violations of conceptual representations: conceptual incongruity (McGhee 1979). An example of humor based on violation of conceptual representations is a cartoon of a picture of a bicycle with square wheels, or an elephant sitting on a tree limb (Dowling 2002).

In Stage 5, at ages 6 or 7 to 10 or 11 years, a general shift in children's humor toward riddles and jokes begins to occur. While the general silliness common in much of the humor in younger children's physical play is still present, there is a gradual reduction in the degree of reliance on physical action for humor. The defining feature of this stage is the acquisition of a new level of cognitive functioning, which permits simultaneous awareness of double meanings of the same word—the key to getting a riddle. (e.g., Q. What are the kissing flowers? A. Tulips.) The shift that occurs in children's humor at about age seven years is more striking than that shown at any other age (McGhee 2002). By seven, most children make the exciting discovery that the same word can have two different meanings, and that one can use this revelation to trick others. As they develop, they begin to understand that humor has a meaning—that jokes must resolve from something absurd into something that makes cognitive sense. The pediatric dentist should consider the child's stage of humor development and design and employ the proper use of age-appropriate humor.

Although the role of humor in health has been emphasized in recent years, little has been written about using humor as a communicative tool with children (D'Antonio 1989), particularly in dentistry (Nevo and Shapira 1986). Since humor reduces the emotional distance between people, it has the potential to improve communication not only with children, but with parents as well (Bennett 1996). Humor can assist the pediatric dentist on all levels by relieving anxiety and pain and establishing a direct path of communication with a new child patient.

### Case 7.11

Sue, aged four years, arrived for her visit accompanied by her older sister Ann, aged seven years, and their mother. Dr. Patty came into the waiting room to greet the patient. She asked Sue what her name was. Sue ignored her. She asked her how old she was; Sue refused to answer. Dr. Patty tried one more time; she complimented Sue on her shoes and asked where she got them. Sue ran behind her mother and refused to speak with the dentist. Sue's mom showed signs of apprehension.

*Case 7.11, Discussion*: Greeting patients is the first part of the dental encounter and experience. It often sets the tone for the entire visit. One of the most critical challenges facing the dentist during the patient's first visit is opening up a direct channel of communication with the child, effectively bypassing the parent and talking directly to the patient. Some of the well-known techniques to open

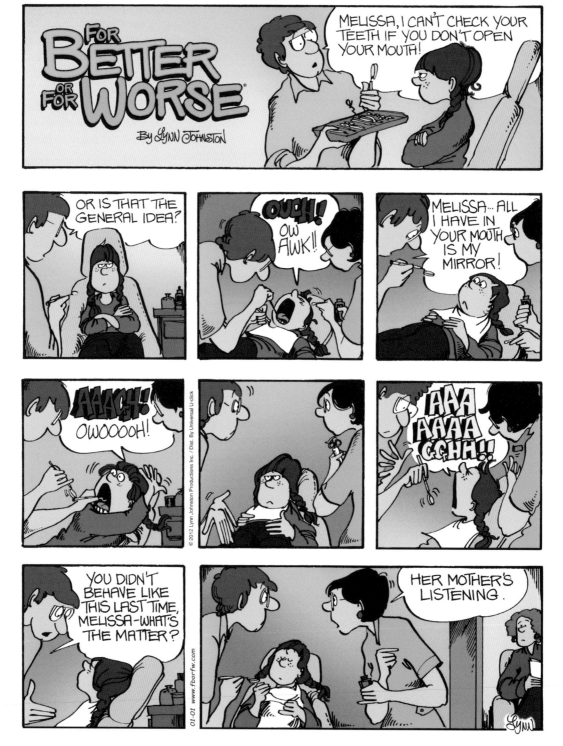

**Figure 7-8** For better or for worse. *Source:* © (1995). Lynn Johnston Prod. Used courtesy of the creator and Universal Uclick. All rights reserved.

communication are complimenting a child about their clothing or asking their name or age. Dr. Patty tried all of these greetings, but Sue refused to communicate with her.

In cases like this, humor can be used to achieve effective communication in several ways. Asking a child their age is often followed by a non-verbal response: they may identify their age by holding up the appropriate number of fingers. At this point, the dentist may employ humor to break the ice by miscalculating the age or exaggerating the age: "Oh, you are already eight!" the child being only four or five. If two siblings are present, and one is obviously taller and older as in the case, the conversation begins: "Who is older?" Addressing the obviously younger child, "Are you older than your sister? I thought you were older but just shorter." Or, as in our case, if the older child answers and identifies herself as Ann, the dentist turns to the younger sibling and asks if her name is also Ann. Most children will immediately answer with a smile and laugh—their name is not Ann! The parent will also laugh in the background, and the child will excitedly reply that her name is Sue. Once the child reacts and answers the dentist, the channel of communication opens. Conversation may continue, "I am happy to meet you. By the way, my name is Dr. Patty, what is your name? I forgot!" Most children now will reply with their name. Most importantly, the effect of humor is cumulative and children relax, expecting more fun to occur. Humor also affects parents, who in turn radiate a relaxed feeling to their children.

Humor can continue. Bennett (2003) suggested asking about the characters with whom children identify, and then making mistakes. "Winnie the Pooh is a horse, right?" While tapping teeth, the dentist can make silly noises. Tap the nose. Get mixed up while counting teeth. During the use of nitrous oxide, the child is instructed to breathe "through your nose and not through your toes, it's hard to breathe through shoes!" Ask the patient, "Do you like pickles, shmickels or tickles?"

Whatever you do, it is important for the dentist to adopt a style that is comfortable and natural. The cumulative humor effect creates a good feeling, and parents and children anticipate returning for their next visit with a smile.

## Parent Presence/Absence

Controversial views exist among pediatric dentists as to the benefit or detriment of parental presence during a child's dental treatment (Figure 7-8).

Since the issue of the "parent in or out" as a general policy was discussed in Chapter 4, it is included here as a legitimate non-pharmacologic technique for child management. Most dentists welcome a parent in the treatment room as long as the child behaves. Dentists are able to demonstrate their expertise to parents when their patients cooperate. The problem arises when the dentist must deal with an uncooperative, defiant child. One treatment modality for such children, which is becoming increasingly common, is treatment with pharmacological agents; however, this may be unnecessary and perhaps detrimental to the overall well-being of the child.

Parental presence/absence is not a rule, but it can be used as a tool for successful patient management (Ahuja S. et al. 2018; Kotsanos et al. 2009; Riba et al. 2018). Consider the following clinical situation and how separation may be used to manage the child.

---

### Case 7.12

Bobby, five years old, appeared for his first dental visit. In the functional inquiry, it was learned that Bobby had visited two other dentists unsuccessfully, leaving the offices without an exam. His mother had mentioned to the dental receptionist that other dentists were incapable of getting him to open his mouth for an examination.

Bobby was now seated on the dental chair. When Dr. Steve asked him to open his mouth, he refused. He also refused to answer questions such as "what's your name?" Ignoring the question, Bobby made a face toward his mother. At this point, his mother jumped into the conversation and answered on his behalf: "Bobby."

Dr. Steve: "How old are you?" Once again, Bobby ignored the dentist. Dr. Steve responded with a stern and disappointed look. Seeing the dentist's reaction, Mommy reassured Bobby: "The dentist won't hurt you! He won't do anything to you! I'll stay with you the whole time!" She moved her chair closer to Bobby and held his hand.

Dr. Steve told Bobby that he must open his mouth so he could count his teeth. Bobby ignored him. When asked again, Bobby screamed. Dr. Steve asked Bobby to stop screaming so that he could hear what he has to say. Bobby looked at his mother. Ignoring the dentist, the child placed his hands on his ears and screamed. Dr. Steve responded in a firm but controlled voice, displaying displeasure with Bobby's behavior: "Bobby, place your hands on your lap! You're expected to behave in here."

The dentist gently tried to move Bobby's hands away from his ears. Immediately, the child's mother interrupted and sternly told the dentist not to touch Bobby. She said with obvious annoyance: "Dr. Steve, Bobby will behave better if you don't get angry with him and use that tone of voice."

***Case 7.12, Discussion***: For a dentist to deliver safe and effective dentistry to a child, a proper pediatric dentistry treatment triangle needs to be established. In the scenario described, this was not the case. The child did not relate to the parent and dentist as a team. Rather, the parent acted as the child's surrogate or protector, shielding him from the dentist. The ultimate authority in the dental office, in the child's view, was the parent, not the dentist. Dr. Steve was up against both Bobby and his mother, reflecting a non-functional pediatric dentistry treatment triangle as denoted by Figure 6-2. A change needs to be made immediately to create a functioning pediatric dentistry treatment triangle. The dentist has to gain control of the situation. The child has to understand that the dentist and parent are on the same team. He needs to pay attention and communicate directly with the dentist. In this type of situation, parental exclusion or separation may be used to re-establish the proper child–dentist–parent relationship. Once a parent is asked to leave the operatory, and the child adjusts to the new relationship, the parent may return. If the child's behavior reverts to the former negativity, the parent again is asked to leave. This scenario may repeat itself one or two times. Everyone has to understand that the parent's role is passive and the dentist is in charge. When this has been established, the parent may remain in the room. Ideally, less aversive management techniques will be effective to recondition the child.

Parents should know what their role is in the operatory. In a case such as this one, it is critical, and the dentist has to educate parents about their role to ultimately achieve positive behavior modification. The parent should be instructed to ignore minor disruptive behavior and refrain from coaxing or pleading with the child to accept dental treatment. When the "game plan" is explained to parents in advance, even reluctant parents will cooperate. Specifically, regarding parental separation, they need to be told to accept the situation when asked to leave, despite the anticipated pleas of their child. They also should be instructed not to ask for a second chance, but rather to leave at the dentist's cue.

Consider the Case 7.12 scenario with some minor changes. Following the initial telephone contact, the receptionist should note that the child is a potential problem and alert the dentist that the child and parent will need special consultation time. The child's age and previous dental history are red flags regarding the type of patient management techniques that may need to be used to obtain proper patient cooperation. Before entering the treatment room, Dr. Steve should have invited Bobby's mother to the bridging room (see chapter 18), leaving Bobby in the play area. A discussion should include the methods of management, including the possibility that the dentist might ask the parent to leave the room for a limited amount of time. The parent must be convinced that she is a key player and is to be envisioned by the child as being in agreement with the dentist. A detailed explanation of TSD and voice control should also be given.

In the previous clinical scenario, none of the non-pharmacologic behavioral management techniques could be employed successfully, since communication had not been established between the patient and the dentist. Further, it is unacceptable to recommend a pharmacologic management procedure without any knowledge of the treatment needs. The use of separation will facilitate and allow the dentist to achieve communication, and then, optimally, patient cooperation.

## Restraint

Protective stabilization, or restraint, in the dental setting is the act of physically limiting the body movements of the child to facilitate dental procedures and decrease possible injuries to the child and/or dentist (Roberts et al. 2010). A wide range of techniques and devices have been used in the past to accomplish restraint, ranging from holding a child's head with one hand to a whole-body wrap, papoose board, or bed sheet (Frankel 1991). The use of protective stabilization, known in the past as *passive restraint*, is an invasive technique. Currently, it is seen by parents as one of the least favorable methods of patient management (see Table 7-4). When parents are presented with two options, one involving restraint and the other no restraint, many opt for the non-restraining mode of treatment delivery. Indeed, studies have shown that more parents consent to general anesthesia than conscious sedation with passive restraint (Allen et al. 1995; Eaton et al. 2005; Patel et al. 2016). However, restraint still has a function in patient management and is part of the armamentarium of some pediatric dentists.

Protective stabilization is mostly used in conjunction with conscious sedation, but it may be indicated in specific clinical situations without sedation. For example, an 18-month-old child appears in the office with a traumatic injury, an extruded upper incisor. A radiograph is needed. An attempt to take the film with the child held by the parent fails. A speedy and harmless solution is to place the child in a restraining device with the parent holding the film in place. The procedure could not be accomplished without any form of restraint.

The use of restraint becomes more complicated when considering an older child, perhaps three to five years of age, who requires comprehensive restorative treatment. The dilemma is, should uncooperative preschoolers be treated with protective stabilization coupled with conscious sedation, or is treatment under general anesthesia the better alternative? A survey by Adair et al. (2004) of behavior management teaching in advanced pediatric dentistry training programs showed that 98% of the programs taught that the use of protective stabilization using a restraining device such as a Pediwrap or papoose board was acceptable for use on the sedated child (see Figure 7-9). However, this is not a universal viewpoint. The exclusion of any form of restraining device has become mainstream practice and the standard of care in many parts of Europe. In the United Kingdom, restraining devices are not acceptable in dental practices under any circumstances (Manley 2004; Morris 2004).

Positive explanations may result in more parents' acceptance of this form of treatment. Kupietzky and Ram (2005)

showed that parents who received a positive explanation about restraint showed higher acceptance levels than parents who received a neutral or noncommittal explanation. Consider this clinical case.

### Case 7.13

A four-year-old child was unsuccessfully treated by a general dentist who used restraint without any pre-medication or local anesthesia. The parents turned to a qualified pediatric dentist for assistance. The child was successfully treated with restraint and conscious sedation. After treatment, the child was asked by his mother how he felt. He answered that he did not like the previous dentist. "Why?" asked the mother. The child answered, "Because he tied me up!" "But this dentist did the same," said the mother. The child answered, "No he didn't, he put a blanket on me and helped me not to move so he could fix my teeth and they won't hurt me anymore." The child was seen subsequently throughout and became an enthusiastic dental patient with good dental health.

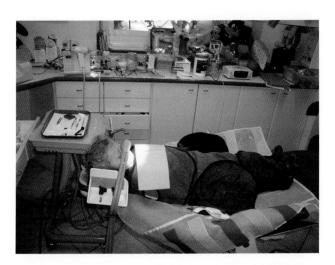

**Figure 7-9** The papoose board with head immobilizer restraint apparatus (Olympic Medical Group, Seattle, WA) used together with a pediatric Rainbow ® wrap (Specialized Care Co., Hampton, NH).

***Case 7.13, Discussion***: Before using medical stabilization, the parents should be given an honest explanation regarding its use. Depending on the age of the child, an explanation should also be given to the patient. "We will use a blanket. It will help you to not move and it will keep you warm." An excellent prop available for the discussion is a doll in a Pediwrap (see Figure 7-10).

The acceptance of restraints by parents, and more importantly their success in helping to instill a positive acceptance of dentistry by the child patient, depends, to a large

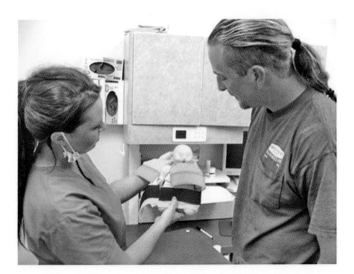

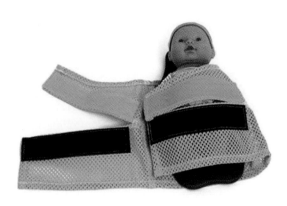

**Figure 7-10** The Protective Stabilization Model and Board Wrap is an adjunct for introducing children to the apparatus. *Source:* Courtesy of Specialized Care Co, Inc. Hampton, NH.

degree, on the frame of mind of the dentist using the techniques. If restraint is used punitively, or out or a sense of anger or frustration, then it is unacceptable (Roberts et al. 2010).

## Hand-over-Mouth (HOM)

When the first edition of this book was written, the HOM technique was generally accepted. However, over the past two decades, it has gradually become less acceptable to parents (Eaton 2005) and to the profession. In 2006, it was no longer endorsed by the American Academy of Pediatric Dentistry guidelines (AAPD 2006). The teaching of HOM in postgraduate programs has also declined dramatically, with only 28% of the programs teaching it as an acceptable technique (Adair et al. 2004). With these attitudes in mind, there was some reluctance on the part of the authors to include this technique with current management procedures. However, a guideline is a standard to help one determine the course of action. It is not legally binding, nor does it restrict practice, and HOM continues to be used today. Oueiss et al. (2010) surveyed members of the AAPD and found that 350 of 704 respondents (50%) believed that HOM was an acceptable technique. Similar findings were obtained by Newton et al. (2004), who surveyed pediatric dental specialists in the United Kingdom. While 60% were of the opinion that HOM should never be used, 40% favored its use under certain conditions. There were other reasons for including HOM in this chapter. In some countries, it is accepted. In others, the acceptability is not even discussed. There are countries where pediatric dentists are legally prevented from using pharmacological approaches, often do not have access to general anesthesia, and have limited alternatives for managing their child patients. For these reasons, it was decided to include HOM in this chapter. It will be discussed by describing the indications for the technique, the technique itself, its psychological rationale, and the controversy surrounding it.

### Indications

If a child's behavior is uncontrolled and the child thrashes about in the dental chair, a potentially dangerous situation develops. There is a possibility that the child may cause physical injury to their person. Controlling this type of behavior may require strong sedation techniques, or perhaps the use of general anesthesia. HOM offers an alternative method. It is an invasive, non-pharmacologic method that is most often used during a first office visit.

The major purpose of the technique is to control the child's behavior after other non-pharmacologic approaches have been tried. It is a method of last resort. It enables the dentist to establish communication so that the child can learn the appropriate responses and expectations. HOM is most effective for gaining the attention of three- to six-year-old children. Before applying the technique, a child should have been prejudged to be of normal intelligence and be able to follow instructions. HOM is not used for children under three years of age who lack the ability to comprehend their situation. The technique is also not used in conjunction with sedation. Children should have a complete awareness of their surroundings when their behavior is modified through this approach.

### Technique

When all avenues of communication have failed and the child's behavior remains uncontrolled, HOM is applied. Control must be considered from two points of view: (1) the explicit emphasis of the technique is control of the child's behavior, and (2) the implied meaning of control is a mastery of emotions by the dentist. The latter can be somewhat difficult following several minutes of kicking, screaming, or fighting. Nevertheless, the dentist's response must be a controlled one. There should be no display of anger or annoyance. The approach must be as unemotional as possible, almost matter-of-fact. Failure to control personal emotions may result in improper behavior management, and thus defeat the dentist's purpose. The critical details of the technique are as follows:

- Place the hand over the child's mouth to muffle the noise.
- Bring your face close to the child and talk directly into the ear.
- Quietly tell the child to stop screaming and listen, and then you will remove the hand.
- Explain that you "only want to talk and look at your teeth."
- Repeat the instructions after a few seconds, adding: "Are you ready for me to remove my hand?"
- Caution the child to be quiet when the hand is removed.

It is difficult to describe all the details of the technique in this section. The dentist's position in close proximity to the child's ear is of major importance (see Figure 7-11). Using a soft, monotone voice makes it necessary for the child patient to become quiet so that instructions are audible. The dentist's directions must be specific. Members of the dental health team also need to understand the technique prior to the situation. The dental assistant must know her role. In some cases, it will be to firmly grasp the child's leg and prevent kicking. In other cases, it will be to intercept the patient's hands so there is no interference with the dentist or scratching of the face. There are several variations of the standard technique. Those interested in learning more about them can obtain the information in earlier writings.

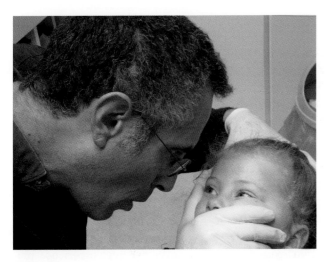

**Figure 7-11** Hand-over-mouth technique is shown with the dentist in close proximity to the child. Use of the technique is highly controversial, but many think it still has a place in pediatric dentistry.

### Rationale for the Technique

HOM or aversive conditioning has a psychological basis. From the behavior modification viewpoint, the laws of learning are applicable to the HOM technique. When a child's behavior is uncontrolled and a hand is placed over the child's mouth to quell the noise, there is a coupling of the active maladaptive act with an unpleasant experience. Immediate punishment of this type lessens the likelihood of the behavior recurring (Azrin et al. 1963). The requirements of an ideal punishing stimulus are it should have a precise physical specification, it should be constantly in contact with the patient, and the patient should not be able to escape or minimize it by unauthorized behavior. HOM meets these requirements.

The temporal relationship has importance in the HOM conditioning treatment. Once the HOM technique is instituted, the child must cooperate. When the hand is removed, if the child begins to fight or cry out, the hand is immediately replaced and the patient is again told that when the hand is removed, he must cooperate, be quiet, open his mouth, and listen to the dentist. The close association between the fighting and crying and the physical restraint is learned quickly and effectively if little or no time is allowed between the response and the stimulus. Chambers (1970), Craig (1972), and Levitas (1974) pointed out that once the desired behavior is elicited by the HOM technique, reward conditioning procedures are instituted immediately. The child is given social verbal reinforcement for behaving properly. Tangible rewards can be given at the end of the visit.

### The Controversy

Whenever the HOM technique has been discussed or demonstrated in the past, there have been strong opposing views regarding its application in the dental environment.

It is difficult to discuss the controversy without considering the historical writing.

In the 1960s and 1970s, HOM was a widely accepted management technique. Leaders in pediatric dentistry supported its use in textbooks at the time (Finn 1973; Kramer 1975; Levitas 1974; McDonald 1963; Wright 1975). There was also evidence of acceptance of the technique in dental practice. A 1972 survey of Diplomates of the American Board of Pediatric Dentistry revealed that 80% of the respondents used physical restraint or some form of HOM for selected cases. Comparable results were found in Craig's study (1972) in the state of Indiana. His survey found that 28 of 35 pediatric dental specialists used HOM in practice.

The technique became controversial, as not everyone was in agreement with the use of HOM. One reason was the apparent harshness of the technique. Some contended that the management method was unscientific and that it could possibly cause psychological trauma to the child patient (Davies and King 1961; MacGregor 1952). No scientific data has ever been presented to support this viewpoint. Indeed, the opinions of psychiatrists and psychologists were opposite, and they advocated for HOM usage (Chambers 1970; Goering 1972).

In the 1980s, the use of HOM became more controversial. Issues were being raised, however, concerning informed consent and the potential for committing battery (Bowers 1982). Shortly thereafter, Schuman (1987) reported that several dentists who had used HOM had been charged with child abuse or criminal assault following routine dental procedures. That same year, HOM was singled out by the Virginia Board of Dentistry as a procedure leading to the report of child abuse against dentists (Virginia 1987). In 1993, Casamassimo opined in an editorial that the technique was harsh, raising further legal concern. Thus, pediatric dentists became very concerned about its use in their practices.

Some clinicians employ only gentle psychological methods for managing children. The majority of pediatric dentists, however, use some restraint at one time or another. Emphatically pushing a hand downward which had been raised inadvertently or intentionally to interfere with treatment or lifting a resisting child and forcibly seating the patient in the dental chair to convey a "no-nonsense" attitude are forms of restraint. These techniques often precede the use of HOM. However, change has gradually occurred in the management of children in pediatric dentistry, and it can be attributed to many factors. Casamassimo et al. (2002) surveyed Diplomates of the American Board to determine some of the changes. Based on their findings, most diplomates were of the opinion that parenting styles had changed, and almost 60% felt that their children's behaviors were worse. The relevant changes in practice procedures were a decrease in the use of restraints and HOM and an increase in sedation usage.

Despite current attitudes, it is likely that some pediatric dentists will continue using restraint and HOM. Barton et al. (1993) contend that, used properly, the technique can be kind and effective. Acs et al. (1990) surveyed utilization of HOM and restraint in postdoctoral pediatric dental education programs and compared their findings to an earlier survey by Davis and Rombom (1979). Interestingly, the Acs survey found a discrepancy in professional standards. It seems that program directors with tenures in excess of 10 years are more likely to teach HOM and/or restraint than their younger colleagues. Hassan et al. (2010) conducted a survey to determine the alternatives for HOM after it was eliminated from the AAPD guidelines. The respondents selected voice control as the first alternative, and minimum to moderate sedation as the second. Since voice control likely had been tried in many vs before using HOM, the only real alternative to HOM is sedation or general anesthesia. Many clinicians consider HOM a much safer method of child management than the pharmacologic techniques.

## Retraining

Retraining, like behavior shaping, fits the learning theorist's model of a behavior modification program. Children's responses to the dental situation are altered in accordance with an established set of rules. Rewards are given for positive behavior to reinforce the learning. Negative behavior may be ignored or punished. Indeed, the theory for retraining and behavior shaping is somewhat similar. The clinical difference, however, is that retraining begins with a child possessing negative expectancies and undesirable responses. The behavior may be the result of a previous dental visit or the effect of improper parental or perhaps peer orientation. If the source of the problem can be determined, it is obviously helpful, for then the problem can be avoided through another technique, or de-emphasized, or a distraction method can be used. These ploys begin the retraining program which eventually leads to behavior shaping.

When encountering negative behavior, the objective is to build a new series of associations in the child's mind. In other words, the goal is to alter the stimulus and response. At the outset, state that "we do things differently here." When the child's expectancy of being hurt is not reinforced, then a new set of expectancies is learned. The child realizes that the dentist has followed through and did not hurt him—the dentist can be trusted. This same child develops a new perception of or relationship to the dental office, the dentist, and dentistry itself. In the language of learning theory, the child patient extinguished an unacceptable behavior learned previously and began to discriminate between this office—where anxieties and fears were not necessarily companions—and the last office, where they were present. The fearful child with anxieties modeled from parents and peers can go back to them and boast about learning something.

Assuming that communication is possible, when beginning the retraining process several ploys can be helpful in revising children's expectancies. Avoidance is possibly the most difficult route, for some procedures simply must be carried out. However, if an immature three-year-old patient who recently underwent a poor dental experience presented with a deep carious lesion, it might be possible to avoid extensive pulp therapy at this time by applying a temporizing medication and utilizing an indirect pulp therapy procedure. This allows the final treatment to be delayed until a more opportune visit. Once the child has been retrained and expectancies have been revised, future treatment becomes much easier. Thus, avoidance at the outset can be a worthwhile strategy.

If older children present with histories of negative behavior, they can be queried about their dislikes. Some children may express an intense dislike for materials such as certain prophylaxis pastes or topical fluorides. It is a simple matter to agree with the child and offer a choice of different brands. The fact that a choice is offered indicates to the child that you have recognized their dislike and that you are prepared to work around the problem. Offering a choice also gives the patient some control of the situation. The techniques of deemphasizing or substituting help to alter the child's expectancies.

A third ploy, distraction, can be used in many ways. Very young children become restless during long procedures. While working, the dentist can tell the child a story, taking the child's mind off the immediate situation. Additionally, through the proper use of the voice, a certain security can be imparted to the child. Counting the number of teeth aloud serves to hold the attention of the young patient during the initial visit. Counting the seconds helps to distract the child who dislikes a fluoride treatment. As mentioned earlier in this chapter, the use of humor in these situations helps to relieve children's anxieties. Thus, there are innumerable ways in which dentists can provide distraction during the course of treatment.

Choice of words during retraining is highly important, no matter how innocuous the procedure. It is not wise to ask, "Would you like me to clean your teeth?" By phrasing the question in this manner, the dentist offers an option that was not intended. A better alternative would have been, "Do you want the fruit- or pepper-mint-flavored toothpaste?" The choice is there, but the procedure is not open to question. Allowing choices gives the child a feeling of control of the situation. It is a key technique for independence training.

There are times when it is necessary to use a form of aversive conditioning in combination with retraining ploys. If an undesirable response occurs, whether inadvertent or intentional, the clinician may say, "No, not that way" or "Stop that" or something similar. The sound of the voice changes from a "matter-of-fact" soft tone to an almost harsh, loud or businesslike tone. Azrin et al. (1963) demonstrated that mild punishment suppresses a response if an alternative response is available for obtaining reinforcement. The child who is a behavior problem at the beginning of the visit will probably receive social aversive conditioning by way of voice control from the operator more often than the child who cooperates from the outset. The end-result, however, should be the same—an amenable child undergoing successful dental treatment.

Retraining children can be very satisfying to a clinician. At the outset, a child may exhibit negative behavior in response to inner anxiety or past experiences. Their fearfulness is generalized to all dentists. Eventually, the child learns that this dental office is different from a previous dental office. There is a different stimulus and response. This learned difference is called *discrimination*. In each case the child visits a dentist, but dentists' cues are different, eliciting different responses. After retraining children, many clinicians develop long-term, close relationships with them.

## Hypnosis in Dentistry for Children

The use of hypnosis as a non-pharmacological behavior management technique for children undergoing dental treatment is not common practice (Al-Harasi et al. 2010). It does not appear in the AAPD's recommendations for best practices chapter on Behavior Guidance for the Pediatric Dental Patient in the American Academy of Pediatric Dentistry's *The Reference Manual of Pediatric Dentistry* (AAPD 2020). This may be due to misconceptions as to how hypnosis actually works. Many health professionals may consider hypnosis as a form of treatment or therapy in its own right and therefore avoid its practice in dentistry (Vingoe 1987). Discussions of hypnosis in dentistry are often misguided and sometimes unclear due to this misunderstanding. Lampshire (1975) in the first edition of *Behavior Management in Dentistry for Children* asks what hypnosis is. He suggested the following as possible explanations: suggestibility, selling sentences, behavior

modification, good bedside manner, faith healing, or systemic desensitization. In fact, these are all terms for hypnosis. However, he went one step further and was bold enough to propose another name for it, *patient management*!

It is important to emphasize that the application of hypnosis in dentistry is different in both purpose and use than the general perception of hypnosis. Lampshire (1975) explains that it is "a means of changing behavior patterns through the dentist's actions or verbal instructions. It is a physical, mental or emotional state of increased awareness." Contrary to common belief, patients do not lose their self-control. Another misconception about hypnosis is that it involves loss of consciousness and weakening of the will. The opposite is true when employing hypnosis as a behavior guidance technique in dentistry. During hypnosis patients remain in complete control for the entire procedure and can decide whether they do or do not wish to cooperate.

Peltier (2014) in his monograph, *Hypnosis in Dentistry*, divides hypnosis into two forms: trance and non-trance.

### Trance Hypnosis

Peltier explains that trance is a state of consciousness that allows special focus. Natural trances occur in everyday life. People drift in and out of various trance states all the time. Children may enter a natural trance while playing a video game or watching a movie. During a class, students may stare out the window and find themselves disassociated from the classroom environment. The focus of attention during a natural trance is of interest to the dentist. People may naturally focus their attention in various ways, and here lies one of the keys of using hypnosis in dental practice. Peltier brings an example of the inconvenience experienced by the driver of a cracked windshield. It may hinder and annoy the driver at first, but before long, the driver will learn to focus on the highway and stare right through the crack. The driver will not even notice the crack. Dentists can assist patients in their focus by using a physical or verbal distraction and thus shift the patient's focus from their anxiety to a more pleasant experience and place. Many children enter the dental office already in a trance. It is up to the dentist to recognize this and utilize it to the benefit of the patient and dental treatment. *Fear* of pain in dentistry is a greater obstacle than the physical experience of pain itself (Kane and Olness 2004). If a patient focuses on the scary aspects of the "painful" dental visit, it will be extremely difficult to work with that patient. Instead, the dentist can assist patients to alter their focus and thus escape the "potential" conceived pain and experience. As Peltier writes: "A dentist can take advantage of naturally occurring states through "utilization" recruiting something in the natural environment to enhance trance." For example, "Whenever you hear the sound of the high speed let that be a signal for you go that special place in your mind imagining that you are on a spaceship drifting in outer space."

### Non-trance Hypnosis

Non-trance hypnosis can be defined as a way of communicating and influencing which bypasses critical-analytical thought (Peltier 2014). Non-verbal messages are more powerful than verbal ones. When you motion to someone with your hand, they walk through a doorway ahead of you. Teachers frequently use 'the lower your voice" technique during classroom lessons thus gaining their pupils attention. In children, non-verbal messages tend to bypass their limitations of critical thinking or belief system. Children are particularly aware of the dentist's non-verbal message or body language. The saying *a smile is worth a thousand words* is very relevant to the pediatric dentist communicating with children. Body language dominates. However, remember this works both ways, a child may be ushered into the treatment room with words of welcome, but the speed of the dentist's voice and rushed physical movements will send a different message. The child will react to the non-verbal message and ignore the verbal one.

Language and in particular the words we choose and how we use them may facilitate the dentist's attempt to achieve this non-trance hypnotic state. Pediatric dentists are trained to be cautious with the words they choose. For example, the word "pain" should be replaced by "discomfort." Peltier writes, "The word 'discomfort' is itself an interesting example of hypnotic communication. There is a principle in hypnosis which asserts that one cannot not think of something. You cannot not think of an elephant. In order to 'not' think of an elephant you have to (positively) think of it and then 'try' to not think of it (that elephant). It really cannot be done. 'Discomfort' contains the word 'comfort' inside of it for many people at some irrational, unspoken level. Discomfort (paradoxically) implies comfort."

Indirect suggestion can successfully be used with a patient without explicitly stating a request or even saying it at all. Adding the word "yet" to the end of a sentence changes its meaning and allows the dentist to bypass the child's analytical thought. For example, "you haven't felt the funny feeling from the funny nose (nitrous oxide) yet"; or "please don't laugh yet, I need to ask you some questions before you begin to laugh and feel funny." Adding the word yet implies they will have that experience. A casual remark like patients being told that they should be proud of themselves and that they will feel better after their treatment can have a significant impact.

Children process information from stories differently than the way they process a direct injunction. By saying "don't do that because you might get hurt" will be less successful than telling a story of a child who did that and got hurt. Pediatric dentists should have a reserve of stories in their hypnotic kit. These can include "today a patient told me that she didn't even feel the pinch (local anesthesia)"; "that little boy in the waiting room said he loved getting his teeth cleaned"; and "I once had a child who bit his lip after treatment while it was numb so be very careful!"

Peltier recommends that all members of the dental practice should model a positive, friendly, safe, comfortable, and can-do attitude. He explains that these attitudes are contagious and send subtle but important messages to the child. Visual and behavioral messages modeled by the dental team are very powerful. The physical behavior of the dentist and staff may create either an atmosphere of safety or danger, of caring or being impersonal. A gentle confident hand on the shoulder or a reassuring smile can send an overwhelmingly positive message that circumvents critical analytic reasoning or resistance.

---

### Case 7.14

Annie, a 4.5-year-old, was waiting for her appointment. Whilst playing in the waiting area, she bumped her head and ran to her mother crying. Her mother promptly kissed her head and gently comforted her daughter. Annie touched her hurting head, stopped crying, and continued playing. The dentist came into the waiting room, smiled and in a calm, warm voice told Annie how glad she was to see her and motioned with her hand for Annie to follow her into the treatment room. The dentist began the consultation by telling her "Today's visit is going to be so much fun! Do you remember what I told you last time about the sleepy juice and Choo Choo train? Soon you're going to relax, when you smell the funny air in the funny nose. But not yet. You might also feel a little discomfort, like when your foot falls asleep. But don't worry it will pass." During treatment, the dentist tells Annie and her mother about another little girl who actually likes coming to get her teeth fixed. At the end of treatment, Annie was told by the dentist "You'll probably feel quite nice when your teeth wake up. You should feel very proud of yourself!"

---

*Case 7.14*, **Discussion:** Many pediatric dentists use hypnosis routinely but are not be aware of it. Try and recognize in the case the elements of hypnosis as discussed above. Pediatric dentists may interact with their patients without use of "formal" hypnosis. They can learn to identify and utilize spontaneous hypnotic states in their patients, with simple techniques such as specific word and language choices, storytelling and suggestion. As a result of work with hypnosis, clinicians may become more aware of the importance of using an encouraging and positive approach with their patients, as well as effective use of body language.

## Summary

There is much to learn about trance and non-trance hypnosis in pediatric dentistry. The most basic question is whether hypnosis can successfully be used on young children. Hypnotic techniques have been found to be particularly effective when used with children between 8 and 12 years of age; however, children as young as 4 years old can be responsive to hypnosis (Olness and Kohen 1996). Most dentists employ hypnosis without even knowing that they are doing so.

## The Use of Magic in Pediatric Dentistry

*Eyal Simchi and Debra Cohen*

*"Magic is nothing but the art of distraction."*

The art of distraction is not just the crux of a magician's craft; it can also be quite beneficial in the field of dentistry as was discussed above. A common dictionary definition of distraction is as follows: "Anything that prevents someone from concentrating on something else." Thus, any action taken to take a child's mind off an impending dental procedure qualifies as a distraction. For example, magic tricks, balloon animals, overhead televisions, singing jingles, popping bubble wrap, and making jokes are all useful forms of distraction that can be used in the dental office to help reduce a child patient's anxiety. Several evidence-based studies prove the effectiveness of distraction. A review of literature (Jiang 2020) illustrates the validity of the technique within the practice, stating, "A positive distraction is a significant environmental feature that introduces positive feelings by diverting attention from stress or anxious thoughts."

Pediatric patients do not come to the dental office with a clean slate. They have often already been through a litany of experiences in the medical field: immunizations, general checkups, and examinations while sick are but a few of the experiences that have the capacity to taint how children view a visit to the dentist. Trying to change the typical perception of a dental office from a place of clinical fear to a place where a patient can feel comfortable certainly proves to be a daunting task. It is therefore crucial to set a positive tone at the beginning of the visit so as to alleviate any lingering anxieties the child has.

The use of magic is not new in the healthcare field. Wiseman and Watt (2018) wrote that "medics and therapists have described performing magic tricks to help reinforce positive health messages, reduce patient anxiety, establish rapport during psychotherapy, deliver life lessons, and gain the cooperation of patients." Magic can be used as a form of distraction, as distraction is a dominant component of magic (Kuhn et al. 2014). A good magician diverts the audience's attention from a point of action so that the action (or magic) can take place. In our role as pediatric dentists, we often use positive reinforcement, guiding conversations from the parts of the visit that may provoke fear to the more fun parts, and use jokes to distract our patients from the fearful clinical aspects. This is akin to the distraction a magician uses, and allows the trick or, in a dental visit, the procedure to take place.

Although there is not a lot of high-quality research using magic in medicine, there is some research focused on the effect of learning how to do magic. One such program, Magic Aid (https://www.magic-aid.org), is a not-for-profit organization that is "dedicated to providing kind and compassionate care to patients through the art of magic." The organization trains healthcare providers how to be "Magic Therapists" who then provide one-on-one magic therapy sessions to patients in their hospital rooms. A program like this can help dentists shape their bedside manner in such a way that the practice of dentistry becomes secondary in the patient's eyes. Armed with such tools, dentists are able to approach their work not only from a clinical and scientific standpoint, but also from a place of great emotional intelligence. One of the most important aspects of behavior management in a pediatric dental office is trust. When a dentist teaches a patient a magic trick, it builds trust between patient and provider because of a shared common secret. Although the research of magic in medicine is not extensive by any means, we are still able to see the amazing effects magic has on patients and how a simple magic trick can pique a terrified patient's interest enough to begin dialog. The cases below demonstrate how to use magic successfully in the dental setting.

### Case 7.15

Multiple dentists saw Kyle, a three-year-old boy. His mother had been told by the previous dentists that Kyle's treatment could only be completed under deep sedation or general anesthesia. Kyle's mother wanted to avoid any type of sedation due to her fear of risks that sedation entails. During his first visit, Kyle was crying uncontrollably, repeatedly saying that he did not want to go to the dentist.

*Case 7.15, Discussion:* In situations like this, the dentist's first goal is to change the negative association the patient has previously established with going to the dentist. To distract him from his fear, the following scenario between the dentist and child may occur.

Dr. S: "Ok we won't go anywhere now. I don't want to go to the dentist either. How about we see a cool trick instead?"

Kyle looks up apprehensively, still crying. Dr S. quickly makes a light appear in his hand and transfers it a few times between his hands (see Box 7-2). Kyle relaxes, slowly. After a minute, Dr S. asks if Kyle wants to try the trick. Kyle nods and reaches out his hand. Dr. S. magically makes the light appear from Kyle's hand. At this point, Kyle is already noticeably calmer. Dr S. and Kyle continue making the light appear and disappear, and Kyle's fear is replaced with excitement. With the previous dread removed, the dentist may now effectively communicate with Kyle. The appointment is able to progress as needed.

Additionally, it is recommended that the dentist initially meet the patient in the waiting room. A well-designed pediatric dental waiting room will have toys and games as well perhaps a large fish tank. Large TV screens and computer tablets are very useful. Keeping the waiting room fun and non-clinical makes it possible to distract patients from the fact that they are in a dental office. When the doctors meet a patient in the waiting room, they should get down to the patient's level, sitting on a small chair or stool. Kneeling down to the patient height helps make the dentist look less intimidating. Being at eye level with the patient can help make them less stressed than when they have to look up to the dentists.

An easy trick to do in the waiting room is "A Fun Magic Coloring Book" (https://www.amazon.com/Fun-Magic-Coloring-Book/dp/B001B1BS9Y) (Box 7-3). This trick

---

**Box 7-2  D'lite magic trick (http://dlite.com/): technique description (Figure 7-12).**

The trick consists of a set of fake thumb sleeves that contains a small LED light at the thumb tip. When the tip is compressed, the circuit is closed and the light goes on. When the tip is released, the light goes off. There are many ways to incorporate this trick into different dental routines. Simply plucking a light out of thin air will quickly catch a patient's eye. Having it appear and disappear from a patient's hand allows them to participate in the trick and also allows the dentist to get a little closer to patients that may be so fearful that they keep a distance from the dentist. During the trick, the patient allows the dentist to look into his mouth to find the missing light.

---

**Box 7-3  Fun Magic Coloring Book: technique description (Figure 7-13).**

The edges of the pages of the book are cut to different lengths to display different pages of the book depending on where the dentist's hand is when flipping through the book. When the dentist flips through the pages by the bottom of the book, only the blank pages are seen. The dentist then asks the patients to pretend to draw some pictures in the magic coloring book. When the dentist moves their hand to the top of the book and flips through the pages, black and white pictures "appear." The dentist then asks the patients to collect all the colors of the rainbow from the children's clothing and throw them into the book. Lastly, the dentist flips through the pages at the center of the book and the previous black and white pictures are now colored with vibrant colors.

---

**Box 7-4  Pencil behind the ear trick: technique description (Figure 7-14).**

For this trick, the child stands to the left of the dentist. The dentist's left hand is extended out, palm upwards. The pen is held in the dentist's right hand as shown in Figure 7-14. The dentist then tells the patient that the pen will disappear. The right hand holding the pen is then brought up to his right ear and swung back down to his left hand two times. While swinging the pen, the dentist is counting out loud as the pen hits his hand "one" then "two." On the third swing, the hand is brought up to the ear, but this time the pen is tucked behind the dentist's right ear, out of sight of the patient. As the hand is brought down for the pen to be press against the left hand, the patient can now see that the pen has disappeared!

---

requires very little "magic talent" and is very user friendly. It allows the dentist to meet the child eye to eye and open a channel of communication.

The "Pencil behind the ear trick" (Box 7-4) is also an easy trick to do anywhere in the office. This trick is fairly easy to learn and does not require the purchase of any props.

Although many of these techniques work very well to mitigate fears, especially in cases where patients have had previously traumatic dental experiences, they may not be enough. Patients who are very frightened will often avoid any communication with the dentist. In situations such as these, it is important for the dentist to do something that can distinguish himself/herself from the

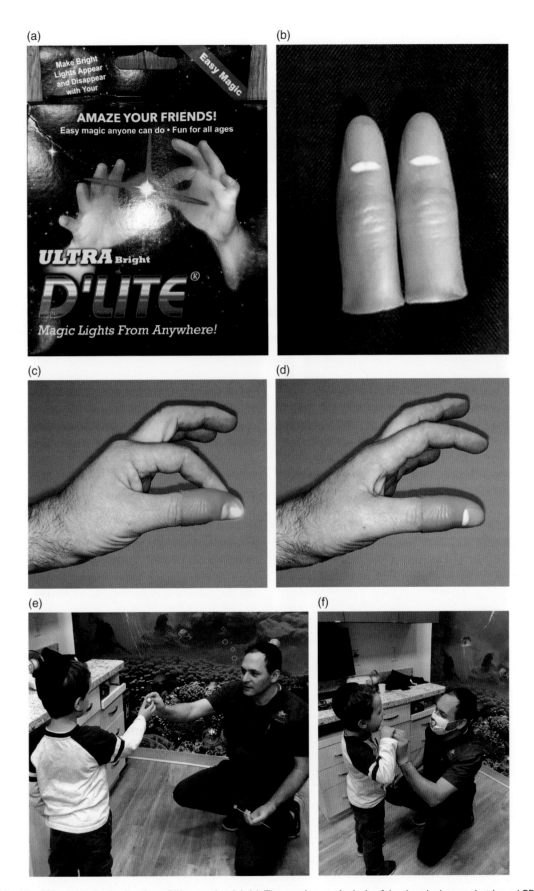

**Figure 7-12** The D'lite trick. Packaging from D'lite magic trick (a). The magic prop includes fake thumb sleeves that have LED lights at thumb tips (b). The D'lite thumb sleeve blends well with dentist's thumb. When the thumb tip is compressed the circuit is closed and the light goes on (c), when it is released the light goes off (d). The trick is performed at first, from a distance in front of the patient (e). Most patients will then allow the dentist to come closer and "look for the magic light in their mouth" (f). *Source:* Riverfront Pediatric.

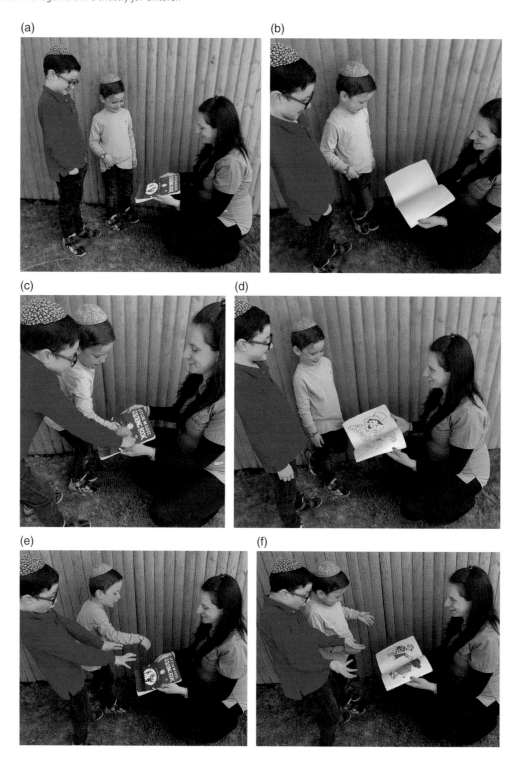

**Figure 7-13** Fun magic coloring book trick. The dentist kneels down to patient's eye level showing them the magic coloring book (a). Next, the dentist flips through the pages of the magic coloring book showing the children that the coloring book is blank (b). The patients are then asked to pretend to draw pictures on the cover of the magic coloring book (c). Black and white pictures "appear" throughout the coloring book to the patients' surprise (d). The patients are then asked to throw all the colors of the rainbow from their clothing into the book (e). The previously black and white pictures are now full of vibrant colors as the children wonder how the magic happened (f). *Source:* Riverfront Pediatric.

(a)

(b)

(c)

(d)

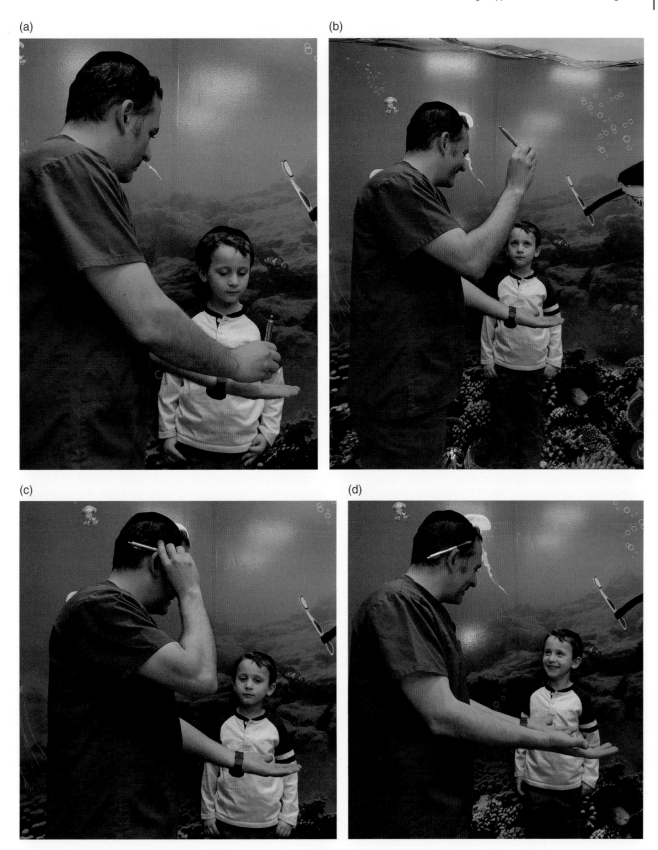

**Figure 7.14** The pencil behind the ear trick. While patient is standing to the left of the dentist, the dentist holds the pen in his right hand and shows the child his "magic pen" while touching the tip of the pen to his left palm (a). He then swings the pen back to his ear twice and as he hits his left palm he counts "one" and "two" (b). On the third swing, the dentist carefully tucks the pen behind his right ear out of the view of the patient (c). The dentist now brings his empty right hand down to his left palm and claps his hands, as a form of distraction, and the pen has magically disappeared amazing the patient (d).

previous dentists the patient has seen. Magic works beautifully! A disappearing pen, magic coloring book or light suddenly appearing out of nowhere is hard to ignore. As the patient's interest is slowly piqued, throwing in some silly jokes and questions can help lighten the mood even more.

---

### Case 7.16

Rayna is a nervous 10-year-old girl who has an infected molar. Her friends told her that the tooth is going to get yanked out. She's already crying when she comes into the operatory but she is okay with discussing her fears.

---

*Case 7.16, Discussion:* The dentist's first goal is to open a window of communication to allow further conversation and allaying of Rayna's fears. The dentist begins by showing Rayna a coin and asks her to guess which hand it will end up in. She guesses wrong every time because the coin has now disappeared. With a quick hand and distractions, he manages to put the coin on his knee under his hands. He then reaches over and plucks it out of her ear. Now Rayna is smiling but she is still nervous. "Do you want to see some more tricks?", the dentist asks. Rayna is now calmer and watching the tricks attentively. Now that she is focused on the magic, the doctor asks, "Should we have the tooth come out magically too?" Using magic to alleviate instilled fears makes her much more open to his suggestions. After magically making the tooth go to sleep, by gently shaking her cheek as he slowly injects the anesthetic, the dentist extracts the infected tooth. As the numbness sets in and increases, Rayna starts to get a little nervous as she realizes that the extraction must be happening soon. "Should we do it normally?" the dentist asks, "Or magically?" "Magically," Rayna quickly answers. The dentist gently tugs on Rayna's ear, and with a loud pop, the previously extracted tooth appears in his hand. "Wow! I'm so proud of myself!" Rayna exclaims. The fear of the appointment has magically morphed into relief (and even excitement) as Rayna tries to figure out the magic.

In conclusion, there are many forms of distraction that can be used to help mitigate a patient's fear and anxiety when going to the dentist. Magic may be used as a fun and exciting way to distract pediatric patients, pique their interest, and start conversation between a fearful patient and dentist.

## Summary

This chapter has dealt with a broad spectrum of non-pharmacologic methods of behavior management. It has described techniques which have evolved in dentistry and has related them to psychology, a science which deals with human behavior. Thus, it has tried to provide an interdisciplinary approach.

There are laws which govern human behavior and concepts that govern learning. Programs most closely following a model will be the most efficient in terms of learning. Those which deviate from the models will be less efficient, with the loss of efficiency directly related to the amount of deviation from the model. With the understanding of such learning principles, pediatric dentistry management becomes more effective. An understanding of these laws cannot help having a positive influence on the daily practice of dentistry and on the lines of communication within the pediatric dentistry treatment triangle. Behavior management is studied by pediatric dentists in some depth. Many general dentists and other dental personnel often receive a cursory introduction to the subject. Hopefully, the writing of this book will help increase general knowledge.

The chapter was divided into seven parts: getting to know your patient, pre-appointment behavior modification, effective communication, non-pharmacologic clinical strategies, retraining, hypnosis, and the use of magic. In some instances, methods such as voice control and modeling overlap were touched upon in more than one part. This was pointed out in the text. In many instances, the referencing was historical. That is the way it is nowadays. Wilson and Cody (2005) searched the literature on behavior management, excluding sedation articles. They found that only 168 articles were published in *Pediatric Dentistry* and the *Journal of Dentistry for Children* over a 30-year period. The number of articles involving clinical studies was less than a third of the total number of articles; 38% were opinion papers and 32% were surveys or descriptions of behavior management in the dental setting. Wilson and Cody concluded that the evidence-based data to support the effectiveness of behavior management techniques in pediatric dentistry is limited and needs further development. The authors of this chapter are in agreement with the conclusion. Averaging less than two clinical studies on behavior management per year over a 30-year period is regrettable. If the management of children in the dental environment is one of the keys to the specialty of pediatric dentistry, then more research is needed.

# References

Acs, G., Burke, M.J., and Musson, C.W. (1990). An updated survey on the utilization of hand over mouth and restraint in postdoctoral pediatric dental education. *Pediatric Dentistry*, 12, 298–302.

Adair, S.M., Rockman, R.A., Schafer, T.E. et al. (2004). Survey of behavior management teaching in pediatric dentistry advanced education programs. *Pediatric Dentistry*, 26, 151–158.

Addelston, H.K. (1959). Child patient training. *Fortnightly Review of the Chicago Dental Society*, 38, 7–9, 27–29.

Adelson, H.K. and Godfried, M. (1970). Modeling and the fearful patient. *Journal of Dentistry for Children*, 37, 476–480.

Ahuja, S., Gandhi, K., Malhotra, R. et al. (2018). Assessment of the effect of parental presence in dental operatory on the behavior of children aged 4–7 years. *Journal of Indian Society of Pedodontics and Preventive Dentistry*, 36, 167–172.

Al-Harasi, S., Ashley, P.F., Moles, D.R. et al. (2010). Hypnosis for children undergoing dental treatment. *Cochrane Database of Systematic Reviews*, Issue 8. Art. No.: CD007154. DOI: 10.1002/14651858.CD007154.pub2

Allen, K.D., Loiben, T., Allen, S.J. et al. (1990). Dentist-implemented contingent escape for management of disruptive child behavior. *Journal of Applied Behavior Analysis*, 25, 629–636.

Allen, K.D., Hodges, E.D., and Knudsen, S.K. (1995). Comparing four methods to inform parents about child behavior management: How to inform for consent. *Pediatric Dentistry*, 17, 180–186.

AlSarheed, M. (2011). Children's perception of their dentists. *European Journal of Dentistry*, 5, 186–190.

American Academy of Pediatric Dentistry (2012). Behavior guidance for the pediatric dental patient. *Reference Manual, Pediatric Dentistry*, 34, 170–182.

American Academy of Pediatric Dentistry (AAPD) (2019). *Behavior guidance for the pediatric dental patient. The Reference Manual of Pediatric Dentistry*. Chicago, Ill.: American Academy of Pediatric Dentistry; pp. 292–310.

Association of Pedodontic Diplomates (1972). Techniques for behavior management–a survey. *Journal of Dentistry for Children*, 39, 368–372.

Ayer, W.H. (1973). Use of visual imagery on needle phobic children. *Journal of Dentistry for Children*, 40, 125–127.

Azrin, N.H., Holz, W.C., and Hake, D.F. (1963). Fixed-ratio punishment. *Journal of the Experimental Analysis of Behavior*, 6, 141–148.

Bailey, P.M., Talbot, A., and Taylor, P.P. (1973). A comparison of maternal anxiety levels with anxiety levels manifested in the child dental patient. *Journal of Dentistry for Children*, 40, 25–32.

Bandura, A. (1977). Social Learning Theory. General Learning Press, New York, USA.

Barton, D.H., Hatcher, C., Porter, R. et al. (1993). Dental attitudes and memories: A study of the effects of hand over mouth/restraint. *Pediatric Dentistry*, 15, 13–19.

Bennett, H.J. (1996). Using humor in the office setting: A pediatric perspective. *Journal of Family Practice*, 42, 462–464.

Bennett, H.J. (2003). Humor in medicine. *Southern Medical Journal*, 96, 1257–1261.

Bowers, L.T. (1982). The legality of using hand-over-mouth exercise for management of child behavior. *Journal of Dentistry for Children*, 49, 257–265.

Brockhouse, R.T. and Pinkham, J.R. (1980). Assessment of nonverbal communication in children. *Journal of Dentistry for Children*, 47, 42–47.

Casamassimo, P. (1993). Editorial: Maybe the last editorial on hand-over-mouth technique? *Pediatric Dentistry*, 15, 233–234.

Casamassimo, P., Wilson, S., and Gross, L. (2002). Effects of US parenting styles on dental practice: perceptions of diplomates of the American Board of Pediatric Dentistry. *Pediatric Dentistry*, 24, 18–22.

Chambers, D.W. (1970). Managing the anxieties of young dental patients. *Journal of Dentistry for Children*, 37, 363–374.

Chambers, D.W. (1976). Communicating with the young patient. *Journal of the American Dental Association*, 93, 793–796.

Craig, W. (1972). Hand over mouth technique. *Journal of Dentistry for Children*, 38, 387–389.

Cunningham, J. (2005). Children's humor (Chapter 5). In: W.G. Scarlett, S. Naudeau, D. Salonius-Pasternak, and I Ponte (Eds.), Children's Play (pp. 93–109). SAGE Publications, Thousand Oaks, California.

D'Antonio, I.J. (1989). The use of humor with children in hospital settings. In: P. McGhee (Ed.), Humor and Children's Development: A Guide to Practical Applications (pp. 157–171). Haworth, New York.

Davies, G.N. and King, R.M. (1961). Dentistry for the Preschool Child. E. and S. Livingston, Edinburgh.

Davis, M.J. and Rombom, H.M. (1979). Survey of the utilization and rationale for hand-over-mouth (HOM) and restraint in postdoctoral pedodontic education. *Pediatric Dentistry*, 1, 87–90.

Dowling, J.S. (2002). Humor: A coping strategy for pediatric patients. *Pediatric Nursing*, 28, 123–131.

Eaton, J.J., McTigue, D.J., Fields, H.W. Jr. et al. (2005). Attitudes of contemporary parents toward behavior management techniques used in pediatric dentistry. *Pediatric Dentistry*, 27, 107–113.

Eysenck, H.J. (1964). Experiments in Behavior Therapy. Pergamon Press, Oxford.

Farhat-McHayleh, N., Harfouche, A., and Souaid, P. (2009). Techniques for managing behaviour in pediatric dentistry: Comparative study of live modelling and tell-show-do based on children's heart rates during treatment. *Journal of the Canadian Dental Association*, 75, 28.

Ferster, C.B. (1964). Reinforcement and punishment in the control of human behavior by social agencies. In: H.J. Eysenck (Ed.), Experiments in Behavior Therapy. Pergamon Press, New York.

Finn, S.B. (1973). Clinical Pedodontics, 4th ed. W.B. Saunders Co., Philadelphia.

Forehand, R. and Long, N. (1999). Strong-willed children: A challenge to parents and pediatric dentists. *Pediatric Dentistry*, 21, 463–467.

Frankel, R.I. (1991). The Papoose Board and mothers' attitudes following its use. *Pediatric Dentistry*, 13, 284–288.

Ghose, L.J., Giddon, D.B., Shiere, F.R. et al. (1969). Evaluation of sibling support. *Journal of Dentistry for Children*, 36, 35–39.

Greenbaum, P.E. and Melamed, B.G. (1988). Parent modeling. *A technique for reducing children's fear in the dental operatory. Dental Clinics of North America*, 32, 693–704.

Greenbaum, P.E., Turner, C., Cook, E.W., et al. (1990) Dentists' voice control: Effects on children's disruptive and affective behavior. *Health Psychol 9*, 546-558.

Goering, P. (1972). To keep the sunlight in a child's life. *Menninger Perspective*, 3, 10.

Hassan, S.O., Ralstrom, E., Miriyala, V. et al. (2010). Alternatives for hand over mouth exercise after its elimination from the guidelines of the American Academy of Pediatric Dentistry. *Pediatric Dentistry*, 32, 223–228.

Ingersoll, B.D., Nash, D.A., and Gamber, C. (1984). The use of contingent audiotaped material with pediatric patients. *Journal of the American Dental Association*, 109, 717–719.

Jiang, S. (2020). Positive distractions and play in the public spaces of pediatric healthcare environments: A literature review. *HERD: Health Environments Research & Design Journal*. https://doi.org/10.1177/1937586720901707

Johnson, R. and Baldwin, D.C. (1968). Relationship of maternal anxiety to the behavior of young children undergoing dental extraction. *Journal of Dental Research*, 47, 801–805.

Kane, S. and Olness, K. (2004). The Art of Therapeutic Communication: The Collected Works of Kay F. Thompson. Crown House Publishing, Ltd, Carmarthen, Wales.

Klingberg, G. (2008). Dental anxiety and behavior management problems in paediatric dentistry—a review of background factors and diagnostics. *European Archives of Paediatric Dentistry*, 1, 11–15.

Kotsanos, N., Coolidge, T., Velonis, D. et al. (2009). A form of "parental presence/absence" (PPA) technique for the child patient with dental behavior management problems. *European Archives Paediatric Dentistry*, 10(2), 90–92. doi:10.1007/BF03321607

Kramer, W.S. (1975). Aversion: A method for modifying child behavior. *Texas Dental Journal*, 93, 22–26.

Kuhn, B.R. and Allen, K.D. (1994). Expanding child behavior technology in pediatric dentistry: A behavioral science perspective. *Pediatric Dentistry*, 16, 13–16.

Kuhn, G. et al. (2014). A psychologically based taxonomy of misdirection. *Frontiers in Psychology*, 5, 1392. DOI: 10.3389/fpsyg.2014.01392. eCollection 2014.

Kuiper, N.A., Martin, R.A., and Olinger, L.J. (1993). Coping humor, stress, and cognitive appraisals. *Canadian Journal of Applied Sciences*, 25, 81–96.

Kupietzky, A. and Ram, D. (2005). Effects of a positive verbal presentation on parental acceptance of passive medical stabilization for the dental treatment of young children. *Pediatric Dentistry*, 27, 380–384.

Lampshire, E.L. (1975). Hypnosis in dentistry for children (Chapter 6). In: G.Z. Wright (Ed.), Behavior Management in Dentistry for Children (pp. 115–128). WB Saunders, Philadelphia.

Lara, A., Crego, A., and Romero-Maroto, M. (2014). Emotional contagion of dental fear to children: the fathers' mediating role in parental transfer of fear. *International Journal of Paediatric Dentistry*, 22, 324–330.

Lawrence, S.M. et al. (1991). Parental attitudes toward behavior management techniques relative to types of dental treatment. *Pediatric Dentistry*, 13, 151–155.

Levitas, T.C. (1974). HOME-hand over mouth exercise. *Journal of Dentistry for Children*, 41, 178–182.

Locker, D., Thompson, W.L., and Poulton, R. (2001). Onset of and patterns of change in dental anxiety in adolescence and early childhood: A birth cohort study. *Community Dental Health*, 18, 99–104.

Loizou, E. (2006). Young children's explanation of pictorial humor. *Early Childhood Education Journal*, 33, 425–431.

MacGregor, S.A. (1952). Practical suggestions on child management. *New Zealand Dental Journal*, 48, 102.

Majstorovic, M., Morse, D.E., Do, D. et al. (2014). Indicators of dental anxiety in children just prior to treatment. *Journal of Clinical Pediatric Dentistry*, 39, 12–17.

Manley, M.C. (2004). A UK perspective. *British Dental Journal*, 196, 138–139.

Martin, R.B., Shaw, M.A., and Taylor, P.P. (1977). The influence of prior surgical experience on the child's dental behavior at the first dental visit. *Journal of Dentistry for Children*, 44, 443–447.

McDonald, R.E. (1963). *Pedodontics*. C.V. Mosby Co., St. Louis.

McGhee, P. (2002). *Understanding and Promoting the Development of Children's Humor: A Guide for Parents and Teachers*. Kendall Hunt Publishing Company, Dubuque Regional, Iowa.

McGhee, P.E. (1979). *Humor Its Origin and Development*. Freeman and Company, San Francisco.

Melamed, B.G., Hawes, R.R., Heiby, E. et al. (1975). Use of filmed modeling to reduce uncooperative behavior of children during treatment. *Journal of Dental Research*, 90, 822–826.

Mora-Ripoll, R. (2010). The therapeutic value of laughter in medicine. *Alternative Therapies in Health and Medicine*, 16, 56–64.

Morris, C.D.N. (2004). A commentary on the legal issues. *British Dental Journal*, 196, 139–140.

Moss, S. (1972). Psychology of communication. Presented at the *Northwestern Pedodontic Teachers Conference*. Chicago.

Murphy, M.G., Fields, H.W., and Machen, J.B. (1984). Parental acceptance of pediatric dentistry management techniques. *Pediatric Dentistry*, 6, 193–198.

Nash, D.A. (2006). Engaging children's cooperation in the dental environment through effective communication. *Pediatric Dentistry*, 28, 455–459.

Nevo, O. and Shapira, J. (1986). Use of humor in managing clinical anxiety. *Journal of Dentistry Children*, 53, 97–100.

Newton, J.T., Patel, H., Shah, S. et al. (2004). Attitudes toward the use of hand over mouth (HOM) and physical restraint amongst paediatric dental specialist practitioners in the UK. *International Journal of Paediatric Dentistry*, 14, 111–117.

Olness, K. and Kohen, D.P. (1996). *Hypnosis and Hypnotherapy with Children*, 3rd ed. Guilford Press, New York.

Oueiss, H.S., Ralstrom, E., Miriyala, V. et al. (2010). Alternatives for hand over mouth exercise after its elimination from the clinical guidelines of the American Academy of Pediatric Dentistry. *Pediatric Dentistry*, 32, 223–228.

Patel, M., McTigue, D.J., Thikkurissy, S. et al. (2016). Parental attitudes toward advanced behavior guidance techniques used in pediatric dentistry. *Pediatric Dentistry*, 38, 30–36.

Peltier, B. (2014). Hypnosis in dentistry (Chapter 23). In: D.I. Mostofsky and F. Fortune (Eds.), *Behavioral Dentistry*, 2nd ed. (pp. 75–85). Wiley-Blackwell.

Riba, H., Al-Shahrani, A., Al-Ghutaimel, H. et al. (2018). Parental presence/absence in the dental operatory as a behavior management technique: A review and modified view. *Journal of Contemporary Dental Practice*, 19(2), 237–241.

Roberts, J.F., Curzon, M.E., Koch, G. et al. (2010). Review: Behavior management techniques in paediatric dentistry. *European Archives of Paediatric Dentistry*, 11, 166–174.

Rosenberg, H.M. (1974). Behavior modification for the child dental patient. *Journal of Dentistry for Children*, 41, 111–114.

Schuman, N.J. (1987). Child abuse and the dental practitioner: Discussion and case reports. *Quintessence International*, 18, 619–622.

Sharma, A., Kumar, D., Anand, A. et al. (2017). Factors predicting behavior management problems during initial dental examination in children aged 2 to 8 years. *International Journal of Clinical Pediatric Dentistry*, 10, 5–9.

Skinner, B.F. (1953). *Science and Human Behavior*. MacMillan Co., New York.

The Virginia Board of Dentistry (1987). The hand over mouth exercise in handling child patients. *Dental Bulletin, Issue* 1.

Tuma, C.F. (1954). How to help your child be a good dental patient: An open letter to parents. *Journal of Dentistry for Children*, 21, 84.

Vingoe, F. (1987). When is a placebo not a placebo? That is the question. *British Journal of Experimental and Clinical Hypnosis*, 4, 165–167.

Venham, L., Goldstein, M., Gaulin-Kremer, E. et al. (1981). Effectiveness of a distraction technique in managing young dental patients. *Pediatric Dentistry*, 3, 7–11.

Welbury, R.R., Duggal, M.S., and Hosey, M.T. (2005). *Paediatric Dentistry*, 3rd ed. Oxford University Press, Oxford.

Wepman, B.J. and Sonnenberg, E.M. (1979). Effective communication with the pedodontic patient. *Journal of Pedodontics*, 2, 13–17.

Wilkins, J. and Eisenbraun, A.J. (2009). Humor theories and the physiological benefits of laughter. *Holistic Nursing Practice*, 23, 349–354.

Wiseman, R. and Watt, C. (2018). Achieving the impossible: A review of magic-based interventions and their effects on wellbeing. *PeerJ*, 6, e6081. https://doi.org/10.7717/peerj.6081

White, L.W. (1974). Behavior modification of orthodontic patients. *Journal of Clinical Orthodontics*, 8, 501–503.

Wilson, S. and Cody, W.E. (2005). An analysis of behavior management papers published in the pediatric dentistry literature. *Pediatric Dentistry*, 27, 331–337.

Wolpe, J. (1969). *The Practice of Behavior Therapy* (p. 15). Pergamon Press, New York.

Wright, G.Z. and Alpern, G.D. (1971). Variables influencing children's cooperative behavior at the first dental visit. *Journal of Dentistry for Children*, 38, 126–128.

Wright, G.Z., Alpern, G.D., and Leake, J.L. (1973). Modifiability of maternal anxiety as it relates to children's cooperative behavior. *Journal of Dentistry for Children*, 40, 265–271.

Wright, G.Z. (1975). *Behavior Management in Dentistry for Children*. W.B. Saunders Co., Philadelphia.

Wright, G.Z., Starkey, P.E., and Gardner D.E. (1983). *Managing Children's Behavior in the Dental Office*. C.V. Mosby Co., St. Louis.

Wright, G.Z. (1979). Management of needle phobic adolescents. *Ontario Dentist*, 56, 22–25.

Wright, G.Z. and Stigers, J.I. (2011). Non pharmacologic management of children's behaviors. In: J.A. Dean, D.R. Avery, and R.E. McDonald (Eds.), *Dentistry for the Child and Adolescent*, 9th ed., p. 32. Mosby Elsevier, Maryland Heights, MO.

Wurster, C.A., Weinstein, P., and Cohen, A.J. (1979). Communication patterns in pedodontics. *Journal of Dentistry for Children*, 48, 159–163.

# 8

# Children with Disabilities

*Gunilla Klingberg*

## Introduction

Disabilities affect many people today. Prevalence varies between different countries and cultures, but it is realistic to assume that up to 20% of all children and adolescents may be affected by a disability or a chronic health condition (Bethell et al. 2008; Merrick and Carmeli 2003). Further, the number of individuals with disabilities is increasing owing to developments in medical health technology, diagnostic tools, and an increase in the number of medical treatment options. For example, more children who have been born preterm survive because of improvements in medical care, but these children also have an increased risk for disabilities.

This chapter will discuss special child patients with disabilities or chronic health conditions and provide examples to assist with their management in the dental office. It will also focus on how the dental team can work together with the child and family to create positive dental appointments and good oral health. As with all child dental patients, caring for the special child involves the pediatric dentistry treatment triangle—the child, the parent or legal guardian, and the dental team. This chapter will provide details about each corner of the triangle. For dental care and treatment to be successful, all three components of the triangle have to collaborate and communicate. Ultimately, the dentist is responsible for the treatment and should acquire appropriate knowledge about the child's diagnosis or disability, as well as an understanding of the psychology of the family.

Before discussing the corners of the triangle, mention must be made of two important international declarations that have direct bearing on special children. The first is the Convention on the Rights of the Child (United Nations 1989), which was ratified by a majority of nations worldwide. The overriding point in the convention is that children have rights. According to the third article in the convention, the "best interest" of the child should be the guiding rule in all decisions involving or affecting children.

The convention has had a significant impact (e.g., child-friendly health care) on the way all children are treated and respected within the health sector. Children have the right to be involved in decisions about treatment, and their points of view should be respected, taking age and maturity into consideration.

The second declaration occurred in 2006 when the United Nations adopted the Convention on the Rights of Persons with Disabilities. Its purpose was "to promote, protect and ensure the full and equal enjoyment of all human rights and fundamental freedoms by all persons with disabilities, and to promote respect for their inherent dignity." The convention noted changing societal views on people with disabilities. Historically, individuals with disabilities have been seen as objects rather than subjects. In the past, society provided help and support for people with disabilities in terms of benevolence and charity. This is no longer an acceptable attitude. The convention strengthened the position of people with disabilities. It stressed that people with disabilities are subjects and individuals like everyone else, and thereby have the same rights for making decisions that influence their lives, including health-related matters. Dental professionals treating children need to be aware of these societal changes in attitude and apply these principles in their practices.

As this chapter deals with children with disabilities, it is important to define "disability." Today, disabilities and chronic conditions are not only looked upon as diagnoses defined in the International Classification of Diseases (ICD). The understanding and classification of disability and chronic health conditions is also based on a bio-psychosocial model, as articulated in the World Health Organization's International Classification of Functioning and Health (ICF), adopted in 2001, and in the Child and Youth Version, ICF-CY, for individuals up to 17 years of age, adopted in 2007. The ICF as a model describes human functioning in terms of body structure, body function, activities, and participation. These functions are influenced

*Wright's Behavior Management in Dentistry for Children*, Third Edition. Edited by Ari Kupietzky.
© 2022 John Wiley & Sons, Inc. Published 2022 by John Wiley & Sons, Inc.

by health condition, environmental factors, and personal factors. Today, the ICF-CY as a classification comprises more than 1600 items related to body structure, body function, activities and participation, and environmental factors. It is universal, allows comparisons of health conditions with different etiologies, and can describe a person's health profile from a bio-psychosocial perspective. This perspective holds interest from a dental standpoint, and studies are currently being undertaken to construct a core set in oral health (Faulks et al. 2013). The ICF and ICF-CY provide a new way of understanding the continuum normal→disability. It focuses on the individual's overall health status instead of focusing only on the specific disability or impairment (Norderyd 2015). By doing so, it becomes evident that anyone can experience a health problem, and thereby a disability.

## The Special Child

Every child is a unique individual. This is true for healthy children with normal development and maturation, even more so for children with disabilities or chronic health conditions. Children and adolescents show great variation in maturity, personality, temperament, and emotions. Additionally, cognitive reasoning, behavioral repertoires, and communicative skills vary, especially in children with disabilities. This leads to a corresponding variation in vulnerability and ability to cope with dental treatment.

The disabled child patient can be special in many different ways. This chapter focuses on children with special needs owing to disability or chronic health conditions, but it is important to acknowledge that there are other reasons for being special. For example, children may have language difficulties because they migrated to a new country, or simply because they are part of an immigrant family that communicates mostly in their native language. Communication is essential and the basis of successful treatment, and if the child or parent does not speak your language, interpretation might be required. Children who live in deprived socioeconomic settings or who have parents with mental or psychiatric illness are other examples that may require special attention from the dentist. And, it must be remembered that not all children develop and mature at the same rate. These children may not necessarily have impairments, but they are late bloomers and communication and treatment may have to be adjusted to their level of maturity rather than to their chronological age. This last example also demonstrates why dentists, especially pediatric dentists, should have knowledge of child development (see Chapter 2). Development and maturation also vary in children with disabilities and medical conditions on an individual basis and can be affected by a poor socioeconomic environment or parental illness.

The best way to learn about a child's capabilities is to ask. A thorough case history is a must, and ideally both the child and the parents should be interviewed. The routine anamnesis for the healthy child should include information about medical diagnoses, medication, family and social contexts, school, and peer-related issues. However, for the special child patient, the interview needs to be more detailed and include specific areas related to the child's condition.

When obtaining a medical history, specifically inquire about the perinatal period and birth. The importance of these developmental periods was emphasized in Chapter 2. Low birth weight or complications like defective saturation or infections can affect nutrition, growth, and development. There are several developmental windows through which all children pass. These windows are open for a limited period of time, and passing through one window, or level, in development provides children with the requirements needed to manage the next level. For example, children born preterm often have difficulties coordinating sucking, swallowing, or breathing, which also may be affected by their medical health status (Delaney et al. 2008). Furthermore, children who have problems in breastfeeding or sucking as newborns may have an increased risk of developing feeding problems. The developmental train typically forecasts that average children learn to manage fluids and to swallow at an early age (Mason et al. 2005). Based on these skills, children will be able to consume more complex food textures, tastes, and temperatures as they mature and their feeding progresses to include new types of foods. Successful managing and swallowing of the bolus has to be preceded by training and handling of other kinds of foods and liquids. Some children with feeding problems, owing to prematurity or medical problems, develop hyper-sensitivity in the orofacial region, which, if untreated, could make it difficult to carry out oral hygiene procedures like toothbrushing, or even to conduct dental examinations (Mason et al. 2005; Rommel et al. 2003).

The perinatal period is also important for tooth mineralization. Hypomineralization and hypoplasia in enamel have been reported as more common in children born preterm; molar incisor hypomineralization (MIH) occurs more frequently in these children. Further, it is probable that dental behavior management problems and dental anxiety are more likely for children born preterm than for others (Brogårdh-Roth 2010).

The medical history should cover all medical issues. Information about periods of hospitalization, medications, and physicians responsible for the child's medical care can become detailed and complex. There are several medical diagnoses and medicines that may impact oral health. The dentist is advised to look up both diagnoses and medications in order to find out if there are any direct implications or interactions in relation to dental care. There are also several rare diagnoses and syndromes that the pediatric dentist may encounter. Apart from textbooks, there are several good databases available via the Internet to learn more about general aspects of the diagnoses, for example, Orphanet and OMIM (Online Mendelian Inheritance in Man), a disomic section that can also be accessed via PubMed. Some countries also have national centers that specialize in the orofacial and odontological aspects of rare diagnoses. One example is the National Resource Centre for Rare Disorders in Sweden (Mun-H-Center), which provides a website and a smartphone app in English.

Other important case history aspects include information about the child's normal life and his/her strengths and weaknesses. For children with disabilities or medical health problems, much time is spent discussing the child's problems and weaknesses. It is equally important to learn about the child's strengths.

Knowledge about the strengths of the child is often useful when trying to individualize the appointment. For example, a child might have problems with sudden or loud noises and is easily frightened, but at the same time could be interested in music and may enjoy specific types of music. This information may be important and useful for the dentist. For example, instead of avoiding noise and being concerned about how the child will react to the sound of suction, the dentist could play music during the treatment or explain the treatment and sounds that will occur in terms of music. Some may think this is farfetched, but when working with a special child patient, it is often necessary to step out of the more traditional role of the dentist. Being successful with special children implies being open to trying new things and being a bit unconventional in the choice of methods from time to time.

It is not always optimal for children to be present while parents and healthcare professionals discuss their problems and limitations. One might try to circumvent the problem by either scheduling a parent appointment without the child or arranging a telephone interview. Apart from not exposing the child to negative information, gaining information in advance from the parents makes it possible for the dentist to be better prepared when meeting the special child patient for the first time. By gathering vital information beforehand, the dentist can fully focus on the child and the interactions at the first visit instead of having to start with the anamnesis.

## The Family

Parents and family constitute the second component of the pediatric dental triangle. Being a parent of a special child is, in many ways, different from being a parent of a healthy child. Living with a child with a disability affects all aspects of family life. It is known to be a powerful stressor for all family members, and several studies have shown that mothers experience more stress and often take more responsibility for the child with a disability or chronic health condition than the rest of the family. The concerns and worries can be life-long. They differ from the more normal worries that all parents have about their children as they grow up. Being a parent of an adult child with a disability will bring concerns about where the child should live, receive adequate help and assistance, and what will happen when the parents are no longer around (Bradshaw et al. 2019; Hallberg et al. 2010).

The family's level of self-reliance (capacity) or reconciliation with having a child with a disability influences how they cope with the child's medical and dental care and how they will manage parenting. It is important that the family balances its subjective feelings of vulnerability and access to support from others. This perspective, emphasizing the need for support, has been reported to increase psychological and physical well-being in families who have a child with a disability (Scheeran et al. 1997). Apart from support from significant others such as relatives and friends, it is important for families to have support and positive responses from professionals within the social sector and healthcare professions, including dentistry (Bradshaw et al. 2019).

Parents and families who are self-reliant and who have become reconciled to their situation tend to develop feelings of confidence in caring for their children. This can gradually lead to their perception of a less stressful and more manageable situation. It will probably affect how they cope with their children's needs in relation to medical and dental treatment, including preventive home care. As prevention of oral diseases requires establishing good rapport with the families, the dental teams need to have good knowledge and insight into the lives of those who have disabilities. In order to achieve this balance, it is important not only to treat the child, but also to consider the whole family (Trulsson and Klingberg 2003).

In a study by Trulsson and Klingberg (2003), parents of children with severe and complex diagnoses were interviewed about issues related to their children's oral health and dental care. The parents identified five qualities they would like to see in dental teams: respect, involvement, continuity, knowledge, and availability. These five qualities might be regarded as a matter of course, but apparently these needs had not been met. Another interesting finding from the interviews concerned the way that the parents described their children's main orofacial or oral health-related problems. According to the participating parents, the main problems were related to nutrition and communication. They also mentioned dental malocclusions, but only in relation to the possibility of improving chewing and speech or decreasing the risk of dental trauma, but not in relation to esthetics. No other oral health issues, such as dental caries and gingivitis, were mentioned by the parents. One could argue that this study dealt with children with very complex diagnoses, but nonetheless, it is apparent that the parents' and dentists' views on what is most important may differ.

## The Dental Team

People with disabilities may be subject to inequality in oral health, in terms of both prevalence of disease and unmet healthcare needs. While most pediatric dentists have training with special child patients, provision of large-scale primary care is only possible through the education and training of all dentists. The literature suggests that it is vital for the dental team to develop the necessary skills and gain experience treating people with special needs in order to ensure access to oral healthcare for all persons (Faulks et al. 2012).

The dental treatment for children with disabilities varies greatly. There are many reasons for this, and some of importance are related to the individual dentist and dental team. Studies have pointed to the fact that many dentists and other members of the dental team feel a professional uncertainty in treating individuals with disabilities (Bedi et al. 2001; Hallberg et al. 2004). Reasons offered for this attitude include the fact that many dentists lack previous knowledge and experience in treating patients with disabilities, and there is little relevant training in either undergraduate or postgraduate programs (Casamassimo et al. 2004; Dao et al. 2005). This is troublesome, as the ambivalent attitudes from dental professionals toward these patients may contribute to less treatment offered to these patient groups (Bedi et al. 2001; Klingberg and Hallberg 2012). Being successful in the dental treatment of special child patients, therefore, depends in large part on the dental team, and specifically on the dentist himself.

Another reason for varying treatment is the economic standard in families. Depending on how dental care and social insurance systems are organized in the country, this will impact dental care for children with disabilities and, in the long-term, the oral health of these children. If pharmacological means are required to treat the patient, it can be

quite costly. The special child patient offers a positive challenge for the dentist and an opportunity to progress and learn more within the profession. Managing and treating the special child patient successfully, and having the child return with a smile on his face, yields immense professional satisfaction. That is what makes working with special child patients so special.

The remainder of this chapter deals with specific disabilities. It will offer some helpful hints for the dentist and the dental team.

## Physical Impairments

Physical impairments constitute a wide group of diagnoses with some having a substantial impact on the child's daily life in terms of reduced motor ability. The clinical manifestations vary widely from quadriplegia to conditions affecting the function of a limb or part of a limb. Some of the physical disabilities may be present at birth, while others may be acquired as a result of trauma or disease. A common diagnosis in this group is cerebral palsy, with four main subtypes: spastic (muscle stiffness), atheotid (slow movements), ataxic (lack of muscular balance and coordination), and mixed (having symptoms of more than one type of cerebral palsy, the most common being spastic-dyskinetic). Other common diagnoses are muscular dystrophies and spina bifida. For all diagnoses that lead to a decrease in physical activity, especially if the muscle tone is altered, there is a risk that body posture will impact the oral cavity both in terms of growth patterns and oral health. A hypotonic patient sitting in a position where the head is not supported will have an increased risk of developing malocclusions because the muscular forces that normally regulate the growth are affected. The tone is too low in the tongue, cheeks, and related structures. The same is true for the opposite condition—hypertonic patients. Patients with spastic problems sometimes present with self-inflicted injuries or bite wounds. These patients can be hard to treat, and the dentist may have to use a bite support or mouth prop to prevent the child patient from involuntary biting during treatment.

### Clinical Considerations

High-quality treatment and good patient management is facilitated if the patient is seated in the dental chair and able to relax. Some patients may have problems moving from their wheelchair to the dental chair. However, the patient should be moved onto the dental chair whenever possible, despite the difficulties that this may entail. To reduce the amount of chair movement, which can heighten a patient's anxiety, some prefer to pre-set the chair in the approximate position before seating the patient. Having the child in the dental chair improves the ergonomic position for the dentist, facilitating treatment and thereby improving quality in dental care. A dental clinic has to be designed to accommodate wheelchairs. (Some ideas for these accommodations can be found in Chapter 17). In many clinics dedicated to the treatment of the special child, sliding equipment and lift systems are available to move the patient to the dental chair.

To make the dental chair more comfortable for patients, different kinds of cushions may be used. A cushion to sit on is very useful for most of the younger patients, as the normal dental chair is designed for an adult's full body length (see Figure 8-1). There are also special cushions available that will support the body for patients with low muscle tone or spasticities. These cushions provide a passive support and should not be confused with restraint. Light Velcro is used to keep the cushions in position. For patients with spastic problems, the cushions are adjusted to help flexing knees and hip joints (ideally to a 90° flexion) and to incline the head to a chin-to-chest position. This position can help to reduce spasticities, which in turn makes it easier for the child to relax. These cushions can also be used for patients with intellectual disabilities or neuropsychiatric disorders. Patients without disabilities may also benefit from the comfort of cushions.

Some children with dysphagia may have an increased risk of aspiration. Therefore, it is highly important for the dental team to be alert and ready to provide good assistance to remove secretions and dental debris during treatment.

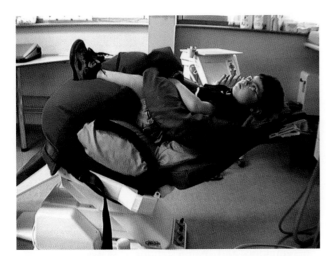

**Figure 8-1** Special cushions to support the body for patients with low muscle tone or spasticities. For patients with spastic problems, the cushions are adjusted to help flexing knees and hip joints (ideally to a 90° flexion) and to incline the head to a chin-to-chest position.

For some children, the problems are so severe that all dental treatment will need to be carried out under general anesthesia.

Sedation often helps to reduce anxiety and assist a child with disability to relax during treatment. Minimum sedation is often sufficient; however, all types of sedation and dosages have to be tailored to the individual child. Nitrous oxide-oxygen sedation should not be used unless the child is able to nose breathe. Apart from being ineffective if not inhaled, exposure to nitrous oxide should be avoided for work environmental reasons. An ASA (American Society of Anesthesiologists) physical status evaluation is extremely important for children with disabilities, and the child's physician should be consulted if any questions arise. For some children, dental treatment cannot be carried out conventionally or under sedation—treatment under general anesthesia may be the only alternative. Access to facilities for general anesthesia varies between different countries; however, it is important to strive for these resources for this group of children. Not having this option may lead to either suboptimal dental care and deteriorated oral health, or no treatment at all. From that perspective, access to general anesthesia is a communal obligation if society wants to ensure these children's right to receive oral health care on the same level as others.

**Editor's Note:** *By cradling a child's head against the operator's body, satisfactory stabilization can often be obtained. Using a rubber dam imparts a feeling of security that may be helpful for managing these children. At times, bite blocks may be used in the mouth. A body wrap may be used to help restrain movements, or sometimes a simple strap over a child's ankles may assist with stabilization. This additional armamentarium serves the purposes of protecting the child, facilitating dental procedures, and providing security. In the development of this chapter, it was recognized that there were regional differences. In Sweden and several other European countries, physical restraints are not culturally accepted and are prohibited by law under any circumstance. It should be emphasized that clinicians in these countries are able to treat patients successfully with extra time devoted to working with the parent and child and without the use of restraints. However, in other countries, some forms of restraints are still used and intended as a benefit to the consenting patient and/ or parent.*

Another form of physical impairment is obesity. The Centers for Disease Control and Prevention (CDC) has categorized obesity as an epidemic with physical, psychological, and social consequences in adults and children (CDC 2009). The prevalence of overweight and obesity is rising in many developed and developing countries and, most worryingly, among children. Currently, 32% of children and adolescents in the United States are overweight or obese

(Ogden et al. 2010). In England, almost a quarter of children now enter primary school either overweight or obese, rising to one in three by 11 years of age. Available data for all other countries indicates a rising trend.

The rise of obesity within populations can have an impact on dental professionals. Problems extend from the effect of obesity directly on dental disease, to medical conditions influencing the development and treatment of dental disease, to the practicality of treating the obese in a conventional dental primary care setting (Reilly et al. 2009). Although the speed of the obesity epidemic has been greater than the recognition of the impending crisis by healthcare services (Levine 2012), many hospitals and dental clinics in developed countries now recognize the need for bariatric equipment such as beds, hoists, wheelchairs, and commodes to take patients weighing more than 350 kg.

Many obese children come from families with lower socioeconomic standards. There are several factors that contribute to overweight and obesity: bad dietary habits, high consumption of fast foods, sucrose-rich beverages, refined wheat bread, little or no physical activity, as well as some genetic influence. Even though dental caries are not always seen in overweight or obese young children, the risk for both caries and gingival inflammation will increase if the weight is not treated. Overweight and obesity affect the ASA evaluation of the patient, and the dentist should be aware of the effect of adiposity on the distribution, binding, and elimination of many commonly used drugs in dentistry. Obesity may complicate the use of pharmacological methods of patient management, and adverse events during sedation for dental procedures have been reported (Kang et al. 2012). There could be increased risk of respiratory depression when midazolam or opioids such as meperidine are administered (Kang et al. 2012). Obese children also have a higher incidence of difficult mask ventilation, laryngoscopy, aspiration, postoperative atelectasis, airway obstruction, bronchospasm, major oxygen desaturation, and overall critical respiratory events (Tait et al. 2008).

Besides attending to the obese child's dental needs, dentists who care for children are in a unique position to help address the childhood obesity epidemic for several reasons (Tseng et al. 2010). First, dentists may see children regularly, providing an opportunity for longitudinal counseling and monitoring of weight status often starting at an early age. Second, dentists have a greater likelihood than pediatricians of seeing older children on a regular basis. Third, dentists are credible sources for dietary counseling. Most dentists who treat children feel that dietary counseling is an important component of oral health.

Perhaps, the most difficult task and significant barrier for overweight and obesity screening among dental professionals is determining the manner in which a child's unhealthy weight status is to be communicated (Tseng et al. 2010). However, showing empathy and tact will enable the dentist to raise the issue and discover whether the child has had any medical weight counseling. If not, the dentist should help to refer the child for medical evaluation. As treatment for obesity and overweight is composed of several different methods that are individually tailored and decided on after careful medical evaluation, the dentist should limit advice to oral health matters.

## Intellectual Disability

According to the American Association on Intellectual and Developmental Disabilities (AAIDD), "intellectual disability" is currently the preferred term for the disability that previously has been referred to as *mental retardation*. This change in terminology is also present in the new DSM-5 manual published in May 2013 (Diagnostic and Statistical Manual of Mental Disorders, Fifth Edition). Intellectual disability is, by the definition from AAIDD, "characterized by significant limitations both in intellectual functioning and in adaptive behavior, which covers many everyday social and practical skills. This disability originates before age 18." Historically, individuals with an intelligence quotient (IQ) under 70 were considered as having an intellectual disability. However, current definitions include both mental functioning and functioning skills in the individual's environment. As a result, a person with a below-average intelligence quotient may not be considered as having an intellectual disability unless they exhibit deficits in two or more adaptive behaviors. Still, the IQ test is a major tool for measuring intellectual functioning, and according to DSM-5, intellectual disability is considered to be approximately two standard deviations or more below the population, which equals an IQ score of about 70 or below. An IQ between 50 and 69 denotes a mild or educable condition, while an IQ under 50 denotes severe intellectual disability. Approximately 3% of the population is affected by intellectual disability and 0.6% is affected to a severe degree.

There are many causes of intellectual disability. The most common causes include genetic deficits (e.g., Down syndrome), perinatal insults (oxygen deficiency before, during, or after birth), infections (such as rubella or meningitis), or trauma affecting the brain.

Since there are different levels of intellectual disability, the symptoms and manifestations vary widely between individuals. Generally, children with intellectual disabilities are slower in acquiring self-care life-skills, have difficulty remembering things, and have delayed language development. There are children with milder forms of intellectual disability that need very little support, and who often become excellent dental patients. At the other end of the spectrum, there are children with severe or profound disabilities who need 24-hour assistance for all situations. These children frequently require general anesthesia or sedation for their dental care. Comorbidity is common in patients with intellectual disability. Many children with intellectual disability have additional health problems, such as other physical impairments, epilepsy, neuropsychiatric problems, and congenital heart defects or syndromes.

### Clinical Considerations

As for all children, the creation of a safe environment for the child patient with an intellectual disability is fundamental for successful dental visits. In order for the child to feel safe, at least three factors have to be fulfilled: (1) a good rapport and relationship between the child, the accompanying person, and the dentist; (2) minimizing the risk of pain during treatment; and (3) helping the child develop a feeling of control. Stepwise introduction using tell-show-do (TSD), sometimes with the help of pedagogic tools like photos or pictures (see the section titled "Autism Spectrum Disorders"), should be performed at a slow pace. The dentist should impart a feeling of control to the patient so that the child knows what is going to happen and feels convinced that the dentist will react or stop if the child signals.

Due to diminished intellectual growth, many children with intellectual disability function with a limited capacity in comparison to other children. Hence, the social functioning of these children is found to be affected, and this is closely related to their degree of impairment. Children and adolescents with intellectual disability need time to feel comfortable in the dental setting, and time has to be invested in these patients. These children also benefit from meeting the same dental team during visits. If this is provided, the dental visits and simple treatments are usually accepted by children with intellectual disability. However, all treatments have to be constantly tailored to the individual patient's capacities and needs. For example, an injection can provoke fear for a child with an intellectual disability, just as it can with any other child, and the numbness following the injection sometimes elicits strong negative reactions. The child with intellectual disability does not understand why this feeling occurs or that it will eventually disappear. Complications such as biting of an anesthetized lip or cheek can occur; the use of periodontal ligament injections when possible may help prevent this common problem.

Many children with intellectual disability will need help from others to carry out basic procedures like toothbrushing, due to their limited or decreased manual dexterity and/or lack of motivation and understanding of the importance of good oral hygiene. This need for assistance often stretches into adulthood.

## Sensory Impairments

This section deals with children possessing varying degrees of auditory and visual impairments. Deficiencies in these senses interfere with communication and may lead to difficulties in patient treatment.

Hearing impairment and deafness occurs in children, although it is much more common in adults and the elderly. There are both congenital and acquired forms, and the level of impairment can vary from mild to total deafness. It should be noted that hearing impairment has comorbidity with other conditions, like intellectual disability, as well as some syndromes. Children who are hard of hearing will find it much more difficult than children who have normal hearing to learn vocabulary, grammar, word order, idiomatic expressions, and other aspects of verbal communication. These deficiencies can affect communication and treatment in dental care. Interpretation using sign language might be necessary and should be offered if available. If not, the dental team should ensure that the appointment is scheduled in a way that allows for extra time. Parents can also be of major assistance in interpreting procedures for their child. They should be invited into the operatory because it may be difficult to explain concepts such as local anesthesia to the deaf child.

Problems related to hearing will affect communication during dental treatment. Ideally, the dentist should know how to communicate with sign language. If this is not the case, it is still possible to learn a few signs that can be helpful during treatment. For example, signs for "open your mouth," "good boy/good girl," and "toothbrush," plus social expressions like "welcome," "good-bye," etc., are beneficial. Sign language is not a universal language, and different verbal language areas and cultural regions can have different signs. Usually, older children who cognitively understand dental treatment can be very good patients. But the dental team has to invest in time and in introduction to accomplish this. Consider the classic tell-show-do (TSD) technique. Verbal communication is an integral part of the procedure, and so the deaf child must be managed differently. In fact, almost all of the communication techniques that are described for the average child cannot be used with the deaf child. For example, as many children with hearing impairments or deafness can use lip reading, the dentist should perhaps avoid wearing a mask during treatment (Champion and Holt 2000).

The use of sedation can be helpful for some children with hearing impairments. If the child with deafness needs extensive dental care, this should preferably be carried out under general anesthesia, especially in younger children. New technology has enabled treatment of deafness—especially congenital forms—by cochlear implants. If the child patient is using a hearing aid device or has a cochlear implant, it is sometimes necessary to adjust the head cushion to find a comfortable position for the child during treatment. Sometimes, the hearing device has to be disconnected if it doesn't function with the noise during treatment, resulting in more difficulties concerning communication.

The deaf child also partially compensates for hearing loss by use of hearing aids, or manual communication (signs and finger spelling). However, too often, these acquired skills are not learned until a child is six or seven years of age, a time when children with normal hearing are learning to read and write. Nonetheless, with gifted children and dedicated teachers, who frequently are the parents, it is often possible to acquire visual communication skills as early as three or four years of age.

### Clinical Considerations

Since normal verbalization is impossible with many deaf children, substitute communication procedures must be used to convey information. The following tips are helpful to communicate with the hearing impaired (Nunn, J.H. 2000):

- Remove masks when communicating with the child and reduce background noise.
- Learn a few basic signs.
- Write essential information on a "magic slate," use picture books to explain things.
- Be sure to face the child when communicating and ensure that the light is not behind you or in the child's eyes.
- Use texting, Typetalk, or some other of form electronic communication that children use today.

Many procedures have been recommended for establishing rapport and communication with children. Although the dentist may not employ all these procedures for the average child, they are highly important in the behavior management of the deaf child. When tipping the dental chair back, for example, the operator should make sure the child knows beforehand what will happen and then maybe touch the patient to impart a feeling of security. A hand mirror is an invaluable aid during most procedures, but the tactile sense also should be used. Children should be allowed to touch the instruments. This is used to great advantage with the average child; it must be used to the

maximum for the deaf child. Use desensitization to introduce new instruments or equipment. For example, when compressed air is used, it should be demonstrated on the operator's cheek or hand, and then on the patient's hand, before it is introduced intra-orally. Since these children learn by touching, they should be allowed as much freedom as the office environment permits. This does not mean being overly permissive; rather, it is intended to allow deaf children to acclimate to the environment. Children have an insatiable curiosity with the gadgetry in the dental office. The deaf child is no exception.

Visually impaired children also present communication problems. Childhood blindness, as defined by the World Health Organization, refers to a group of diseases and conditions occurring in childhood or early adolescence which, if left untreated, result in blindness or severe visual impairment. The estimated prevalence of blindness in children varies from 0.3/1,000 in wealthy countries to 1.2/1,000 in poorer countries (Gilbert 2001).

Blindness can be found in conjunction with other conditions, such as deafness or intellectual disability. As with other conditions, evaluation of the child's intellectual capacity and a clear understanding of intrinsic limitations is extremely important before approaching the patient. When intellectual disability or deafness is found in conjunction with blindness, even the most primitive communication with the afflicted child may be difficult and unproductive. In these instances, referral to a specialist with broad experience with children having disabilities is advisable.

Like many other conditions, blindness occurs in varying degrees and in specific circumstances. Some children may have partial sight. Others may have had normal sight and then lost it. When this occurs after five years of age, children may retain a visual frame of reference. However, without minimal visual experiences, these children out of necessity become highly verbal. Through verbalization, they try to identify objects and understand everyday happenings.

There are different levels of visual function, and the dentist should always check with the parents as to the level of the child's impairment.

### Clinical Considerations

Since TSD, the "show" portion of behavior shaping is greatly limited or impossible with visually impaired or blind children, the other aspects of education and conditioning in dental office procedures must be stressed. These children compensate for the lack of visual input by increased use of the auditory, tactile, and olfactory senses. Therefore, new procedures must be carefully explained, maximizing sensory perceptions other than sight. All new sounds and smells should be identified. The children should be allowed to feel new objects, and these objects should be named whenever possible. By the process of exploring with their fingers, blind children develop a great tactile sensitivity. They also tend to be rather passive and inactive because movement is obviously more hazardous and requires more effort for them. They require more stimulation to venture into unknown experiences. Thus, the show technique is accomplished for the blind child with more effort from the dental team in a manner that is different from that used for the sighted child.

A new technique, using audiovisual tactile performance technique, was developed by Hebbal and Ankola (2012) for training visually impaired children in oral hygiene maintenance. This special education technique follows a pattern: children are informed about the importance of teeth and a brushing method; children then feel teeth on a model and brush the model; once mastered, the children feel and brush their own teeth. The study demonstrated that visually impaired children could maintain an acceptable level of oral hygiene when taught using a special customized method. It is often difficult to treat blind children and extensive treatment may require sedation and/or general anesthesia. Therefore, the focus should be on disease prevention.

## Neuropsychiatric Disorders

Neuropsychiatric disorders include several diagnoses like autism and attention deficit hyperactivity disorder (ADHD) and are expected to affect at least 5% of the child population (Gillberg 1995). The diagnoses are based on a specific set of symptoms describing the main domains of problems experienced by the individual person. A person's diagnosis may change over time, as problems and symptoms change with individual development (Gillberg and Coleman 2000). There have been some changes of the definitions and naming of the different diagnoses in the new version of the DSM, DSM-5 (*Diagnostic and Statistical Manual of Mental Disorders*, Fifth Edition) that was published in May 2013 (American Psychiatric Association). One of new features is that autism spectrum disorders (ASDs) now will incorporate several previously separate diagnoses, whereas DSM-4 included pervasive developmental disorders, a spectrum of disorders from Asperger's syndrome (mild) to autism (more challenging symptoms).

### Autism Spectrum Disorders

According to DSM-5, the individual should meet four different criteria in order to be diagnosed with ASD: persistent deficits in social communication and social interaction across contexts, not accounted for by general developmental delays; restricted, repetitive patterns of behavior, interests, or activities; symptoms must be present in early childhood (but may not become fully manifest until social demands exceed limited capacities); and symptoms together limit and impair everyday functioning (American Psychiatric Association).

### Clinical Considerations

The literature reports no differences in prevalence of caries between children with ASD and others, providing there is no other underlying medical condition. A probable reason for this is that families or caregivers are able to provide a good diet for the child, with a low intake of cariogenic items. However, there are reports of more plaque and gingivitis compared with dental records of healthy children. The reason may again be related to families or caregivers, as many children and adolescents with ASD are dependent on help from others to carry out oral hygiene procedures. Brushing the teeth of children and adolescents with ASD is often difficult.

If the dental team knows beforehand that the child has been diagnosed with ASD, it is advisable to discuss the case history and treatment with the parents before the first visit. This could be achieved by either contacting the family by phone or scheduling a separate appointment with the parents alone. One advantage of having the parents visit the clinic before the child's appointment is that they might feel more comfortable when they bring their child—they easily find their way, know where to park, and already know the dentist. Additionally, parental input may be more important for ASD child patients than for average children.

Interviews with parents should focus on the child's strengths, what the child likes, appropriate rewards, and whether or not the child speaks and if not, the best way to communicate. It is also important to find out about the child's fears, particularly things like noise or a strong light. Children with ASD are often overly sensitive to sounds, tastes, smells, and sights. In the dental treatment situation, children with ASD need help to understand and focus on the treatment. Many children feel comfortable with established rituals, which can be used for treatment. It is important for the patient to meet the same dentist and preferably the same assistant or dental hygienist in order to get to know the personnel and learn to trust them. Several appointments are often necessary for an introduction to dental care. As for most patients with neuropsychiatric disorder, children with ASD need help to both understand and to focus on the treatment situation. Reducing incoming visual and auditory stimuli is often helpful. This will be discussed further when describing the management of patients with ADHD.

As many children with ASD have difficulty with abstract reasoning, the communication should be modified to suit the individual patient. Use concrete language and eliminate abstract concepts. Many children with ASD are quite literal and often misunderstand abstract sayings like "it's raining cats and dogs" or "take my hand." It is wise to be clear and objective in communication. Just tell the child what you want to achieve, give simple directions, and skip the small talk. Avoid detailed explanations and nonverbal cues—the child will often be happier with very concrete information. For example, you fix a tooth because it is broken. The reason behind the cavity is not important.

The introduction to examination or treatment may be carried out over a number of appointments spaced one or a few days apart. Alternatively, several short appointments sequentially on the same day may be used. A stepwise introduction to gradually more stress-provoking items and parts of a normal dental visit is carried out. It is important to allow sufficient pause between the steps if that is what the child requires. Praising and rewarding the child is essential, and it should immediately follow good cooperation.

Many children and adolescents with ASD and other neuropsychiatric disorders use pictures or photographs as an aid in communication. The dentist can easily create this type of individually customized aid by using a digital camera and a printer. The set of photos should include pictures of the dental clinic, as well as the dentist and the staff whom the patient will meet. A photo of an open mouth will symbolize "open your mouth," and other useful pictures can depict a toothbrush, equipment for prophylaxis, a mirror, the operatory lamp, and the dental chair. The photographs can be arranged in a photo album in the sequence the patient will see them at the appointment (Bäckman and Pilebro 1999). The album also can be used as a pedagogic tool both at home when preparing for the visit and during the appointment as an aid to communicate what will happen next. Knowing what will happen is probably one of the most important factors to reduce anxiety and prevent behavior management problems in all children. For children with neuropsychiatric disorders, it may be more difficult to ensure that the child fully understands what will happen and that he/she feels at ease with that information. Pedagogic tools like the photos in the album or written social stories describing the expected course of events are very useful and function as an itinerary or travel plan for the appointment. Parents can help with this, as they know what their child will experience during the dental appointment and they will be better prepared to support and encourage their child both before and during the visits.

In most instances, parents should be encouraged to remain with their child during treatment. Many dentists acknowledge that most parents can be helpful, as they signal that the treatment is satisfactory. Further, the children feel safe having someone as a support in the special or strange situation. Undoubtedly, there are exceptions to parental presence. Some fearful or dental phobic parents will not be supportive to the child, and there could be parents who refuse to be present. In some instances, the dentist may not want the parent present during treatments like oral surgery.

The introduction to treatment can be carried out by a dental assistant or hygienist. Once the child is judged to feel safe with all introductory steps, an examination appointment is scheduled with the dentist, preferably with the same personnel who performed the introduction.

Photographs are used during this appointment to show the child the different steps in treatment. Using the same photos and having the same hierarchy of treatment steps helps the child to cooperate and feel safe, even when meeting a new member of the dental team. The album signals that "this is the way we do things here and you, the patient, can rely on us." This kind of aid is also useful when treating other patients, like patients with ADHD, intellectual disability, or even young or anxious children (Bäckman and Pilebro 1999). Photographs also can serve as tools or aids for toothbrushing at home. For this purpose, photos could show what will be used to brush the teeth, toothpaste, a helping parent, and, for some patients, illustrations of tooth surfaces to be cleaned (Pilebro and Bäckman 2005).

It is usually possible to carry out a dental examination with a mirror and probe and to perform preventive measures like toothbrushing, polishing, and applying topical fluorides after this kind of special introduction to dental care. But for a majority of children with ASD, it is more problematic to take radiographs or restorative treatment. Not all children can be managed with nonpharmacologic techniques. Some patients do well with light sedation, while others do not. For the latter, general anesthesia is often required for comprehensive dentistry. Knowing that a child may require a general anesthetic for treatment, every effort should be made to help the patient remain healthy. The preventive care should preferably include both chair-side prevention and enhanced self-care, and it can be conducted by dental hygienists and/or trained dental assistants. To enhance the dental care, ASD children are scheduled for frequent recall appointments to maintain contact and ensure successful experiences. There are also specific issues concerning communication and environment to minimize the risk for behavioral problems. They will be elaborated upon in the next section.

## Attention Deficit Hyperactivity Disorder

This is a relatively common disorder affecting around 7% of children and adolescents (Thomas et al. 2015). Hence, it is something that all dental healthcare personnel are likely to meet. More boys than girls are diagnosed, although girls, who show fewer observable symptoms—such as hyperactivity—are supposedly under-diagnosed. The etiology is not fully understood, but it is regarded as a highly heritable disorder in most cases of familial origin. Parents with ADHD have a greater than 50% probability of having a child with ADHD. A majority of children with ADHD have at least one close biological relative who presents with symptoms of ADHD. However, the disorder can also be acquired, and some individuals have a combination of genetic and acquired ADHD. ADHD can be considered a disorder of neurotransmitter function, with particular focus on the neurotransmitters dopamine and norepinephrine. Inattention, hyperactivity, and impulsivity are the main problems in ADHD, and the diagnosis can be of a combined type (most common) in which the individual exhibits symptoms in all domains. Treatment includes both medication (mainly with methylphenidate or amphetamine) and psycho-educative strategies with didactic programs for parents and teachers.

There is much disagreement regarding the oral health status of children with ADHD. However, it appears that there is a slight increase in risk for dental caries, especially as reports point to higher frequency of food and beverage intakes and a lower frequency of toothbrushing in children and adolescents with ADHD (Blomqvist et al. 2007).

## Clinical Considerations

Reports indicate more dental behavior management problems and more dental anxiety in children with ADHD (Blomqvist et al. 2006). The reason for this is not fully understood, but it is likely that many children with ADHD have difficulties adjusting their level of activity to the demand of the dental setting. Many children and adolescents with ADHD behave and function at a lower age level in the dental setting. If the dental team does not understand the reason behind the child's behavior and does not adapt the treatment and demands to the child's capacities, there is an obvious risk for behavioral problems. Forcing a child to accept treatment is never a good idea. Instead, children with ADHD are often successfully managed when given an appropriate introduction to the treatment. The chances of a successful appointment are enhanced if the child feels safe and trusts the dental team. To achieve this, the dentist must allow himself sufficient time for the treatment. An environment that helps the child focus on the dental treatment must be provided, thus facilitating acceptance of treatment.

As for all special child patients, preventing oral health problems and promoting a positive attitude and acceptance of dental care should have the highest priority. Try to reduce disturbing visual and auditory noise to help the child focus on the treatment. To help the child concentrate, reduce unnecessary sensory input by turning off the radio or music, closing the door to the treatment room to reduce background noise and disturbances, and removing visual distractors like toys or books. This might seem strange, as it counters the working of most dental offices. However, one of the problems for children with ADHD is to select and filter the incoming stimuli. They drown in too much input. The same caution applies to communication. Dentists and other health professionals often think that conversation and small talk is beneficial for the patient. While this is true for many patients, this is not the case for children with neuropsychiatric disorders. Like children with ASD, those with ADHD need to be informed as to what will happen during the treatment. Again, using photos can be helpful. Further, they need to know who they will meet and who will do the treatment, the length of the treatment procedure, and finally, what will happen afterward. Using direct and objective guidance during the treatment helps the child to focus. It is far better to direct the child by saying "Sit in the chair," rather than "Would you like to sit in the chair?" (Blomqvist et al. 2007). The first statement is a direct instruction, whereas the latter statement could be interpreted as a question. A child may well reply to the question with a "No, I don't want to." In that case, it is next to impossible to proceed with the planned treatment without encountering problems.

At this time, readers should have recognized similarities in the approach to many different disabilities. Many of the techniques used to manage children with ASD are the same used for other neuropsychiatric disorders including ADHD, for children with intellectual disabilities, and for other children with special needs or anxiety. The key is to select what works best for the individual child.

## Homecare for Children with Disabilities

Children with disabilities and chronic medical conditions spend lots of time meeting doctors and healthcare professionals due to their medical circumstances. Good oral health is particularly important in this regard as to reduce the need for multiple dental appointments. Children with disabilities have been reported to have experienced oral discomfort and pain more often than their healthy peers and have their teeth brushed less often than others

(Krekmanova et al. 2016). This illustrates that homecare for this special population is essential but not always easy for parents and caretakers to succeed with.

As dental caries is the major dental problem for children, homecare should focus on this. Unfortunately, the scientific evidence of most pediatric dental treatment, including dental care for children with disabilities, shows major knowledge gaps (Mejàre et al. 2015). Exceptions are preventives measure (fluoride toothpaste and possibly fissure sealants) where the quality of evidence is high or moderate. Based on this and the multiple primary studies behind it, toothbrushing twice a day using fluoride toothpaste forms the foundation of home preventive care. In order to succeed in doing this, the parents and caretakers need information, instruction, and support. As for all children, parents are responsible for their children's oral hygiene and toothbrushing, but depending on age and capacity, children are more and more involved, and for some adolescents with disabilities, the young individual should eventually also have full responsibility.

The dental team should help the parents to establish a routine for oral hygiene procedures every morning and evening. It is advisable to use a soft toothbrush that is not too big. An ordinary brush may suffice, but there are also alternatives in the market with multiple sets of bristles (e.g., the Superbrush® and Collis Curve®; see Figure 8-2). These are designed to brush the occlusal as well as the lingual and buccal sides of the teeth simultaneously. For many patients, a powered electric toothbrush may be helpful. This has to be introduced step by step, as some children object to the sensation and noise.

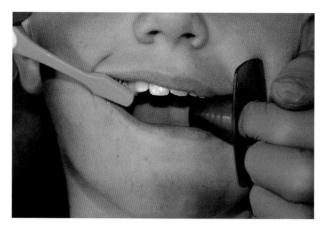

**Figure 8-3** A prop is often useful to facilitate toothbrushing.

Depending on the child's capacity, diagnosis, and layout of the bathroom, it may be easier to carry out toothbrushing using a changing table or with the parent sitting with the child on the lap outside of the bathroom. Parents should be advised to stabilize the body and head by gently having the child lean on them. In this way, involuntary and sudden head movements may be avoided or controlled. In order to enhance visibility of the teeth while brushing, parents should be instructed by the health professional and shown how to retract lips and cheeks. The use of a bite support (or mouth prop) can be useful preventing the child from chewing on the toothbrush and making it easier for the caregiver to brush on the other side (Figure 8-3). For older children and adolescents, a cheek retractor may be a helpful tool, especially if the person brushes himself/herself.

## Concluding Remarks

Meeting patients with disabilities is not always easy, and carrying out dental treatment is even more difficult. While this is something that dental professionals have to accept, we also must be sure that it does not color our views, and care must be taken to avoid discrimination against this large group of individuals.

Research has shown that there are several possible barriers keeping children with disabilities from receiving oral health care on the same premise as others. The barriers involve factors that are related to the child patient, the family, and the medical and dental health professionals. The problem is that the oral health of children with disabilities is not a priority issue, and that no one seems to take an overriding responsibility for this area (Klingberg and Hallberg 2012). Many of the barriers have been identified in this chapter.

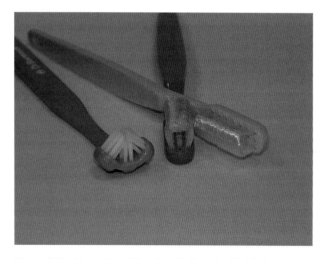

**Figure 8-2** Manual toothbrushes designed with bristles arranged to enable simultaneous cleaning of occlusal as well as buccal and lingual surfaces. A Superbrush® on the left and two Collis Curve® brushes on the right.

There is a risk that children with disabilities will not have the same access to dental care or receive the same dental treatment as others. If unattended, this will lead to inequalities in oral health—that is unacceptable. This can be changed. A first step is to learn more about all children— how they develop and mature physically, emotionally, and cognitively. Secondly, one should learn more about disabilities and how different diagnoses affect oral and general health. Finally, practice with an open mind. Dentists who are motivated to treat special children will find it both stimulating and rewarding.

## References

American Association on Intellectual and Developmental Disabilities. http://www.aaidd.org/intellectual-disability/definition Accessed July 2020.

American Psychiatric Association. DSM-5 Development. http://www.dsm5.org/Pages/Default.aspx. Accessed July 2020.

Bäckman, B. and Pilebro, C. (1999). Visual pedagogy in dentistry for children with autism. *ASDC Journal of Dentistry for Children*, 66, 325–331, 294.

Bedi, R., Champion, J., and Horn, R. (2001). Attitudes of the dental team to the provision of care for people with learning disabilities. *Special Care in Dentistry*, 21, 147–152.

Bethell, C.D., Read, D., Blumberg, S.J. et al. (2008). What is the prevalence of children with special health care needs? Toward an understanding of variations in findings and methods across three national surveys. *Maternal and Child Health Journal*, 12, 1–14.

Blomqvist, M., Holmberg, K., Fernell, E. et al. (2006). Oral health, dental anxiety, and behavior management problems in children with attention deficit hyperactivity disorder. *European Journal of Oral Sciences*, 114, 385–390.

Blomqvist, M., Holmberg, K., Fernell, E. et al. (2007). Dental caries and oral health behavior in children with attention deficit hyperactivity disorder. *European Journal of Oral Sciences*, 115, 186–191.

Bradshaw, S., Bem, D., Shaw, K. et al. (2019). Improving health, wellbeing and parenting skills in parents of children with special health care needs and medical complexity – a scoping review. *BMC Pediatrics*, 19, 301.

Brogårdh-Roth, S. (2010). The preterm child in dentistry. Behavioural aspects and oral health. PhD Thesis. Malmö University, Sweden.

Casamassimo, P.S., Seale, N.S., and Ruehs, K. (2004). General dentists' perceptions of educational and treatment issues affecting access to care for children with special health care needs. *Journal of Dental Education*, 68, 23–28.

Centers for Disease Control and Prevention (CDC) Obesity and overweight. https://www.cdc.gov/obesity/index.html. Accessed July 2020.

Champion, J. and Holt, R. (2000). Dental care for children and young people who have a hearing impairment. *British Dental Journal*, 189, 155–159.

Child Friendly Healthcare. https://www.coe.int/en/web/children/child-friendly-healthcare. Accessed July 2020.

Dao, L.P., Zwetchkenbaum, S., and Inglehart, M.R. (2005). General dentists and special needs patients: Does dental education matter? *Journal of Dental Education*, 69, 1107–1115.

Delaney, A.L. and Arvedson, J.C. (2008). Development of swallowing and feeding: prenatal through first year of life. *Developmental Disabilities Research Reviews*, 14, 105–117.

Faulks, D., Freeman, L., Thompson, S. et al. (2012). The value of education in special care dentistry as a means of reducing inequalities in oral health. *European Journal of Dental Education*, 16, 195–201.

Faulks, D., Norderyd, J., Molina, G. et al. (2013). Using the International Classification of Functioning, Disability and Health (ICF) to describe children referred to special care or paediatric dental services. *PLoS One*, 8, e61993.

Gilbert, C. (2001). New Issues in Childhood Blindness. *Community Eye Health*, 14, 53–56.

Gillberg. C. (1995). Epidemiological overview. In: C. Gillberg (Ed.), Clinical Child Neuropsychiatry (pp. 4–11). Cambridge University Press, Cambridge.

Gillberg, C. and Coleman, M. (2000). The Biology of the Autistic Syndromes, 3rd ed. Mac Keith, London.

Hallberg, U., Oskarsdóttir, S., and Klingberg, G. (2010). 22q11 deletion syndrome—the meaning of a diagnosis. A qualitative study on parental perspectives. *Child: Care, Health and Development*, 36, 719–725.

Hallberg, U., Strandmark, M., and Klingberg, G. (2004). Dental health professionals' treatment of children with disabilities: a qualitative study. *Acta Odontologica Scandinavica*, 62, 319–327.

Hebbal, M. and Ankola, A.V. (2012). Development of a new technique (ATP) for training visually impaired children in oral hygiene maintenance. *European Archives of Pediatric Dentistry*, 13, 244–245.

Kang, J., Vann, J.Y., Jr., Lee, J.Y. et. al. (2012). The safety of sedation for overweight/obese children in the dental setting. *Pediatric Dentistry*, 34, 392–396.

Klingberg, G. and Hallberg, U. (2012). Oral health—not a priority issue: A grounded theory analysis of barriers for young patients with disabilities to receive oral health care on the same premise as others. *European Journal of Oral Sciences*, 120, 232–238.

Krekmanova, L., Hakeberg, M., Robertson, A. et al. (2016). Perceived oral discomfort and pain in children and adolescents with intellectual or physical disabilities as reported by their legal guardians. *European Archives of Paediatric Dentistry*, 17, 23–30.

Levine, R. (2012). Obesity and oral disease—a challenge for dentistry. *British Dental Journal*, 213, 453–456.

Mason, S.J., Harris, G., and Blissett, J. (2005). Tube feeding in infancy: Implications for the development of normal eating and drinking skills. *Dysphagia*, 20, 46–61.

Mejàre, I.A., Klingberg, G., Mowafi, F.K. et al. (2015). A systematic map of systematic reviews in pediatric dentistry – what do we really know? *PLoS One*, Feb 23;10(2):e0117537.

Merrick, J. and Carmeli, E. (2003). A review on the prevalence of disabilities in children. *The Internet Journal of Pediatrics and Neonatology*, 3(1). DOI: 10.5580/29 ac.

Mun-H-Center. National Orofacial Resource Centre for Rare Disorders. https://www.mun-h-center.se/en/. Accessed July 2020.

Norderyd, J. (2015). Oral health, medical diagnoses, and functioning profiles in children with disabilities receiving paediatric specialist dental care – a study using the ICF-CY. *Disability and Rehabilitation*, 37, 1431–1438.

Nunn, J.H. (2000). Paediatric dentistry: Are we dealing with hearing-impaired children correctly? *British Dental Journal*, 189, 151–154.

Ogden, C.L., Carroll, M.D., Curtin, L.R. et al. (2010). Prevalence of high body mass index in US children and adolescents, 2007-2008. *Journal of the American Medical Association*, 303, 242–249.

Online Mendelian Inheritance in Man® (OMIM®) https://omim.org/. Accessed July 2020.

Orphanet. http://www.orpha.net/consor/cgi-bin/index.php?lng=EN. Accessed July 2020.

Pilebro, C. and Bäckman, B. (2005). Teaching oral hygiene to children with autism. *International Journal of Paediatric Dentistry*, 15, 1–9.

Reilly, D., Boyle, C.A., and Craig, D.C. (2009). Obesity and dentistry: A growing problem. *British Dental Journal*, 207, 171–175.

Rommel, N., De Meyer, A.M., Feenstra, L. et al. (2003). The complexity of feeding problems in 700 infants and young children presenting to a tertiary care institution. *Journal of Pediatric Gastroenterology and Nutrition*, 37, 75–84.

Scheeran, T., Marvin, R.S., and Pianta, R.C. (1997). Mother's resolution of their child's diagnosis and self-reported measures of parenting stress, marital relations, and social support. *Journal of Pediatric Psychology*, 22, 197–212.

Tait, A.R., Voepel-Lewis, T., Burke, C. et al. (2008). Incidence and risk factors for perioperative adverse respiratory events in children who are obese. *Anesthesiology*, 108, 375–380.

Thomas, R., Sanders, S., Doust, J. et al. (2015). Prevalence of attention-deficit/hyperactivity disorder: a systematic review and meta-analysis. *Pediatrics*, 135(4), e994–e1001.

Trulsson, U. and Klingberg, G. (2003). Living with a child with a severe orofacial handicap: experiences from the perspectives of parents. *European Journal of Oral Sciences*, 111, 19–25.

Tseng, R., Vann, W.F. Jr., and Perrin, E.M. (2010). Addressing childhood overweight and obesity in the dental office: Rationale and practical guidelines. *Pediatric Dentistry*, 32, 417–23.

United Nations. Convention on the Rights of Persons with Disabilities. https://www.un.org/development/desa/disabilities/convention-on-the-rights-of-persons-with-disabilities.html Accessed July 2020.

United Nations (1989). Convention on the Rights of the Child. https://www.ohchr.org/en/professionalinterest/pages/crc.aspx. Accessed July 2020.

World Health Organization. International Classification of Diseases (ICD). https://www.who.int/classifications/icd/en/. Accessed July 2020.

World Health Organization. International Classification of Functioning, Disability and Health (ICF). https://www.who.int/classifications/icf/cn/. Accessed July 2020.

# 9

# Local Anesthesia

*Ari Kupietzky and Steven Schwartz*

## Introduction

One of the most important and challenging aspects of child behavior management is pain control. Children who undergo early painful experiences during dental procedures are likely to carry negative feelings toward dentistry into adulthood. Therefore, it is important that clinicians make every effort to minimize pain and discomfort during dental treatment. The successful children's dentist must master the skill and art of administering the most painless injection possible. Some clinicians will try to avoid the administration of local anesthesia; however, this often results in poor clinical practice. As a consequence of no local anesthesia, a rubber dam will rarely or never be used and cavity preparations may be left shallow, with the end result far from optimal. In addition, there are times when an anticipated "minor" procedure becomes a major procedure and the patient is placed in a painful situation because of the lack of dental anesthesia.

On the other hand, one of the greatest single fears of the pediatric dental patient is "the needle" (Eichenbaum and Dunn 1971). Childhood fears emanate from many sources, and some can be extremely obscure. One possible cause of general dental anxiety may be previous exposure to invasive medical care in early childhood (Karjalainen et al. 2003). A review (Sokolowski et al. 2010) on needle phobia presented several publications suggesting that the fear of needles may result after a negative experience at a physician's or dentist's office. Many childhood fears are learned and may be the result of early childhood conditioning (i.e., "shots" administered from infancy). The average child will receive 21 vaccines in up to six to seven injections before the age of six years. Children may not be voluntarily cooperative during these immunization procedures, and sometimes they may be physically restrained. Ost (1991)

examined subjects with injection phobia and showed that 56% could trace their fear back to negative conditioning from a healthcare experience. The mean age onset was eight years and often correlated with a first-time-healthcare–related appointment. This study also determined that 24% of the subjects could trace their phobias to having seen another child, often a sibling, have a negative experience to needles.

As a consequence of these conflicting concerns—the dentist wanting to control pain with local anesthesia and the child fearing the pain of the needle—injection procedures present an almost constant challenge to the dentist's skills. Thus, the aims of this chapter, which covers an important aspect of behavior management, are (1) to discuss factors associated with administering injections and (2) to review the most commonly used local anesthetic techniques for children. The chapter will not present every type of local anesthesia, nor will it include detailed techniques. It will focus instead on the most commonly used injections, with an emphasis on how to administer local anesthesia with minimum pain and maximum effect.

## Administration of Local Anesthesia

It is extremely important for the dentist to have an effective system for the administration of local anesthesia. Children are very sensitive to body language. Pediatric patients can detect uncertainty or hesitation, which can lead to difficulty. If the dentist's approach, and that of the assistant's, are not confident and well-timed, the child may easily sense their attitude and resist every effort that they make. Considerable skill is needed for administering local anesthesia to children while avoiding behavior problems. Some of the following clinical procedures, which have been

*Wright's Behavior Management in Dentistry for Children*, Third Edition. Edited by Ari Kupietzky.
© 2022 John Wiley & Sons, Inc. Published 2022 by John Wiley & Sons, Inc.

developed over the years, are widely accepted and highly successful with children. Others, however, are debatable.

## Preparation of Patient

Preparation of the patient prior to injection consists of two components: mental and physical.

Mental preparation begins with explaining the anesthesia administration process to the child in terminology that they can understand. The child may be sitting upright in a non-threatened position. Consider the following narrative:

> "Today I'm going to put your tooth to sleep, wash some germs out of your tooth and fix your tooth and make it all better. When your tooth falls asleep your lip and tongue will feel fat and funny for a little while. You will not look funny or fat. You will just feel funny and fat.
>
> To make your tooth fall asleep, I am going to use sleepy juice. Only your tooth will go to sleep, not you! The sleepy juice doesn't taste so good, so as soon as I put it next to your tooth, I will wash it away with some water. Oh, and while I put the juice next to your tooth I will give you a little pinch. A pinch only hurts a little. Not a lot. Let's pretend to do it. Not for real, just pretend. I'm going to show you everything I do so you can see how easy this is."

The dentist asks the child to pinch her arm. Some children may hesitate, but after a little coaxing, they will happily proceed to pinch the dentist. At this point, the dentist may turn around and, with a smile, inform the accompanying parent that kids love this part of the procedure. During the pinch, the dentist says: "That hurt me, but not a lot. It hurt very little. I do not need to cry for such a little pinch."

The dentist now takes the child's arm and gently pinches the skin. The slight amount of pain created will not upset most children, and the child has now learned an objective association for the expectation of the injection, "the pinch." The dentist proceeds to gently pinch the cheek or gingiva adjacent to the tooth and immediately spray water, demonstrating the feeling of the intraoral pinch and subsequent washing away of the bitter sleepy juice. The dentist then says, "you are a good boy (or girl) and I am sure you can stand a little pinch like that." An overwhelming majority of children will agree and will cooperate during the injection.

## Chair Position

Some authors have suggested giving injections, particularly mandibular blocks, with the patient in a somewhat upright position, resulting in the patient's mandible being

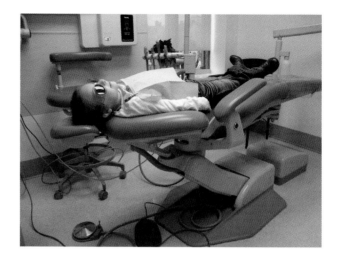

**Figure 9-1** Most pediatric dentists prefer to deliver local anesthetics with the patient in a supine position.

approximately parallel to the floor and the clinician's elbow close to the body. Most pediatric dentists prefer to deliver local anesthetics with the patient in a supine position (Figure 9-1). This is especially true for those using custom-made benches, as shown in Chapter 18. The anatomical positions and injections are essentially the same. However, when the child is in the supine position, the mandible is at approximately a 30° angle to the floor, and the clinician's elbow will be high, with the arm nearly parallel to the floor. The patient is positioned with the head and heart parallel to the floor and the feet slightly elevated. Positioning the patient in this manner reduces the incidence of syncope that can occur as a result of increased anxiety. In addition, the patient's sudden movements are more easily controlled.

"It will be much easier for me to see your teeth if you lay back, so I will give you a ride and make the chair go back. Before I give you the pinch, I will practice with you again and explain everything." Repeating the explanation and pinch while the child is reclined may not be necessary with all children. In addition, if the child has been holding a hand mirror, it should be taken by the assistant with the promise that it will be shortly returned.

## Assembling the Syringe

There is debate among clinicians as to whether the syringe and its components should be assembled in or out of view of the patient. The majority of pediatric dentists attempt to keep anesthetic syringes out of the sight of child patients (Starkey 1983). Proponents of assembling the syringe out of the patient's sight assert that most children have developed a fear of the injection during prior visits to the pediatrician, and the slightest suspicion that they are getting an injection will set them off. This is especially true when told stories by

(a)

(b)

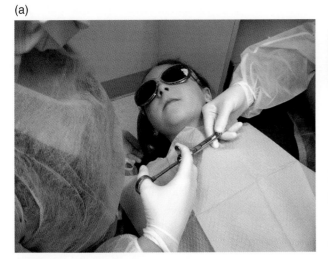

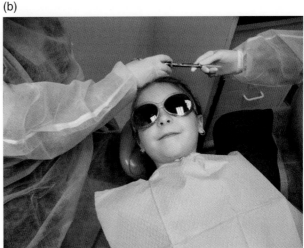

**Figure 9-2** With the proper technique, the child need not ever see the syringe. It is always passed and held in blind spots, away from the patient's view: under the child's chin (a) and behind her head (b).

older siblings and friends. In addition, the word "injection" has not been used. From the perspective of the child, he or she is simply getting a special pinch with sleepy juice. Introducing the syringe may complicate the process. In addition, some children may insist on removing the cap, thus exposing the needle. With proper technique the child need not ever see the syringe, which is always passed and held in blind spots, away from the patient's view (Figure 9-2).

Proponents of assembling the syringe in view of the patient assert that doing so acts as a desensitization technique. The patient has the opportunity to touch and feel the individual, non-threatening components, reducing patient apprehension linked to prior injections. Clinicians who opt to show the syringe and its assembly in view of the patient may use the following narrative during syringe assembly.

"I'm going to make the tooth go to sleep and feel fat and funny with my sleepy juice. The sleepy juice is kept in this little glass jar." (Allow the child to hold the cartridge.) "We place the jar in a special water sprayer," (allow the child to hold the syringe) "and we place a plastic straw at the end of the water sprayer." (Allow the child to hold the covered needle.)

### Case 9.1

Jack, a six-year-old boy, is seated in the dental chair for his first restorative appointment. The dentist explains to Jack that she will be putting his tooth to sleep by pinching the cheek near the tooth and, at the same time, squirting sleeping juice around the tooth. Jack becomes excited and upset. He asks the dentist: "Are you going to give me a shot? I don't want a shot. Shots hurt. Show me the shot!"

*Case 9.1, Discussion*: **Option 1.** The dentist answers: "I am not giving you a shot, only a pinch." The child suddenly moves and sees the syringe. He screams: "You are a liar! You are giving me a shot!" The boy manages to jump off the chair and run out of the room. A severe behavior problem ensued, and no amount of talk from the dentist made any difference to the child. The parents opted to switch to another dentist.

**Option 2.** The dentist answers: "As I told you before, I am going to give you a little pinch and put your tooth to sleep. Let's pretend and pinch your cheek. See? It only hurts a little. Now let's do it for real." Jack answers: "How do you squirt the sleepy juice? Show it to me!" Dentist: "I am like a magician. Magicians never reveal their tricks. Maybe later, if you are a good patient, I will show you how I do it." Most patients will not ask to see the syringe at the end of their treatment.

**Option 3.** The dentist answers: "Yes, I am going to give to you a shot, if that is what you want to call it. I know how to give a shot in a special way so that it does not hurt a lot, only a little. I don't call it a shot, I call it a pinch." Jack answers: "Show it to me!" The dentist shows Jack the covered syringe.

There are unlimited ways to successfully manage the above scenario. However, it is obvious that Option 1 is not one of them. The dentist lied to the child, thereby losing all credibility. In Option 2, the dentist never acknowledged that a shot would be given, yet she did not deny it either. She never stated that she would not be giving an injection. In many instances, the child will receive the injection, never aware of it being a "shot"—just an uncomfortable pinch. The child was worried about the shot, not the pinch.

Jack had been adversely preconditioned to injections. His fear of the shot might have emanated from his experience with vaccinations. He disliked them and remembered crying. Although he returned from his first dental appointment excited and pleased, he became very anxious in anticipation of the next visit. He had told his best friend in kindergarten how much fun the visit was. The friend responded by warning him of his next visit, when the dentist would give him a shot.

## Administration of the Anesthetic

There are two important goals which one must accomplish during anesthetic administration: controlling and limiting movement of the patient's head and body and communicating with the patient to draw their attention away from the minor discomfort that may be felt during the injection process. Most clinicians prefer to keep the uncapped needle out of the patient's line of sight. The child should not be asked to close her eyes, as that is usually a sign that something bad or painful is about to occur. In addition, pain perception may be enhanced with eyes closed. Instead, the assistant should pass the uncapped syringe behind the patient's head (Figure 9-2). Once the assistant has handed the syringe to the dentist and has freed her hands, she positions them over the patient. The assistant should not actively restrain or even touch the child's arms unless an attempt is made by the patient to lift her arms to reject treatment (Figure 9-3). Just touching the arms, as if to restrain, may cause apprehension in the child and, at that moment, the youngster may attempt to resist physically.

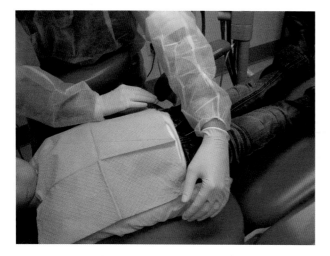

**Figure 9-3** The assistant should not actively restrain or even touch the child's arms unless an attempt is made by the patient to lift her arms to reject treatment.

Instead, the dental assistant should position her hands above the child's hands to intercept any untoward movement.

### Stabilization

Before placing the syringe in the mouth, the patient's head should be stabilized. There are two basic positions for stabilizing the patient's head. A behind-the-patient position is assumed for injecting the quadrants that are contralateral to the clinician's favored hand and the anterior regions (i.e., right-handed clinicians injecting the left side, left-handed clinicians injecting the right side). The clinician stabilizes the patient's head by supporting the head against the clinician's body with the less favored hand and arm. He stabilizes the jaw by resting the fingers against the mandible for support and retraction of the lips and cheek.

For injections on the same side as the clinician's favored hand (i.e., right side for right-handed clinicians and left side for left-handed clinicians), the clinician assumes a more forward position—eight o'clock for right-handed clinicians and four o'clock for left-handed clinicians (Figure 9-4a and b). The clinician stabilizes the patient's head and retracts the soft tissues with the fingers of the weaker hand resting on the bones of the maxilla and mandible.

### Communication and Distraction

The clinician speaks with the patient in a reassuring manner during anesthesia administration. The subject matter can range from describing the process using child-friendly terminology, to praise, to storytelling, to singing, or, if the clinician is totally unimaginative, counting. Avoid words like shot, pain, hurt, and injection and substitute them with words like cold, warm, weird, fat, and funny.

"The sleepy juice may feel real cold. So what I'll do is count, and by the time I reach five the water will warm up."

Two distraction techniques, which may be employed, are described. The child is asked to say "la, la, la, la" during the pinch. Not "ah, ah, ah, ah" but "la, la, la, la." The patient also may be asked to raise the left or right leg during the injection. After depositing the desired amount of anesthetic, the syringe is withdrawn and the needle safely recapped.

Finally, the mouth is rinsed with water from the triple syringe, thus eliminating any blood from view: "Does the sleepy juice taste bitter? Let me rinse it away. Here is some water. Swallow the water. Wow, what a great helper you are." Include a specific compliment: "You were very still."

The assistant may return the hand mirror to the child. "Your tooth and cheek feel fat and funny, but you look the

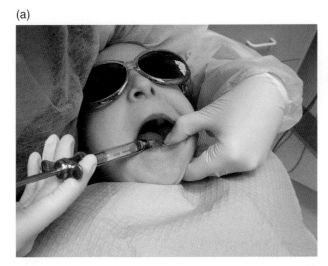 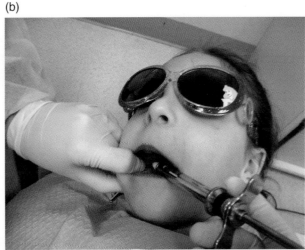

(a) (b)

**Figure 9-4** A behind-the-patient position is assumed for injecting the contralateral quadrants to the clinician's favored hand (i.e., right-handed clinicians injecting the left side). The clinician stabilizes the patient's head by supporting the head against the clinician's body with the less favored hand and arm (a). For injections on the same side as the clinician's favored hand (i.e., right side for right-handed clinicians), the clinician assumes a forward position of eight o'clock (b).

same." The child looks in the mirror and sees that all appears normal, although the mouth does indeed feel strange.

### Case 9.2

Dr. H. planned to administer a mandibular block to a six-year-old patient. The child sat still while the dentist took the injection syringe from the dental assistant and gave the injection. Dr. H. then said, "You are a good helper."

*Case 9.2, Discussion*: Dr. H. was fortunate that the patient was highly cooperative. Had the child not been an ideal patient, the injection might not have gone as smoothly. Two oversights occurred. First, Dr. H. offered little support to the child during the injection. Sometimes, a dentist becomes anxious about an injection or concentrates on the procedure and almost forgets the patient. The dentist must not be silent during the injection process. A continuous flow of verbal reinforcement should take place throughout the procedure. The voice contact distracts and supports the child. Silence seems to promote the development of apprehension and anxiety in children.

Second, the dentist's compliment to the child was vague. To reinforce cooperative behavior appropriately, verbal praise should be specific. During the injection, the dentist could have said: "You are a good helper. You are sitting still and opening wide. That really helps. Thank you." This makes the constant patter more meaningful.

### Topical Anesthesia

Topical anesthetics are available in gel, liquid, ointment, patch, and pressurized spray forms. Topical anesthetics are effective to a depth of 2–3 mm and are limited in their effect to reduce the discomfort of the initial penetration of the needle into the mucosa: they offer little benefit when performing a mandibular block. The benefits of topical anesthetics may not be entirely pharmacological; a psychological advantage may ensue. A number of investigations have compared topical anesthetics with placebo intraorally with conflicting results (Meechan 2008). Some show positive benefits from the use of topical anesthesia before needle insertion and others do not. There is no evidence that topical anesthetics have any value in reducing the discomfort of regional block administrations, such as inferior alveolar nerve block injections (Meechan 2002). In addition, their disadvantages include a disagreeable taste that may be a cause of patient discomfort, sometimes eliciting crying even before the actual injection is given. In addition, the length of application time may increase apprehension of the approaching procedure in the pediatric patient. The application duration time is a crucial factor governing effectiveness (beyond a placebo). The onset times of topical anesthetics range between thirty seconds and five minutes. Many clinicians do not wait for the anesthetic to take effect; they proceed with the injection almost immediately after placing the topical. In a survey on local anesthesia, Kohli et al. (2001) reported that two-thirds of the responding pediatric dentists waited a minute or less. In addition, most practitioners responded that patients disliked the taste, consistency, and the warm or burning sensation of the topical anesthetics. A majority of the respondents (86%) always used a topical anesthetic, while 9% sometimes used a topical anesthetic, 4% rarely used a topical anesthetic, and 1% reported that they never used a topical anesthetic. Another reason for the widespread use of topical anesthetic may be the expectation of the accompanying parent, who presumes that its use is crucial for a painless injection. However, if a child has been referred due to behavior problems and the previous dentist used a topical anesthetic, it might be best to avoid it.

Benzocaine is a very common topical anesthetic. It is not known to produce systemic toxicity in adults, but can produce local allergic reactions. However, the Food and Drug Administration announced in April 2011 that "Topical benzocaine sprays, gels, and liquids used as anesthesia during medical procedures and for analgesia from tooth and gum pain may cause methemoglobinemia, a rare but serious and potentially fatal condition." Children younger than two years appear to be at particular risk. In the most severe cases, methemoglobinemia can result in death. Patients who develop methemoglobinemia may experience signs and symptoms such as pale gray- or blue-colored skin, lips, and nail beds; headaches; lightheadedness; shortness of breath; fatigue; and rapid heart rate.

### Application of Topical Anesthetic

Use a 2 × 2 gauze to dry the tissue and remove any gross debris around the site of needle penetration. The effectiveness of the topical will be enhanced when applied onto dry mucosa. Retract the lip to obtain adequate visibility during the injection. Wipe and dry the lip to make retraction easier. "I'm wiping your tooth and gums with my little washcloth to make sure everything is clean."

Apply a small amount of topical only at the site of preparation, thus avoiding anesthetizing the pharyngeal tissues. The topical anesthetic should remain in contact with the soft tissue for one to two minutes. "Now I'm rubbing (goofy, cherry, bubble gum) tooth jelly next to your tooth. If it begins to feel too warm or goofy let me know and I'll wash it away with the special water."

### Needle Selection

Controversy centers on both the gauge and length of needles. The most common gauges are 25-, 27-, and 30-gauge. Needles come in three lengths: long, short, and ultrashort. Gauge refers to the diameter of the lumen of the needle; the smaller the number, the greater the diameter of the lumen. For example, a 30-gauge needle has a smaller internal diameter than a 25-gauge needle. There is a trend among dentists toward the use of smaller-diameter needles

on the assumption that they are less traumatic to the patient. Proponents of large gauges claim that these needles yield better aspiration and may cause less pain during initial penetration of the mucosa, believing that needles with a smaller diameter result in less injection pain than wider-diameter needles. Studies have refuted both points. Trapp and Davies (1980) and Delgado-Molina et al. (2003) reported that no significant differences existed in the ability to aspirate blood through 25-, 27-, and 30-gauge dental needles. On the contrary, the studies concluded that there is increased resistance to aspiration of blood through a thinner needle (e.g., 30-gauge) compared with a larger-diameter needle (e.g., 27- or 25-gauge). With regard to pain experienced by the patient, numerous studies have reported that patients are unable to differentiate among 23-, 25-, 27-, and 30-gauge needles—no significant differences in the perception of pain produced by them were reported (Reed et al. 2012).

Pain associated with dental anesthesia results mostly from the pressure caused when the anesthetic solution is injected into the mucosa—especially during the first few seconds—and less so from the actual needle penetration. The pressure produced is greater when using high gauges than with lower gauges. Needle deflection along the axis of the bevel and breakage must also be considered when choosing the gauge. The smaller the diameter of the needle, the more it deflects. Thus, 30-gauge needles deflect significantly, whereas 25-gauge needles essentially do not deflect at all. Likewise, 25-gauge needles very rarely, if ever, break during an intraoral injection. This is an important advantage when treating a child who may make sudden movements. Malamed et al. (2010) reported that 99% of the needles that do break are 30-gauge needles. In his classic textbook, *The Handbook of Local Anesthesia*, he recommends using the smallest gauge (largest diameter) needle available, which allows for easier aspiration, less deflection of the needle as it perforates the soft tissue, and less chance of breakage at the hub.

Traditionally, clinicians were taught to decide on the length in relation to the type of injection (block or infiltration), the size of the patient, and the thickness of the tissue. Although a long needle has been recommended for inferior alveolar injections, short needles seem to offer better control to the dentist dealing with children. The long needle recommendation relates to the possibility of needle fracture. Proponents of long needles claim that after a needle fracture, a portion of the needle is exposed for easy removal. However, in the event of this rare happenstance, fracture usually occurs at the hub. In addition, it is never recommended to insert a short needle to the hub. Thus, long needles seem to offer little advantage over short ones, and the authors recommend the short needle for all local anesthetics (excluding the intraligamental injection for which extra short needles are indicated) for children, regardless of their age and the type of injection.

### Injection Rate

Another aspect of anesthetic technique that is often mentioned but has not been quantified is the injection rate. Most educators recommend slow injections because a rapidly expelled solution causes discomfort. But how slow is "slow?" Based on videotaped procedures, Wright et al. (1983) calculated that a slow injection takes approximately 45 seconds, using an entire 1.8 ml cartridge. In most pediatric cases, two-thirds of a cartridge are sufficient, the injection time being 30 seconds or less. Malamed (2012) recommended an injection time of one minute or more. However, the authors' experience with pediatric patients is not to prolong the injection procedure. Kohli et al. (2001) reported in their survey of American Academy of Pediatric Dentistry (AAPD) members that 56% of the respondents inject a cartridge in less than 30 seconds. The majority (89%) reported their injection time as being under one minute. A more recent study reported the average injection time of local anesthesia given to 147 children aged 4–11 years as being 48 seconds (Versloot et al. 2005).

### Testing for Anesthesia

An important aspect of clinical practice, particularly following a mandibular block administration, is determining the presence of profound anesthesia. When children are asked for signs or symptoms of anesthesia, their responses are often unreliable. Sometimes, by simply observing the child patient sitting in the dental chair and watching the mouth movements, an experienced dentist will intuitively know that the injection has taken effect. Asking a child "Are you numb?" usually will not provide the answer. Most children cannot express the feeling of numbness or understand its meaning. The clinician has to point to non-anesthetized areas and have the child compare them to the anesthetized region, saying, "Tell me where it feels funny." Many dentists have been trained to routinely probe anesthetized areas with an explorer. This does not necessarily indicate profound block anesthesia, and it causes delays in the procedure, which can build apprehension in the child patient. Another approach following a mandibular block is to observe the external signs carefully, question the patient, evaluate for positive responses, and then proceed, placing the rubber dam clamp if restorative dentistry is to be performed. While placing the clamp, the dentist should watch the child's reactions, particularly the eyes. If profound anesthesia has been obtained, there will be no flinching and the procedure can continue. On the other hand, if there is any discomfort, steps can be retraced and appropriate measures taken.

### Initial Injection

The first operative visit is undoubtedly the most significant in the dental experience of the child. It may very well be the key to his dental future. Some dentists hold the view that if a choice is to be made between a mandibular block and a maxillary supraperiosteal (commonly known as local infiltration) injection for the child's first local anesthetic experience, the mandibular block should be chosen because of the profound anesthesia that it produces. The authors' clinical impression is that the best choice is the maxillary supraperiosteal injection. This injection is made with virtually no discomfort, and there is minimal risk of missing the target area. Many children in pediatric dental practices receive supraperiosteal injections without realizing that they have been given.

## Basic Injection Technique

The anesthetic injection begins by stretching the tissue taut at the administration site (Figure 9-5). When possible, bring the tissue over the needle. Insert the needle 1–2 mm into the mucosa with the bevel oriented toward bone (Figure 9-6). Inject several drops of anesthetic before advancing the needle. While injecting, wiggle the patient's cheek. Slowly advance the needle toward the target while injecting up to a 1/4 cartridge of anesthetic to anesthetize the soft tissue ahead of the advancing needle so that the needle is constantly moving into anesthetized tissue. Aspirate. The depth of insertion will vary with the type of injection; however, one should never insert a needle in its entirety to the hub. Although it is a rare occurrence, retrieving a broken needle fully embedded in soft tissue is extremely difficult. After confirming a negative aspiration, the injection process should take under one minute. Continue injecting during needle retrieval. The clinician should be careful not to inject a greater amount of anesthetic than recommended for the patient's weight. Continue to speak to the patient throughout the injection process. Close observation of the patient's eye and hand movements, along with crying, will alert the clinician to patient discomfort.

Upon completion of treatment and dismissal of the patient, the clinician says to the patient with the accompanying adult present: "You were a terrific helper. You sat still and we finished quickly. We are a good team! I'm

(a)

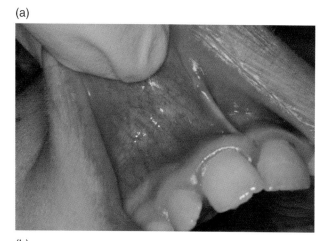

(b)

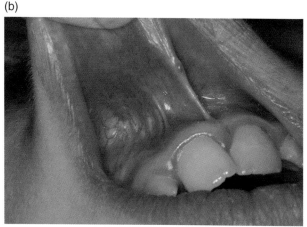

(c)

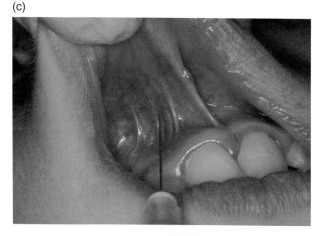

**Figure 9-5** The anesthetic injection begins by stretching (a) the tissue taut at the administration site (b). When possible, bring the tissue over the needle (c).

giving you an extra special sticker that says 'Careful! Tooth, tongue, lips asleep.' Although we're finished with today's treatment, your tooth will be asleep and your lip and tongue will feel fat and funny for another hour. Don't eat until your lip and tongue no longer feel fat and funny."

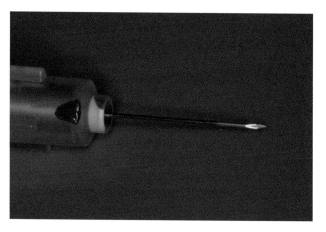

**Figure 9-6** The needle's bevel should always be oriented toward the bone. Some needles have a marking on the bevel side to help the clinician orientate the needle properly.

Some children who did not cry during treatment may begin to do so after treatment, complaining of "pain" and telling the parent that their mouth hurts. Showing the child the mouth in a mirror will help alleviate concerns that the area is swollen. At this point, the dentist should repeat that the child's mouth is numb and the feeling the patient is experiencing is not pain, but rather numbness. A child who has never had an anesthetic may ask what the word "numb" means. A possible explanation is as follows: "Do you remember when you sat on your foot and your foot went to sleep? Well, that is sort of what numb feels like. Your mouth is asleep. Don't worry, it will wake up soon and feel regular."

## Specific Injection Techniques

The most common injection techniques used in pediatric dentistry are presented in the following pages. Detailed descriptions will be omitted; however, clinical tips from a patient management perspective, specific for the pediatric patient, will be reviewed.

### Inferior Alveolar Nerve Block

The inferior alveolar nerve block (IANB) is indicated when deep operative or surgical procedures are undertaken for mandibular primary and permanent teeth. While a supraperiosteal injection (infiltration) may provide adequate anesthesia for the primary incisors and molars, it is not as effective for providing complete anesthesia for the mandibular permanent molars. In addition, it provides profound pulpal anesthesia and may be indicated when pulpal treatment is anticipated. A major consideration for IANB in the pediatric patient is that the

(a)

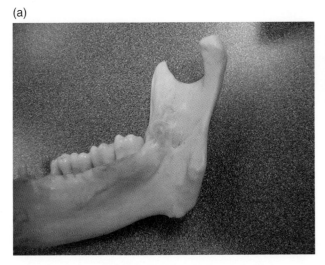

(b)

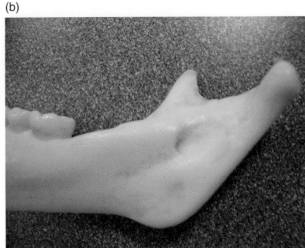

**Figure 9-7** A major consideration for inferior alveolar nerve block in the pediatric patient is that the mandibular foramen is situated at a lower level (below the occlusal plane) than in an adult (a). Thus, the injection is made slightly lower and more posteriorly than in an adult (b).

mandibular foramen is situated at a lower level (below the occlusal plane) than in an adult. Thus, the injection is made slightly lower and more posteriorly than in an adult (Figure 9-7).

Physical position can be an important factor when the dentist is injecting children, particularly when administering a mandibular block. To accomplish the mandibular injection for the right side of the mandible, the right-handed dentist approaches the face from the front. The left thumb is placed with the middle of the thumbnail at the coronoid notch and lightly over the deep tendon of the temporalis muscle (Figure 9-8). The pterygomandibular raphe is medial to the thumb. The needle penetrates the tissue at the middle of the thumbnail and is thus carried between the deep tendon of the temporalis laterally and the pterygomandibular raphe medially, entering the mandibular sulcus at the level of the lingular notch. Unfortunately, this injection provides the dentist with little control over a child's head movement.

On the opposite, or the left side of the arch, the right-handed operator's arm may be placed over the head of the patient and the left thumb on the anterior border of the ramus, with the forefinger just anterior to the mandibular angle and the middle finger just above the mandibular angle. Again, the mandibular sulcus will be at the center of the triangle formed by the tips of these two fingers and the thumb. When the right-handed operator administers a left mandibular block and places the left forearm over a child's forehead, this technique controls head movements and helps to keep the syringe out of the child's view. For these reasons, when given a choice between right and left sides, many dentists prefer beginning with the left mandibular block.

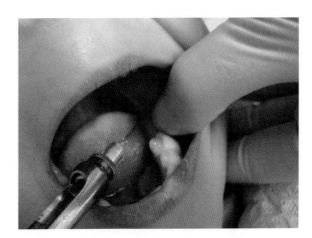

**Figure 9-8** On the left side of the arch, the right-handed operator's arm may be placed over the head of the patient and the left thumb on the anterior border of the ramus, with the forefinger just anterior to the mandibular angle and the middle finger just above the mandibular angle.

Technique:

- Lay the thumb on the occlusal surface of the molars, with the tip of the thumb resting on the internal oblique ridge and the ball of the thumb resting on the retromolar fossa. Support the mandible during the injection by resting the ball of the middle finger on the posterior border of the mandible.
- The barrel of the syringe should be directed between the two primary molars on the opposite side of the arch.
- The best way to visualize the lateral positioning of the needle prior to penetrating soft tissue is to look for the depression seen on the immediate lateral aspect of the pterygomandibular raphe while asking the patient

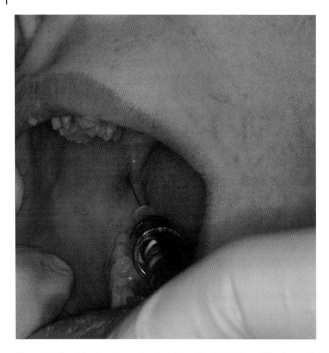

**Figure 9-9** The best way to visualize the lateral positioning of the needle prior to penetrating soft tissue is to look for the depression seen on the immediate lateral aspect of the pterygomandibular raphe while asking the patient to open as wide as possible and pulling the cheek taut.

to open as wide as possible and pulling the cheek taut (Figure 9-9).

- Inject a small amount of solution as the tissue is penetrated.
- Advance the needle 4 mm while injecting minute amounts (up to a 1/4 cartridge).
- Stop and aspirate.
- If aspiration is negative, advance the needle 4 mm while injecting minute amounts (up to a 1/4 cartridge).
- Stop and aspirate.
- The average depth of insertion is about 15 mm (varies with the size of the mandible and the age of the patient). Deposit about 1 ml of solution around the inferior alveolar nerve.
- If bone is not contacted, the needle tip is located too posteriorly. Withdraw it until approximately 1/4 length of the needle is left in the tissue, reposition the syringe distally so it is over the area of the permanent molar and repeat as above.
- If bone is contacted too early (less than half the length of a long needle), the needle tip is located too anteriorly. Withdraw it until approximately 1/4 length of the needle is left in the tissue; reposition the syringe mesially over the area of the cuspid and repeat as above.
- The needle is withdrawn and recapped.
- Wait one minute before commencing dental treatment.

## Lingual Nerve Block

Successful anesthesia of the inferior alveolar nerve will result in anesthesia of the lingual nerve with the injection of a small quantity of the solution as the needle is withdrawn. The clinician must not assume effective anesthesia is attained if the patient only exhibits tongue symptoms. She must also exhibit lip and mucosa symptoms.

## Long Buccal Nerve Block

The long buccal nerve provides innervation to the buccal soft tissues and periosteum adjacent to the mandibular molars. For the removal of mandibular permanent molars, it is necessary to anesthetize the long buccal nerve. It is contraindicated in areas of acute infection.

For other procedures, a separate injection for buccal anesthesia is not always necessary in children before the eruption of the second permanent molars, the ramus being narrower in young children. After mandibular block anesthetic, the buccal tissue usually becomes anesthetized—probably a result of anesthetized nerve fibers that emanate from the mental foramen and enervate the buccal mucosa. Expelling the anesthetic solution on penetration and withdrawal probably affects some of the buccal enervating nerve fibers.

Technique:

- With the index finger, pull the buccal soft tissue in the area of the injection taut to improve visibility.
- Direct the needle toward the injection site with the bevel facing bone and the syringe aligned parallel to the occlusal place and buccal to the teeth.
- Penetrate the mucous membrane at the injection site distal and buccal to the last molar.
- Advance the needle slowly until mucoperiosteum is contacted.
- The depth of penetration is 1–4 mm.
- Aspirate.
- Inject approximately 1/8 of a cartridge over 10 seconds.
- The needle is withdrawn and recapped.

### Case 9.3

Carol, aged three years, is a very active youngster who requires restoration of the mandibular left first and second primary molars. She needs shallow occlusal restorations in both teeth. Carol's dentist believes that the teeth should be anesthetized but is concerned that administering a mandibular block anesthetic to the active child may be difficult.

*Case 9.3, Discussion*: Giving the active young child a mandibular block injection may be difficult, and it also has three other disadvantages. First, this is Carol's initial experience with dental anesthesia, and long-lasting numbness in the tongue and buccal mucosa could adversely affect her permanent attitude. Second, it can be difficult to render a painless block injection to a highly active child, and the dentist obviously wants Carol to experience minimal discomfort. Third, with long-lasting anesthetic, the active youngster may traumatize the soft tissues postoperatively. Thus, the concern of the dentist in this case is legitimate. The dentist should consider using buccal supraperiosteal (infiltration) anesthesia in place of a mandibular block injection. Two main advantages of this approach are the ease of administration and the minimal period of time that the child patient's mouth is anesthetized. The dentist injects up to 1 ml of local anesthetic solution in the mucobuccal fold adjacent to the mandibular primary tooth to be restored. In addition, the papilla should be anesthetized on the buccal, followed by penetration of the needle to the lingual side. In addition, anesthesia may be supplemented by an intra-ligamental injection (Figure 9-10).

The supraperiosteal anesthesia technique is useful for minor operative procedures. The problem with this technique is that profound mandibular anesthesia cannot be reliably achieved. Starkey suggests that the technique works best for young children (up to five years of age) who require restoration of mandibular first primary molars, cuspids, and incisors. In older children, or in the region of the second primary molars, bone is denser.

## Anesthetizing the Palatal Tissues

Palatal tissue anesthesia has traditionally been indicated for procedures involving manipulation of the palatal tissues, such as extractions, gingivectomy, and labial frenectomy. However, the authors recommend its routine use when treating maxillary molars. It may also be necessary when treating incisors. Unfortunately, it is one of the most traumatic and painful procedures experienced by a dental patient during treatment. The following techniques should help to reduce patient discomfort and, in a small number of cases, eliminate it entirely. Malamed (2012) recommended that the clinician forewarn the patient that there might be discomfort so that they are mentally prepared. If the experience is atraumatic, the patient bestows the "golden hands" award on the clinician. If it is painful, the clinician can console the patient with "I'm sorry. I told you that it might be uncomfortable" (avoid using the word "hurt").

The steps in atraumatic administration of anesthesia in all palatal areas are as follows:

- Provide adequate topical anesthesia (at least two minutes) in the injection area. The applicator should be held in place by the clinician while applying sufficient pressure to cause blanching. Alternatively, clinicians who do not use topical anesthesia apply finger pressure for a few seconds at the injection site. This may reduce the pain caused by the initial penetration of the needle.
- Use pressure anesthesia at the injection site before and during needle penetration and solution deposition. The pressure is maintained with a cotton applicator or with a finger with enough pressure to cause blanching.

(a)

(b)

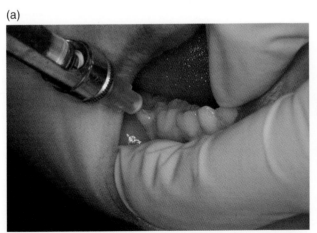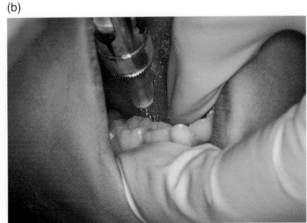

**Figure 9-10**   The dentist injects up to 1 ml of local anesthetic solution in the mucobuccal fold adjacent to the mandibular primary tooth to be restored. In addition, the papilla should be anesthetized on the buccal, followed by penetration of the needle to the lingual side (a). Anesthesia may also be supplemented by an intra-ligamental injection (b).

(a)

(b)

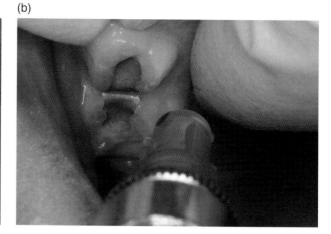

**Figure 9-11**   For palatal injections, the use of an ultrashort needle will result in less deflection and greater control (a). A finger rest will aid in stabilizing the needle (b).

- Maintain control over the needle. The use of an ultrashort needle will result in less deflection and greater control. A finger rest will aid in stabilizing the needle (Figure 9-11).
- Inject a minimum amount of anesthetic solution. Because of the density. Because of the density of the palatal soft tissues and their firm adherence to the hard palate, there is little room to spread during solution deposition. A small quantity of solution reduces tissue pressure and results in a less traumatic experience. During the injection, ask the patient to raise a leg off of the chair.

---

### Case 9.4

Mark, aged three years but small for his age, is a well-behaved child who requires restorative treatment on two central incisors. Strip crowns will be placed. All carious lesions are of moderate depth. The child is sedated with conscious sedation. The dentist is debating whether or not local anesthesia should be used. She is considering labial and palatal injections.

---

*Case 9.4, Discussion:* Although dentists treating children should always anesthetize for restorative treatment, there are exceptions. With proper technique, caries removal can be achieved with minimum pain in this region. Tooth preparation for a strip crown is minimal. In most instances, indirect pulp capping will be the treatment of choice, avoiding pulpal pain. In addition, the child is sedated and attention to correct doses of local anesthesia must be made, taking into consideration the weight of the child and the interaction with the sedative.

The actual injection may be just as painful as the restorative procedure. It takes considerable skill to administer a pain-free anterior injection. Even those dentists possessing this skill worry about hurting the child patient. In addition,

the palatal injection, which can be painful, should be avoided when possible. In most instances, a labial injection will suffice.

If the dentist anticipates pulpal treatment or possibly a complication which may involve extraction, local anesthesia is mandatory. For the supraperiosteal injection on the facial side for the primary anterior teeth, the soft tissues are retracted to reveal the junction of the firmly fixed gingival mucosa and the loose or movable alveolar mucosa. A topical anesthetic may be applied to the area, with the puncture point located in the movable alveolar mucosa, very close to the junction with the gingival mucosa. The dentist deposits a drop or two of solution immediately and then waits a few seconds before advancing the needle to a point opposite the apex of the tooth. In the primary dentition, the needle will usually not be advanced more than a millimeter or two. Note that in Figure 9-12, in the primary dentition, the apex of the teeth will be very near the point of insertion of the needle. Following labial anesthesia, palatal anesthesia may be accomplished by applying digital pressure to the palate opposite the involved teeth and inserting the needle under the finger with the bevel of the needle flat against the mucosa on the side of the papilla. A very small amount of anesthesia solution is deposited. Blanching will occur and is a sign of proper technique.

### Supraperiosteal Injections (Local Infiltration)

Supraperiosteal injection (commonly known as *local infiltration*) is indicated whenever dental procedures are confined to a localized area in either the maxilla or mandible. The more appropriate term for this type of anesthesia is "supraperiosteal" rather than "infiltration" because supraperiosteal indicates the placement of the anesthetic, whereas infiltration refers to the technique of injecting the

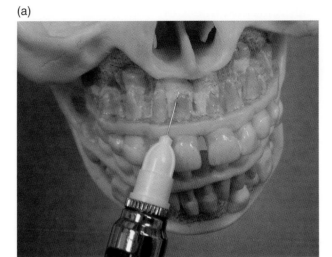

(a)

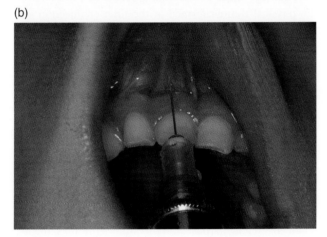

(b)

**Figure 9-12** In the primary dentition, the apex of the teeth (a) will be very near the point of insertion of the needle at the level of mucobuccal fold (b).

solutions directly into the tissues to be treated. The terminal endings of the nerves innervating the region are anesthetized. The indications are pulpal anesthesia of all the maxillary teeth (permanent and primary), mandibular anterior teeth (primary and permanent), and mandibular primary molars when treatment is limited to one tooth or two teeth. It also provides soft tissue anesthesia as a supplement to regional blocks. It is contraindicated in areas where dense bone covers the apices of the teeth (i.e., the permanent first molars in children). It is not recommended for larges areas due to the need for multiple needle insertions and the necessity to administer larger total volumes of local anesthetic that may lead to toxicity.

A number of studies have reported on the effectiveness of injecting local anesthetic solution in the mucobuccal fold between the roots of the primary mandibular molars (McDonald 2011). When comparing the effectiveness of

mandibular infiltration to mandibular block anesthesia, it was generally agreed that the two techniques were equally effective for restorative procedures, but the mandibular block was more effective for pulpotomies and extractions than mandibular infiltration. The mandibular infiltration should be considered in situations where one wants to perform bilateral restorative procedures without anesthetizing the tongue. Bilateral anesthesia of the tongue is uncomfortable for both children and adults.

Technique:

- Retract the cheek so the tissue of the mucobuccal fold is taut.
- Apply topical anesthetic.
- Orient the needle bevel toward the bone.
- Penetrate the mucous membrane mesial to the primary molar to be anesthetized, directing the needle to a position between the roots of the tooth. Slowly inject a small amount of anesthetic while advancing the needle to the desired position and injecting about a 1/2 cartridge of anesthetic.
- If lingual tissue anesthesia is necessary (rubber dam clamp placement), then one can inject anesthetic solution directly into the lingual tissue at the free gingival margin, or one can insert the needle interproximally from the buccal and deposit anesthesia as the needle is advanced lingually.
- The needle is withdrawn and recapped.
- Wait one minute before commencing treatment.

### Case 9.5

Sara, a five-year-old, required a large restoration on her maxillary second primary molar. The dentist deposited 1 ml of local anesthetic supraperiosteally and between the buccal roots of the tooth to be restored. During the cavity preparation, Sara cried and complained of pain. The dentist re-anesthetized the child, who continued to complain, "It hurts." Was Sara misbehaving?

***Case 9.5, Discussion:*** The dentist will need to determine if the child's reaction is indeed due to pain or perhaps a behavior management issue. In order to rule out pain, the dentist needs to be confident that the anesthesia technique used was correct.

Sometimes, it can be difficult to discern actual pain from an avoidance tactic. In this case, however, the possibility of inadequate anesthesia should be considered. Although most dentists probably use supraperiosteal anesthesia for operative procedures on maxillary second primary molars, bone thickness is a problem. The second primary molar roots lie deep within the zygomatic process of the maxillary bone. If a supraperiosteal injection is to be effective, the anesthetic solution must penetrate a considerable amount (about 1 cm) of bone. Therefore, for more profound anesthesia, a posterior superior injection is desirable. Anesthesia in this region is not a problem in adults because the forward growth of the maxilla carries the second premolar anterior to the zygomatic process of the alveolar bone. In adults, a supraperiosteal injection provides adequate anesthesia because the second premolar has only a thin layer of alveolar bone overlying its buccal root.

The possibility that the anesthesia given to Sara may have been inadequate is quite probable. Supraperiosteal injections often have to be made over both the mesial and distal roots to anesthetize the middle and superior nerve branches. When performing restorative dentistry on the maxillary first permanent molar, two buccal injections are needed for profound anesthesia. In addition to a tuberosity injection, a supraperiosteal injection is required over the mesial buccal root, since this root is innervated by the middle superior alveolar nerve. A single injection midway between the buccal roots does not routinely yield profound anesthesia. For the maxillary second permanent molar, only a tuberosity injection is necessary.

For the sake of continued discussion, the same case occurs, but both buccal injections were given and Sara starts crying hysterically as the high-speed drill touches the tooth.

In this case, the dentist is confident that the injection has taken effect. Sara is reacting to the sound of the drill. She expects pain. The child was previously treated without local anesthesia and associated the activation and sound of the high-speed drill to pain. Whenever the previous dentist used it, it hurt. A patient's apprehension can often cause local anesthetic failure (Kaufman et al. 1984). Nerve conduction may be blocked successfully from a neurophysiological perspective, but as soon as the patient anticipates or hears the sound of the drill, she perceives pain. The patient will need to be reconditioned. As soon as Sara experiences a painless procedure, she will understand and cooperate. This problem can be resolved by discussing the procedure with the child and explaining that every dentist is different and today's appointment will be better than her previous one.

To avoid this scenario, the dentist should always begin procedures involving a high-speed without initial contact with the tooth. Rather, he should activate it next to the tooth without contact, which emits the characteristic sound, thus isolating the sound of the drill from the cutting of tooth structure. If the parent is present, let the parent know this without alerting the patient to the test. If the child starts to complain of pain, the dentist shows the child with the aid of a mirror that the drill is not touching the tooth. The child is reassured that all will be all right. The drill is once again used, not touching the tooth at first, and finally cutting the tooth begins.

## Supplemental Injection Techniques

### Periodontal Ligament Injection (Intraligamentary Injection)

The periodontal ligament (PDL) injection has been used for a number of years as either a method of obtaining primary anesthesia for one or two teeth or as a supplement to infiltration or block techniques. The technique's primary advantage is that it provides pulpal anesthesia for 30–45 minutes without an extended period of soft tissue anesthesia and is, therefore, extremely useful when bilateral treatment is planned. It is useful in pediatric or disabled patients when there is concern of postoperative tissue trauma to the lip or tongue. Intraligamental anesthesia delivered by a high-pressure syringe is often associated with damage to the periodontal tissue, which results from the physical trauma formed at the time of injection and from the cytotoxic effects of the anesthesia. Damage heals within a few weeks. This is of particular concern to the pediatric dentist treating primary teeth.

In their study, Brannstrom et al. (1984) suggested that developmental disturbances to the underlying permanent tooth buds might occur. A high-pressure intraligamental anesthesia injection was used to anesthetize 16 monkey primary teeth. Teeth in the contralateral positions were not injected and served as controls. Hypoplasia or hypomineralization defects developed in 15 permanent teeth, but in none of the controls. The position of the enamel lesions indicated that the disturbance occurred at the same time on all affected teeth. Based on this study's findings, the use of intraligamental anesthesia on primary teeth with a developing permanent tooth bud has been contraindicated (Moore et al. 2011). However, a clinical study by Ashkenazi et al. (2010) using a computerized syringe system for delivery of intraligamental anesthesia concluded that it does not damage the underlying permanent dental bud in children four years or older. In any event, its use may be beneficial to the pediatric dentist when treating permanent molars. This is also a good technique for removing lower bicuspids bilaterally for orthodontic treatments. Since it is injected into a site with limited blood circulation, the technique is also advantageous for treating patients with bleeding disorders.

The PDL technique is simple, requires only a small amount of anesthesia, and produces instant anesthesia. Two devices were developed for this technique and were very popular for a period, the PERIPRESS (PERIPRESS®, Universal Dental Implements, Edison, NJ) syringe/pen and the Ligmaject syringe (Ligmaject, IMA Associates, Boston, MA). However, the authors' experience allows for the use of a standard syringe fitted with an ultrashort needle. The ultrashort needle is placed in the gingival sulcus on the mesial surface and advanced along the root surface until resistance is met. Initial finger pressure is applied on the attached gingiva. In multi-rooted teeth, injections are made mesially and distally. If lingual anesthesia is needed, the procedure is repeated in the lingual sulcus. Approximately 0.2 ml of anesthetic is injected.

Considerable effort is needed to express the anesthetic solution, placing a great deal of pressure on the anesthetic cartridge with the possibility of breakage. There are syringes specifically designed to enclose the cartridge and provide protection from breakage. Since so little anesthetic solution is necessary, Malamed (2012) suggested that when using a conventional syringe, expressing half the contents of the cartridge prior to injection will reduce the pressure exerted on the walls of the cartridge and reduce the likelihood of breakage.

## Computer-controlled Anesthetic Delivery System

"The Wand" also known as *CompuDent* (Milestone Scientific Inc, Livingston, NJ.), is a computer-controlled local anesthetic delivery system. The latest version of the Wand is called the *single tooth anesthesia system*. The system consists of a conventional local anesthetic needle inserted into a disposable pen-like syringe. A foot-controlled microprocessor controls the delivery of the anesthetic solution through the syringe at a constant flow rate, volume, and pressure. Studies with children have shown contradicting results. Some reported lower pain ratings for injections with the Wand® in comparison to injections with the traditional syringe (Allen et al. 2002; Gibson et al. 2000; Palm et al. 2004). Others found no differences between the two injection methods (Asarch et al. 1999; Ram and Peretz 2003). A recent systematic review and meta-analysis (Smolarek et al. 2020) concluded that there is no difference in the perception of pain and disruptive behavior in children subjected to computerized or conventional dental local anesthesia. A disadvantage of the system which is especially important when treating a child patient is the extended injection time of computerized systems. The injection time of the Wand is much longer than that of the traditional method, so children who already react negatively to an injection seem to be in distress longer with the Wand system. Versloot et al. (2008) reported the mean injection time with the Wand being three times as long as with the traditional syringe. The authors' experience is that with proper technique, the traditional syringe can be used successfully with most, if not all, patients.

## Intraosseous Anesthesia

Computerized intraosseous (IO) anesthesia in the dental setting is a relatively new concept for delivering dental anesthesia with few pediatric studies available (Sixou and Barbosa-Rogier 2008, 2009, Sixou and Marie-Cousin 2015; Smail-Faugeron et al. 2019). The IO injection allows placement of a local anesthetic solution directly into the cancellous bone adjacent to the tooth to be anesthetized. Since the IO anesthesia technique aims for the apices of the teeth to be treated, profound and immediate anesthesia can be predictability achieved. The computerized technique includes both computerized needle rotation and anesthetic solution delivery system. Proponents of this technique claim that because infiltration injections with lidocaine solutions are not effective for anesthesia of the mandibular molar teeth due to the thickness of the cortical plate, infiltration anesthesia in the posterior mandible is contraindicated, and the IO injection may overcome this problem by allowing direct access to the cancellous bone. However, with pediatric patients, mandibular local infiltration may be successful since the mandible is less compact, and the cortex is crossed by many canals (Salomon et al. 2012). The authors' experience is that even with adults, mandibular infiltration coupled with intraligamental injections may be employed with varying degrees of success. The IO involves three steps: gingival anesthesia, followed by perforation of the cortical plate by drilling a small hole through the cortical plate and subsequent penetration into the cancellous bone to the appropriate depth, and finally injection into the cancellous bone and needle withdrawal. This process may be considered by some clinicians as being over-complicated and not appropriate for use in pediatric patients. However, perhaps situations in which profound anesthesia is required and may prove difficult to achieve with a standard mandibular block such as a permanent first molar with molar incisor hypomineralisation (Dixit and Joshi 2018) or acute pulpitis (Farhad et al. 2018; Verma et al. 2013) might dictate the use of IO. The technique requires caution as prolonged rotation of the perforator drills in the bone can cause excessive heat, which can lead to bone necrosis (Woodmansey et al. 2009).

## Vibrating Devices

As mentioned above, wiggling the cheek during administration of local anesthesia is recommended. The action achieves distraction which may aid in delivering a pain-free injection. In addition, vibrating the cheek or the surrounding mucosa tissues may reduce the sensation of pain, as postulated by the gate control theory of pain management, which suggests that pain can be reduced by simultaneous activation of nerve fibers through the use of vibration. Vibrating stimuli are mediated by large, myelinated fibers which inhibit small pain fibers presynaptically in the dorsal horn of the spinal cord (Melzack and Wall 1973). Therefore, stimulating the larger diameter

A-beta fibers by application of pressure or vibration can interrupt nociceptive signals, thereby "closing the gate" and reducing the perception of pain (Elbay et al. 2016).

Commercial devices have been made available to produce vibrations during dental injections. Some are designed to be attached to the syringe, and others are placed on the surrounding mucosa of the injection site. Research evaluating both the effectiveness and patient acceptance of the devices has shown mixed results (Chaudhry et al. 2015; Elbay et al. 2015; Elbay et al. 2016; Hassanein et al. 2020; Hegde et al. 2019; Raslan and Marsi 2017; Tung et al. 2018). Some studies reported that children actually preferred traditional injections without the additional vibrating device (Elbay et al. 2015; Elbay et al. 2016; Raslan and Marsi 2017).

## Complications

### Postoperative Soft Tissue Injury

Accidental biting or chewing of the lip, tongue, or cheek is a problem seen in very young pediatric and disabled patients. Soft tissue anesthesia lasts longer than pulpal anesthesia and may be present for up to four hours after local administration. The most common areas of trauma are the lower lip and, to a lesser extent, the tongue, followed by the upper lip (Figure 9-13).

Several preventive measures can be followed:

- Advise the patient and accompanying adult about the possibility of injury if the patient bites, sucks, or chews on the lips, tongue, and cheek. If not clearly forewarned, a parent may accuse the dentist of creating the resulting damage during the operative session.
- The sensation created by the local anesthesia will be new to most children. They should be reassured that it will go away within an hour or two. They also should delay eating and avoid hot drinks until the effects of the anesthesia have totally dissipated.
- Sedated children may fall asleep after being discharged and cause damage. Parents should be instructed to observe the child during the ride home.
- Reinforce the warning with patient stickers.

### Anesthetic Toxicity (Overdose)

While rare in adults, young children are more likely to experience toxic reactions because of their lower weight. Most adverse drug reactions occur within 5–10 minutes of injection. Overdoses of local anesthetics are caused by high blood levels of anesthetic as a result of an inadvertent intravascular injection or repeated injections. Local anesthetic overdose results in excitation, followed by depression of the central nervous system and, to a lesser extent, of the cardiovascular system.

(a)

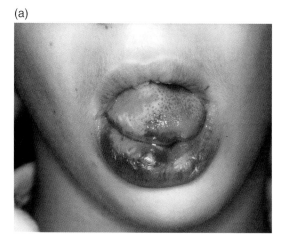

(b)

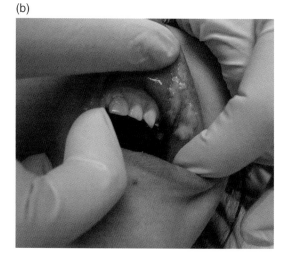

**Figure 9-13** The most common areas of trauma are the lower lip (a) and, to a lesser extent, the tongue, followed by the upper lip (b).

Early subjective symptoms of the central nervous system include dizziness, anxiety, and confusion and may be followed by diplopia, tinnitus, drowsiness, and circumoral numbness or tingling. Objective signs include muscle twitching, tremors, talkativeness, slowed speech, and shivering, followed by overt seizure activity. Unconsciousness and respiratory arrest may occur. The initial cardiovascular system response to local anesthetic toxicity is an increase in heart rate and blood pressure. As blood plasma levels of the anesthetic increase, vasodilatation occurs, followed by depression of the myocardium with a subsequent fall in blood pressure. Bradycardia and cardiac arrest may follow.

Local anesthetic toxicity is preventable by following proper injection technique—i.e., aspiration during slow injection. Clinicians should know maximum recommended dosages (MRD) based on weight. If lidocaine topical anesthetic is used, it should be factored into the total administered dose, as it can infiltrate into the vascular system. After injection, the patient should be observed for any possible toxic response as early recognition and intervention are the keys to a successful outcome. One cannot over-emphasize the universal importance that all dental practitioners treating children should consistently calculate a weight-based MRD of both local anesthetics and sedative agents. Additionally, clinicians should adjust downward the doses of local anesthetic when sedating children with drugs that are known to cause respiratory depression. For example, it has been well-documented that sedation with opioids and other CNS depressant agents like chloral hydrate may increase the risk of local anesthetic toxicity due to their synergistic CNS depressing effects, especially in children (see Chapter 13). In addition, local anesthetic toxicity reactions may be masked by the administration of benzodiazepines during sedation, thus making it more difficult for the practitioner to recognize a local anesthetic overdose. The two most common local anesthetic solutions used in pediatric dentistry are 2% lidocaine with 1/100,000 epinephrine and 3% mepivacaine (used in children when vasodepressor is contraindicated). The maximum dosage of both lidocaine and mepivacaine is 2.0 mg/lb (4.4 mg/kg), and the maximum total dosage is 300 mg.

Referring to Table 9.1, it is possible to approximate the maximum recommended dosage and amount of local anesthetic agents for patients of specific weight and type of anesthetic. For example, to calculate the maximum amount of lidocaine 2% with 1:100,000 epinephrine and the number of cartridges that can be safely administered to a 30-pound patient, the clinician would perform the following calculations.

A quick approximation using Table 9-1:

**Table 9-1** Quick dosage chart.

| | | | AAPD Maximum Recommended Dosages | | |
|---|---|---|---|---|---|
| | | | 2% Lidocaine<br>Epinephrine 1:100,000<br><br>4.4 mg/kg[*]<br>2.0 mg/lb[*]<br>MRD 300 mg[*]<br><br>36 mg/1.8 ml cartridge<br><br>**every 8 kg = 1 cartridge**<br>**every 20 lbs = 1 cartridge** | 3% Mepivacaine<br>With or without vasoconstrictor<br><br>4.4 mg/kg[*]<br>2.0 mg/lb[*]<br>MRD 300 mg<br><br>54 mg/1.8 ml cartridge<br><br>**every 12 kg = 1 cartridge**<br>**every 30 lbs = 1 cartridge** | 4% Articaine<br>Epinephrine 1:100,000<br><br>7.0 mg/kg<br>3.2 mg/lb<br>MRD 500 mg<br><br>72 mg/1.8 ml cartridge<br><br>**every 10 kg = 1 cartridge**<br>**every 22 lbs = 1 cartridge** |
| **Age** | **Kg** | **Lbs** | Maximum number of 1.8 ml cartridges | | |
| | | | 2% Lidocaine | 3% Mepivacaine | 4% Articaine |
| 1+ yrs | 7.5 | 16.5 | 0.9 | 0.6 | 0.7 |
| 2–3 yrs | 10.0 | 22.0 | 1.2 | 0.8 | 1.0 |
| | 12.5 | 27.5 | 1.5 | 1.0 | 1.2 |
| 4–5 yrs | 15.0 | 33.0 | 1.8 | 1.2 | 1.5 |
| | 17.5 | 38.5 | 2.1 | 1.4 | 1.7 |
| 6–8 yrs | 20.0 | 44.0 | 2.4 | 1.6 | 2.0 |
| | 22.5 | 49.5 | 2.8 | 1.8 | 2.2 |
| 9–10 yrs | 25.0 | 55.0 | 3.1 | 2.0 | 2.4 |
| | 27.5 | 60.5 | 3.4 | 2.2 | 2.7 |
| | 30.0 | 66.0 | 3.7 | 2.4 | 2.9 |
| 11+ yrs | 32.5 | 71.5 | 4.0 | 2.6 | 3.2 |
| | 35.0 | 77.0 | 4.3 | 2.9 | 3.4 |
| | 37.5 | 82.5 | 4.6 | 3.1 | 3.7 |
| | 40.0 | 88.0 | 4.9 | 3.3 | 3.9 |

[*] *Note:* The clinical guidelines in the American Academy of Pediatric Dentistry 2020 Reference Manual recommend reduced dosages as compared to the manufacturers' maximum recommended dosages (MRDs) by weight and maximum total dosages for lidocaine (7.0 mg/kg, 3.2 mg/lb and 500 mg maximum total dosage) and mepivacaine (6.6 mg/kg, 3.0 mg/lb and 400 mg maximum total dosage).Source: Based on American Academy of Pediatric Dentistry (2020).

## Pediatric local anesthetic dose limits by volume

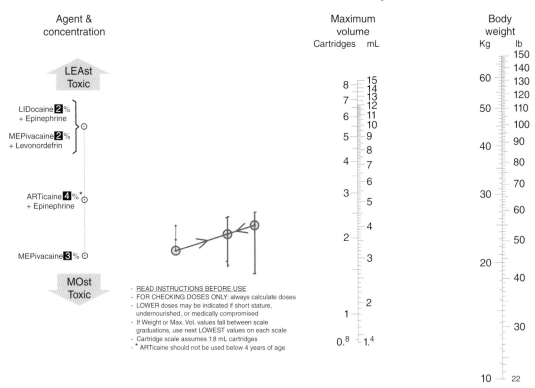

**Figure. 9.14** Nomogram for calculating maximum recommended dose (MRD) of local anesthetic by volume for pediatric dentistry. A straight-line drawn from the agent and concentration to the child's body weight (kilograms or pounds) will intersect the central axis to indicate the MRD by volume (milliliters or cartridges). *Source:* Williams et al. (2017). © 2019 by the American Academy of Pediatric Dentistry and reproduced with their permission.

30 lb divided by 20 (every 20 lb = 1 cartridge)

   = 1.5 cartridges

An exact calculation using the maximum dosage:

Maximum dosage (mg / lbs) × weight (lbs)

   = Maximum total dosage (mg)

     2.0 × 30 = 60 mgs

Maximum total dosage (mg) √ mg / cartridge

   = Maximum cartridges

     60 ÷ 36 = 1.67 cartridges

Thus, for a 30-pound child, the maximum safe administration is 1.67 cartridges of lidocaine 2% with 1:100,000 epinephrine. The quick approximation of 1.5 cartridges is clinically insignificant when compared to 1.67 cartridges, given that most cartridges do not have markings allowing for accurate dispensing of the anesthetic.

The clinician should be aware of the drug interaction between local anesthetic and sedative agents when administering enteral or parenteral sedatives for behavior management. The action of the sedative has an additive depressive effect on the central nervous and cardiovascular systems and can initiate overdose consequences.

Another simplified method to easily calculate the MRD is using a graphical aid (nomogram), as presented in Figure 9.14 (Williams et al. 2017). The nomogram may be laminated for repeated use or may be printed onto individual sheets of paper; drawing a line across the axes simultaneously performs the calculation and provides a permanent record for filing in patient notes. The nomogram may be enlarged to afford greater legibility and accuracy; however, it is essential that the original proportions (aspect ratio) be maintained, or the chart will produce erroneous calculations.

### Case 9.6

Steve, a 36-pound (16.4 kg), four-year-, one-month-old male patient presented to a dental clinic for extensive restorative treatment involving three quadrants. The patient's medical history included obstructive sleep apnea, and he was reported as being congested on the day he presented for dental treatment. Steve was placed in a papoose board and was administered three cartridges of 2% lidocaine (108 mg, 6.6 mg/kg) within three minutes. After a few minutes, the child appeared to fall asleep. Within 15 minutes of beginning treatment, the dental assistant noticed that the patient's tongue was purple. He was unwrapped from the papoose. The patient's vital signs were checked, and there was no detectable pulse or breathing. Cardiopulmonary resuscitation was started, and the paramedics were called. Paramedics arrived within four minutes of the call and assumed the resuscitative efforts. The patient was intubated, after which a volume of thick, mucous-filled fluid was suctioned from his airway. When the paramedics' efforts to resuscitate the child were unsuccessful, the child was transported to the local children's hospital, where he was pronounced dead.

*Case 9.6, Discussion*: Tragically, unlike the other cases presented in this chapter, this case is an accurate description of an actual overdose that occurred. It was presented as a closed malpractice insurance claim (Chicka et al. 2012). One unexpected finding was that 41% of claims involved the administration of an overdose of a local anesthetic agent, ranging from 118% to 356% of the MRD. The widespread use of local anesthesia in dentistry is generally very safe and

effective (Townsend et al. 2020). Serious adverse reactions involving children are usually the result of dose-dependent toxicity reactions. The study's findings suggest that there continues to be local anesthetic overdoses, resulting in significant morbidity and mortality in children.

The child in this case received one cartridge more than he should have:

$$2.0 \times 36 = 72 \text{ mgs, maximum total dosage (mg)}$$

$\div$ mg/cartridge
= Maximum cartridges, $72 \div 36 = 2$ cartridges.

### Allergic Reactions

Although allergic reactions to injectable amide local anesthetics are rare, patients may exhibit a reaction to the bisulfite preservative added to anesthetics containing epinephrine. Patients may also exhibit allergic reactions to benzocaine topical anesthetics. Allergies can manifest in a variety of ways, including urticaria, dermatitis, angioedema, fever, photosensitivity, and anaphylaxis.

The cases and selected texts have been adapted with permission from Paul E. Starkey's chapter on local anesthesia for children in *Managing Children's Behavior in the Dental Office* (G.Z. Wright, P.E. Starkey, Gardner D.E; C.V. Mosby Company, St. Louis MS 1983).

## Disclaimer

This information is not intended to be a comprehensive list of all medications that may be used in all emergencies. Drug information is constantly changing and is often subject to interpretation. While care has been taken to ensure the accuracy of the information presented, the authors are not responsible for the continued currency of the information, errors, omissions, or the resulting consequences.

Decisions about drug therapy must be based upon the independent judgment of the clinician, changing drug information, and evolving healthcare practices.

## References

Allen, K.D., Kotil, D., Larzelere, R.E. et al. (2002). Comparison of a computerized anesthesia device with a traditional syringe in preschool children. *Pediatric Dentistry*, 24, 315–320.

American Academy of Pediatric Dentistry (AAPD), (2020). *Use of local anesthesia for pediatric dental patients. The Reference Manual of Pediatric Dentistry*. Chicago, Ill.: American Academy of Pediatric Dentistry, pp. 318–323.

Asarch, T., Allen, K., Petersen, B. et al. (1999). Efficacy of a computerized local anesthesia device in pediatric dentistry. *Pediatric Dentistry*, 27, 421–424.

Ashkenazi, M., Blumer, S., and Eli, I. (2010). Effect of computerized delivery intraligamental injection in primary molars on their corresponding permanent tooth buds. *International Journal of Paediatric Dentistry*, 20, 270–275.

Brannstrom, M, Lindskog, S., and Nordenvall, K.J. (1984). Enamel hypoplasia in permanent teeth induced by periodontal ligament anesthesia of primary teeth. *Journal of the American Dental Association*, 109, 735–736.

Chaudhry, K., Shishodia M., Singh, C. et al. (2015). Comparative evaluation of pain perception by vibrating needle (VibrajectTM) and conventional syringe anesthesia during various dental procedures in pediatric patients: A short study. *International Dental & Medical Journal of Advanced Research*, 1, 1–5.

Chicka, M.C., Dembo, J.B., Mathu-Muju, K.R. et al. (2012). Adverse events during pediatric dental anesthesia and sedation: A review of closed malpractice insurance claims. *Pediatric Dentistry*, 34, 231–238.

Delgado-Molina, E., Tamarit-Borrás, M., Berini-Aytés, L. et al. (2003). Evaluation and comparison of 2 needle models in terms of blood aspiration during truncal block of the inferior alveolar nerve. *Journal of Oral and Maxillofacial Surgery*, 61, 1011–1015.

Dixit, U.B. and Joshi, A.M. (2018). Efficacy of intraosseous local anesthesia for restorative procedures in molar incisor hypomineralization-affected teeth in children. *Contemporary Clinical Dentistry*, 9(Suppl. 2), S272–S277.

Eichenbaum, I.W. and Dunn, N.A. (1971). Projective drawings by children under repeated dental stress. *ASDC Journal of Dentistry for Children*, 38, 164–173.

Elbay, M., Elbay, Ü.Ş., Yıldırım, S. et al. (2015). Comparison of injection pain caused by the DentalVibe Injection System versus a traditional syringe for inferior alveolar nerve block anaesthesia in paediatric patients. *European Journal of Paediatric Dentistry,* 16, 123–128.

Elbay, U.Ş., Elbay, M., Yildirim, S. et al. (2016). Evaluation of the injection pain with the use of DentalVibe injection system during supraperiosteal anaesthesia in children: A randomised clinical trial. *International Journal of Paediatric Dentistry*, 26, 336–345.

Farhad, A., Razavian, H., and Shafiee, M. (2018). Effect of intraosseous injection versus inferior alveolar nerve block as primary pulpal anaesthesia of mandibular posterior teeth with symptomatic irreversible pulpitis: a prospective randomized clinical trial, *Acta Odontologica Scandinavica*, 76(6), 442–447. DOI: 10.1080/00016357.2018.1428826.

Gibson, R.S., Allen, K., Hutfless, S. et al. (2000). The Wand vs. traditional injection: a comparison of pain related behaviors. *Pediatric Dentistry*, 22, 458–462.

Hassanein, P.H., Khalil, A., and Talaat, D.M. (2020). Pain assessment during mandibular nerve block injection with the aid of dental vibe tool in pediatric dental patients: A randomized clinical trial. *Quintessence International*, 51, 310–317. DOI: 10.3290/j.qi.a44145.

Hegde, K.M., Neeraja, R., Srinivasan, I. et al. (2019). Effect of vibration during local anesthesia administration on pain, anxiety, and behavior of pediatric patients aged 6-11 years: A crossover split-mouth study. *Journal of Dental Anesthesia and Pain Medicine*, 9, 143–149. DOI: 10.17245/jdapm.2019.19.3.143. Epub 2019 Jun 30.

Karjalainen, S., Olak, J., Soderling, E. et al. (2003). Frequent exposure to invasive medical care in early childhood and operative dental treatment associated with dental apprehension of children at 9 years of age. *European Journal of Paediatric Dentistry*, 4, 186–190.

Kaufman, E., Weinstein, P., and Milgrom, P. (1984). Difficulties in achieving local anesthesia. *Journal of the American Dental Association*, 108, 205–208.

Kohli, K., Ngan, P., Crout, R. et al. (2001). A survey of local and topical anesthesia use by pediatric dentists in the United States. *Pediatric Dentistry*, 23, 265–269.

Malamed, S.F., Reed, K.L., and Poorsattar, S. (2010). Needle breakage: Incidence and prevention. *Dental Clinics of North America*, 54, 745–756.

Malamed, S. (2012). Handbook of Local Anesthesia, 6th ed. Mosby Elsevier, Missouri, U.S.A.

McDonald, R.E., Avery, D.R., Dean, J.A. et al. (2011). Local anesthesia and pain control for the child and adolescent. In: J. Dean, D. Avery, and R. McDonald (Eds.), McDonald and Avery's Dentistry for the Child and Adolescent, 9th ed. (pp. 243–244). Mosby Elsevier, Missouri, U.S.A.

Meechan, J.G. (2002). Effective topical anesthetic agents and techniques. *Dental Clinics of North America*, 46, 759–766.

Meechan, J.G. (2008). Intraoral topical anesthesia. *Periodontology* 2000, 46, 56–79.

Melzack, R. and Wall, P.D. (1973). Pain mechanisms: A new theory. *Science*, 150, 971–979.

Moore, P.A., Cuddy, M.A., Cooke, M.R. et al. (2011). Periodontal ligament and intraosseous anesthetic injection techniques: Alternatives to mandibular blocks. *Journal of the American Dental Association*, 142(Suppl. 3), 13S–18S.

Ost, L.G. (1991). Acquisition of blood and injection phobia and anxiety response patterns in clinical patients. *Behaviour Research and Therapy*, 29, 323–332.

Palm, A.M., Kirkegaard, U., and Poulsen, S. (2004). The wand versus traditional injection for mandibular nerve block in children and adolescents. Perceived pain and time of onset. *Pediatric Dentistry*, 26, 481–484.

Ram, D. and Peretz, B. (2003). The assessment of pain sensation during local anesthesia using a computerized local anesthesia (Wand) and a conventional syringe. *Journal of Dentistry for Children*, 70, 130–133.

Raslan, N. and Marsi, R. (2017). A randomized clinical trial to compare pain levels during three types of oral anesthetic injections and the effect of Dentalvibe on injection pain in children. *International Journal of Paediatric Dentistry*, 28, 102–110.

Reed, K.L., Malamed, S.F., and Fonner, A.M. (2012). Local anesthesia Part 2: Technical considerations. *Anesthesia Progress*, 59, 127–137.

Salomon, E., Mazzoleni, S., Sivolella, S. et al. (2012). Age limit for infiltration anaesthesia for the conservative treatment of mandibular first molars. A clinical study on a paediatric population. *European Journal of Paediatric Dentistry*, 13(3 Suppl), 259–262.

Sixou, J.L. and Barbosa-Rogier, M.E. (2008). Efficacy of intraosseous injections of anesthetic in children and adolescents. *Oral Surgery Oral Medicine Oral Pathology Oral Radiology Endodontics*, 106, 173–178.

Sixou, J.L., Marie-Cousin, A., Huet, A. et al. (2009). Pain assessment by children and adolescents during intraosseous anaesthesia using a computerized system (QuickSleeperTM). *International Journal of Paediatric Dentistry*, 19, 360–366.

Sixou, J.L. and Marie-Cousin, A. (2015). Intraosseous anaesthesia in children with 4% articaine and epinephrine 1:400,000 using computer-assisted systems. *European Archives of Paediatric Dentistry*, 16, 477–481.

Sokolowski, C.J., Giovannitti, J.A., and Boynes, S.G. (2010). Needle phobia: Etiology, adverse consequences, and patient management. *Dental Clinics of North America*, 54, 731–744.

Smail-Faugeron, V., Muller-Bolla, M., Sixou, J.-L. et al. (2019). Evaluation of intraosseous computerized injection system (QuickSleeper™) vs conventional infiltration anaesthesia in paediatric oral health care: A multicentre, single-blind, combined split-mouth and parallel-arm randomized controlled trial. *International Journal of Paediatric Dentistry*, 29, 573–584. https://doi.org/10.1111/ipd.12494.

Smolarek, P.D.C., Wambier, L.M., Siqueira Silva, L. et al. (2020). Does computerized anaesthesia reduce pain during local anaesthesia in paediatric patients for dental treatment? A systematic review and meta-analysis. *International Journal of Paediatric Dentistry*, 30, 118–135. https ://doi.org/10.1111/ipd.12580.

Starkey, P.E. (1983). Local anesthesia in children. In: G.Z. Wright, P.E. Starkey, D. E. Gardner (Eds.), Managing Children's Behavior in the Dental Office, 123–143. The C.V. Mosby Company, St. Louis, Missouri, USA.

Townsend, J.A., Spiller, H., Hammersmith, K. et al. (2020). Dental local anesthesia-related pediatric cases reported to U.S. poison control centers. *Pediatric Dentistry*, 42(2), 116–122.

Trapp, L.D. and Davies, R.O. (1980). Aspiration as a function of hypodermic needle internal diameter in the in-vivo human upper limb. *Anesthesia Progress*, 27, 49–51.

Tung, J., Carillo, C., Udin, R. et al. (2018). Clinical performance of the DentalVibe® injection system on pain perception during local anesthesia in children. *Journal of Dentistry for Children*, 85, 51–57.

Verma, P.K., Srivastava, R., and Ramesh, K.M. (2013). Anesthetic efficacy of X-tip intraosseous injection using 2% lidocaine with 1:80,000 epinephrine in patients with irreversible pulpitis after inferior alveolar nerve block: A clinical study. *Journal of conservative dentistry*, 16, 162–166. https://doi.org/10.4103/0972-0707.108202

Versloot, J., Veerkamp J.S.J., and Hoogstraten, J. (2005). Computerized anesthesia delivery system vs. traditional syringe: comparing pain and pain-related behavior in children. *European Journal of Oral Science*, 113, 488–493.

Versloot, J., Veerkamp, J.S., and Hoogstraten, J. (2008). Pain behaviour and distress in children during two sequential dental visits: Comparing a computerised anaesthesia delivery system and a traditional syringe. British Dental Journal, Jul 12; 205(1), E2; discussion 30–1. DOI: 10.1038/sj.bdj.2008.414. Epub 2008 May 23.

Williams, D., Splaver, T., and Walker, J. (2017). A nomogram for calculation of maximum recommended dose by volume of local anesthetic in pediatric dentistry. *Pediatric Dentistry*, 39, 150–154.

Wright, G.Z., Starkey, P.E., and Gardiner, D.E. (1983). *Managing Children's Behavior in the Dental Office.* In: Chapter 11 Local anesthesia for children, pp. 125. The C.V. Mosby Company.

Woodmansey, K.F., White, R.K., and He, J. (2009). Osteonecrosis related to intraosseous anesthesia: Report of a case. *Journal of Endodontics*, 35, 288–291.

# 10

## Introduction to Pharmacological Techniques: A Historical Perspective

*Gerald Z. Wright and Ari Kupietzky*

This introduction provides a brief chronologic history of pediatric dental sedation, beginning with the 1970s. It focuses on changes that have occurred in the United States in the last 40 years, as Americans have led the changes. Knowing what has transpired in the past helps to understand current regulations and practices.

IThe American Academy of Pediatric Dentistry (AAPD) uses the terms *minimal*, *moderate*, and *deep* to categorize sedations (Coté, and Wilson 2019) . These are different degrees of central nervous system depression, each corresponding to a level of sedation relaxation. However, in the first edition of this book, Musselman and McClure (1975) categorized drugs differently. They opined that decisions concerning the type of drug and the suitable route of drug administration may be made, in part, on the basis of the level of a child's cooperative behavior. They classified sedation as two types: *preventive premedication* and *management medication*. A preventive premedication is used when a child is stressed by the dental situation but is still communicative. There are different types of behaviors—scared, timid, and apprehensive—that could be considered candidates for a preventive medication. Management medication is used for children who are unable to control their behavior or for those lacking in cooperative ability. The dentist would find it difficult or impossible to obtain adequate radiographs on these children. Verbal communication may have little meaning for them.

These sedation categories are rarely used today, but it is sometimes helpful to think of the drug you are about to use in this way. Consider the following case.

### Case 10.1

Jill, aged four years, was a healthy child requiring four quadrants of dentistry. At the initial examination, the child appeared cooperative, but the dentist recognized her apprehension. When the napkin was placed on Jill's chest, a very rapid heartbeat was felt. The child's eyes followed every movement of the dental team. She talked incessantly and laughed forcefully, as if trying to camouflage her concern.

Despite these observations, the dentist elected to treat Jill with behavior shaping, a non-pharmacologic approach. Performing dentistry quadrant by quadrant, the dentist achieved good patient cooperation at the first and second restorative appointments. At the third visit, the child cried at the injection but eventually calmed down. When the time arrived for the fourth appointment, Jill's parent had to forcibly bring her to the office. The child cried continuously and hysterically, refusing the injection.

*Case 10.1, Discussion*: The case illustrates an excellent example of when a preventive medication might be used. The child was obviously apprehensive at the first visit, and her behavior changed from cooperative to highly uncooperative by the fourth appointment. If the child had received a preventive medication, a more favorable outcome may have resulted. A contemporary example of a preventive medication is nitrous oxide inhalation analgesia. Thinking in terms of the child's cooperative behavior is a useful way of guiding drug selection.

*Wright's Behavior Management in Dentistry for Children*, Third Edition. Edited by Ari Kupietzky.
© 2022 John Wiley & Sons, Inc. Published 2022 by John Wiley & Sons, Inc.

In 1975, numerous sedation agents were being used in private practices and teaching venues. To determine which sedation agents to include in the original edition of this book, a survey of members of the American Board of Pedodontics (now AAPD) was undertaken (Wright and McAulay 1973) to determine: (1) which drugs were used by the members, and (2) what the common methods of drug administration were. The survey concluded that hydroxyzine (Atarax and Vistaril) was the most popular sedating agent when used alone.

Hydroxyzine, a minimal sedation agent, can serve as an excellent preventive medication. It is best used for children three to six years of age and those who are timid, apprehensive, or highly anxious. However, the drug by itself likely will not be sufficient. Success in patient management requires both pharmacological and non-pharmacological techniques; the individual dentist's training and experience makes the difference in choice and efficacy of techniques employed (Phero 1993). This is especially true when using a minimal or preventive medication. Indeed, since a patient's awareness may be somewhat dulled, greater emphasis is placed on using a very good non-pharmacologic approach. As the sole sedating agent, hydroxyzine has limited success with older children, but nowadays, it is often used in combination with other agents. When used with nitrous oxide, its antiemetic effect can be advantageous.

Chloral hydrate was the next most popular drug when used alone, and it was usually employed as a management medication. In 1975, pediatric dentists were still trying to determine the proper dosage. There was little agreement. Maximum suggested dosages for a four-year-old child ranged from 750 mg to 1000 mg (Sim 1975) and sometimes as high as 1250 mg (Smith 1977). While historically there was confusion as to the correct dosage, it did not prevent its use, and deep sedations often were obtained with the limited monitoring that was available at that time. Chloral hydrate is no longer manufactured commercially in the United States, but it remains available at local pharmacies and in other countries. For this reason, it has been included in this book.

When it came to drugs used in combination, promethazine (Phenergan) and meperidine (Demerol) were the most popular. When children were "strongly apprehensive," the combination of Phenergan and Demerol were used widely as a management medication. The 1975 survey reported that 35% of American Board of Pediatric Dentistry (ABPD) members administered medication intramuscularly. The injections were likely for meperidine.

The Wright and McAulay survey also found that only 44% of pediatric dentists were using nitrous oxide at the time. In 1996, Wilson reported that 89% of AAPD members were using nitrous oxide, doubling its usage over a span of 20 years. Similar trends are revealed by consecutive surveys undertaken by Houpt (1985, 1993, 2002) as part of the Project on Usage of Sedative Agents by Pediatric Dentists. Because nitrous oxide—oxygen inhalation analgesia—is now highly popular, an expanded chapter has been devoted to its application in pediatric dentistry.

In 1973, the survey revealed that slightly more than 10% of pediatric dentists administered drugs submucosally. The majority of pediatric dentists administered Nisentil (alphaprodine HCl) in this way. The drug was synthesized by Ziering and Lee in 1947 and was used by physicians in obstetrics for many years. Although Nisentil is not used in dental practice today, it has great historical importance, as its use led to major changes in pediatric dental sedation practices.

Pediatric dentists used Nisentil to control the behavior of difficult child patients, particularly those three to six years of age. The drug acted rapidly, with a peak effect of 5–10 minutes. It was similar to Demerol, but 2.5 times more potent. Its side effects included respiratory depression, nausea, and vomiting. Like Demerol, its effects could be reversed with a narcotic antagonist. In 1980, Nisentil was suddenly withdrawn by the manufacturer Roche Laboratories, a division of Hoffman-LaRoche.

The American Academy of Pediatric Dentistry (AAPD) voiced its concern to Roche Laboratories about the sudden withdrawal of Nisentil. Many pediatric dentists were outraged, as they relied on the drug to manage their patients. To deal with the Nisentil issue, a symposium was held in Los Angeles in 1981 and its proceedings were published in a special issue of *Pediatric Dentistry* the following year. Chen (1982), representing Roche Laboratories, cited four cases of adverse experiences with the drug. Children of ages 28 months to 4 years died or suffered cerebral damage due to anoxia. Key information extracted from 7,372 cases gathered from the files of 12 dentists using Nisentil was as follows: patients ranged from 2 to 12 years of age, drug efficacy was rated between 2.8 and 2.9 (3 max), dosage was 5–15 mg in most cases, and severe adverse reactions occurred in 8/7,372 cases.

Aubuchon (1982) also presented an important report at the symposium. Basing his findings on 2,911 questionnaires, his main conclusions were: a narcotic sedative technique was the most popular means of sedating pediatric patients, narcotic sedations had an adverse risk reaction of 1:5,000 as compared to a risk of 1:20,000–30,000 for non-narcotic agents, and an alphaprodine sedation is as safe or safer than a meperidine sedation. Creedon (1982) and Troutman and Renzi (1982), citing their experiences and case reports, provided further support for the use of Nisentil. The symposium panel concluded that although there were other drugs available for pediatric dental sedation, none were as effective as Nisentil. Two outcomes of the symposium were that: (1) better education was needed for practitioners choosing to use sedation medication, and (2) there needed to be a set of guidelines to establish a basic standard of care for these procedures. Until that time, there were no formal sedation guidelines.

Shortly thereafter, the AAPD Board of Directors appointed an ad hoc committee charged specifically with developing and writing the guidelines. The committee consisted of appointed members from the AAPD and representatives from American Society of Dentistry for Children, American Academy of Pediatrics, and Roche Laboratories. In 1983, the committee presented the guidelines to the AAPD members, leading to controversy and fury. Many objected to the content of the guidelines—they viewed them as possible regulation of their practices—and serious opposition was heard. Subsequently, the guidelines underwent further changes and presentations at AAPD annual meetings. Input was also obtained from the Academy of Pediatrics section on Anesthesiology, the American Dental Society of Anesthesiology, and the American Association of Oral and Maxillofacial Surgery. In the end, the guidelines were the result of a consensus of opinions, and the final document was entitled "Guidelines for the Elective Use of Conscious Sedation, Deep Sedation and General Anesthesia." Following a few minor changes at the behest of the American Academy of Pediatrics, the guidelines were jointly published in the July 1985 issue of *Pediatrics* and in the December 1985 issue of *Pediatric Dentistry*. Those guidelines are the basis for guides today. It is interesting to reflect upon this period of time. If Nisentil had not been withdrawn, how long would it have taken for pediatric dentistry to have sedation guidelines?

The guidelines focused on details which theoretically act to protect and promote the welfare of children who required sedation. From the practitioner's viewpoint, the guidelines could be perceived as mediating major change in practice. For instance, maintaining time-based records of sedation may be misconstrued as a significant logistical problem.

- Who in the operatory is to be trained to record physiological parameters?
- What should be on the data gathering form?
- When is it really necessary to record monitored parameters?
- What do the guidelines offer in providing guidance to these questions?

Sedation guidelines are not static: they need to be dynamic and require modification on a periodic basis. Fortunately, the AAPD had the foresight to recognize the potential need for modification, and in 1992, the subcommittee on sedation convened to evaluate all aspects of the guidelines. They were revised further in 1996, 2000, 2005, 2008, and 2011. Guidelines also have to be adjusted to satisfy the laws of various states, provinces, or nations.

While sedation usage was increasing, it was very difficult to determine the effectiveness of the guidelines. Consequently, Davis (1988) surveyed Diplomates of the ABPD. He found that the two most important reasons for the increase in sedation usage were that (1) 54% of pediatric dentists claimed they now treated more difficult patients, and (2) many (32%) felt the need to provide more efficient care due to economic pressures. Interestingly, 12% felt that they were now better prepared to use conscious sedation and 39% decreased their sedation usage because of the difficulty in complying with the AAPD guidelines. The latter two findings suggested that the guidelines were beginning to have a positive effect.

Compliance with the guidelines was slow. Houpt (1993) found that practitioners who used sedation monitored their patients in a variety of ways. Most evaluated by the color of their patient's appearance, but only 54% used a precordial stethoscope and only a third of practitioners took blood pressure. On the other hand, pulse rate was taken by 83%, respiration was monitored by 80%, and 69% used a pulse oximeter. What was difficult to determine in this report was whether the monitoring was appropriate for the types of sedation administered.

Six years after the guidelines were published, further need for changes was evident based upon survey responses from 95% of pediatric dentistry program directors. A survey report by Wilson (2001) found an increase in conscious sedation lecture hours, as compared to earlier data. It was also found that midazolam was the most frequently used sedative, and there was an increase in emergency preparedness. In some cases, there were no changes. Oral administration remained the predominant route and, importantly, the precordial stethoscope, pulse oximeter, and blood pressure cuff were the most commonly used monitors. The anticipated sedation depth and sedation agents were key factors in choosing these monitors.

While the use of sedation to treat children was increasing, not everyone in the 1990s was in favor of the increase. Griffin and Schneiderman (1992) questioned the need to sedate and suggested that before sedating, pediatric dentists should consider:

- the urgency of treatment,
- deferral of treatment until the use of non-pharmacologic techniques is appropriate, and
- weigh the benefit versus the risk.

Studying and adhering to guidelines is critical—they assist clinicians to deliver safe sedation to their child patients. A recent (and disturbing) report (Chicka et al. 2012) of 17 closed malpractice cases revealed that in all cases, guidelines were not observed. Overdoses and instances of inadequate monitoring were found in anesthesia cases for pediatric dental patients, and nine cases resulted in death or permanent brain damage. While there will undoubtedly always be untoward incidents such as these, there is no excuse for disregarding the guidelines.

The foregoing is a brief summary of the history of pediatric sedation. It reveals how the area of pediatric dental sedation has changed, and it is still changing. Considering recent surveys, Johnson et al. (2012) reported change. From 1,219 survey returns, they found that 63% of the respondents practiced conscious sedation primarily to help provide care for patients who were difficult to manage. That is quite different than earlier findings that showed economics to be one of the prime reasons for sedation. Those who did not practice conscious sedation gave exposure to liability as the main reason. Years ago, that was not a major consideration. Wilson and Nathan (2011) followed up on the 2001 survey of program directors. They found varying experiences in training programs, and they concluded that there was a need to strengthen competencies in sedation practices in academic programs. In earlier years, there was no mention of competencies. Thus, sedation in pediatric dentistry is continually changing. That challenges the practitioner to keep up with the changes.

The shifts in sedation practices within pediatric dentistry reflect the many changes occurring within modern society. Traditionally, widely acceptable behavior management techniques such as tell-show-do and other more aversive methods were used by pediatric dentists. However, due to evolving societal norms, their use is slowly being phased out. In May 2006, the AAPD eliminated the hand-over-mouth exercise technique from its clinical guidelines on behavior management. Pediatric dentists are also hesitant to use other techniques. Today, many parents refuse to be separated from their child, and others will not allow voice control, stating, "We never raise our voices to our children, why should we allow you to do so?"

Without the ability to use these time-proven techniques, pediatric dentists will often find their hands tied when confronting a defiant, uncooperative, and/or over-indulged child who is perhaps accompanied by over-protective parents. Casamassimo et al. (2002) reported the effects of changing parenting styles on dental practices in the United States. The majority of pediatric dentists (92%) indicated that parenting style changes were probably (54%) or definitely (38%) responsible for changes in patient management. Respondents felt that parenting styles had changed because parents were less willing to set limits, less willing to use physical discipline, unsure of their roles as parents, too busy to spend time with their children, and too self-absorbed or materialistic. Practitioners reported using much less assertive behavior management techniques due to these changes. Adair et al. (2004) also found that the great majority of practitioners believed that parenting styles had changed during their years in practice, and that these changes may have contributed to an increase in behavior management problems in the dental setting. Thus, a trend within the profession is to use sedation and general anesthesia more frequently as a means of treating many young children in the dental office that in previous years may have been successfully treated non-pharmacologically. Anesthesiologists also have detected this change. Olabi's survey (2012) concluded that the use of dental anesthesiologists for administration of deep sedation and general anesthesia appears to be an emerging trend in pediatric dental practice. In 2019, dental anesthesiology became the tenth dental specialty (joining dental public health; endodontics; oral and maxillofacial pathology; oral and maxillofacial radiology; oral and maxillofacial surgery; orthodontics and dentofacial orthopedics; pediatric dentistry; periodontics; and prosthodontics) recognized by the National Commission on Recognition of Dental Specialties and Certifying Boards in the United States. It is amazing that within such a relatively short period of time, the acceptance of general anesthesia by parents has drastically changed (see Table 7-4): in 1991 (Lawrence et al. 1991), it was rated as being the least acceptable of all techniques; in 2005 (Eaton et al. 2005), it was ranked as the third-most acceptable; and in 2016, it moved forward to the second-most acceptable of all techniques (Patel et al. 2016). To expect today's dentist to achieve the administration of uncompromised and proper dental treatment without the use of aversive patient management or pharmacotherapy techniques is unrealistic. This is the rationale that prompted the decision to include chapters describing sedation and general anesthesia techniques.

## References

Adair, S.M., Waller, J.L., Schafer, T.E. et al. (2004). A survey of members of the American Academy of Pediatric Dentistry on their use of behavior management techniques. *Pediatric Dentistry*, 26, 159–166.

American Academy of Pediatric Dentistry. (2006). Guideline on behavior guidance for the pediatric dental patient. Reference Manual 2006–07. *Pediatric Dentistry*, 28, 97–105.

Aubuchon, R.W. (1982). Sedation liabilities in pedodontics. *Pediatric Dentistry*, 4, 171–180.

Casamassimo, P., Wilson, S., and Gross, L. (2002). Effects of changing U.S. parenting styles on dental practice: Perceptions of diplomats of the American Board of Pediatric Dentistry. *Pediatric Dentistry*, 24, 18–22.

Chen, D.T. (1982). Alphaprodine HCl: Characteristics. *Pediatric Dentistry*, 4, 158–163.

Chicka, M.C., Dembo, J.B., Mathu-Muju, K.R. et al. (2012). Adverse events during pediatric dental anesthesia and sedation: A review of closed malpractice insurance claims. *Pediatric Dentistry*, 34, 231–238.

Coté, C.J. and Wilson, S. (2019). Guidelines for monitoring and management of pediatric patients before, during, and after sedation for diagnostic and therapeutic procedures. *Pediatric Dentistry*, 41, 259–260.

Creedon, R.L. (1982). Alphaprodine in 20 years of practice experience. *Pediatric Dentistry*, 4, 187–189.

Davis, M.J. (1988). Conscious sedation practices in pediatric dentistry: A survey of members of the American Board of Pediatric Dentistry College of Diplomates. *Pediatric Dentistry*, 10, 328–329.

Eaton, J.J., McTigue, D.J., Fields, H.W. Jr. et al. (2005). Attitudes of contemporary parents toward behavior management techniques used in pediatric dentistry. *Pediatric Dentistry*, 27, 107–113.

Griffin, A.L. and Schneiderman, L.J. (1992). Ethical issues in managing the noncompliant child. *Pediatric Dentistry*, 14, 178–181.

Houpt, M. (1989). Report of project USAP: The use of sedative agents in pediatric dentistry. *Journal of Dentistry for Children*, 56, 302–309.

Houpt, M. (1993). Project USAP the use of sedative agents in pediatric dentistry: 1991 update. *Pediatric Dentistry*, 15, 36–40.

Houpt, M. (2002). Project USAP-2000. Use of sedative agents by pediatric dentists: A 15-year follow-up survey. *Pediatric Dentistry*, 24, 289–294.

Johnson, C., Weber-Gasparoni, K., Slayton, R.L. et al. (2012). Conscious sedation attitudes and perceptions: A survey of American Academy of pediatric dentistry members. *Pediatric Dentistry*, 34, e132–137.

Lawrence, S.M., McTigue, D.J., Wilson, S. et al. (1991). Parental attitudes toward behaviour management techniques used in pediatric dentistry. *Pediatric Dentistry*, 13, 151–155.

Musselman, R.J. and McClure, D.B. (1975). Pharmacotherapeutic approaches to behavior management. In: G.Z. Wright (Ed.), Behavior Management in Dentistry for Children (p. 147). W.B. Saunders Co., Philadelphia, PA, USA.

Olabi, N.F., Jones, J.E., Saxen, M.A. et al. (2012). The use of office-based sedation and general anesthesia by board certified pediatric dentists practicing in the United States. *Anesthesia Progress*, 59, 12–17.

Patel, M., McTigue, D.J., Thikkurissy, S. et al. (2016). *Pediatric Dentistry*, 38, 30–36.

Phero, J.C. (1993). Pharmacologic management of pain, anxiety, and behavior: Conscious sedation, *deep sedation and general anesthesia. Pediatric Dentistry*, 15, 429–433.

Sim, J.M. (1975). Pharmacotherapeutic approaches to behavior management. In: G.Z. Wright (Ed.), Behavior Management in Dentistry for Children (pp. 165–195). W.B. Saunders Co., Philadelphia, PA, USA.

Smith, R.C. (1977). Chloral hydrate in dentistry for children with handicaps. Master's Thesis, University of Iowa, Iowa City.

Troutman, K.C. and Renzi, J. Jr. (1982). The efficacy of alphaprodine in pedodontics. *Pediatric Dentistry*, 4, 181–161.

Wilson, S. (1996). A survey of the American Academy of Pediatric Dentistry membership: Nitrous oxide and sedation. *Pediatric Dentistry*, 18, 287–293.

Wilson, S. (2001). Conscious sedation experiences in graduate pediatric dentistry programs. *Pediatric Dentistry*, 23, 307–314.

Wilson, S. and Nathan, J.E. (2011). A survey of sedation training in advanced pediatric dentistry programs: Thoughts of program directors and students. *Pediatric Dentistry*, 33, 353–360.

Wright, G.Z. and McAulay, D.J. (1973). Current premedicating trends in pedodontics. *Journal of Dentistry for Children*, 40, 185–188.

# 11

## Sedation for the Pediatric Patient

*Stephen Wilson*

## Introduction

The behavior of children in a dental setting is an interesting window through which many domains, including, among others, biological, genetic, psychosocial, cognitive, and emotional are expressed either imperceptibly or overtly in a relatively short period of time. Not only is child behavior interesting in this setting, it can be enormously challenging to consistently manage and, as desired, permanently modify so the outcome skillfully and beneficially favors the various needs of the child, parent, and the clinical team. Only a few short decades have witnessed a multitude of significant changes associated with the pharmacological management of children for dental and medical procedures. As alluded to in the previous chapter, there are many possible reasons for the change. Importantly, these include the development, acceptance, and implementation of sedation guidelines and their updates by professional groups and the unpredictable but constantly evolving professional, regulatory, and societal influences affecting behavioral guidance techniques, including sedation practices (Wilson and Houpt 2016). There seems to be a tendency, however, for pediatric dentists to practice pharmacological management of children in a similar vein to that in which they were trained (Houpt 2002). Thus, the practice of sedation in the United States probably has retained much from the past. Ironically, recent evidence suggests sedation training in graduate and residency programs in the United States may not be fully compliant with guidelines and accreditation standards (Morin et al. 2016).

One aspect of pharmacological management that remains constant is the quest for the "magic bullet." The "magic bullet" is thought of as a single sedative agent or concoction of sedative agents that when given to a child patient (1) will ensure that the child is peaceful in demeanor and responds favorably during the procedure; (2) harbors enough working memory to retain the impression of a "pleasant" experience at the dental office; (3) is minimally affected by invasive dental interventions from physiological, behavioral, and emotional perspectives; and (4) is always safe in the hands of the clinician. So far, the only "magic bullet" that comes close but does not fully satisfy this idyllic state is that of general anesthesia (GA). One might predict that the future will see such a "magic bullet," but not in the same heuristic conceptualization that we currently embrace. Rather, it may involve the use of some selective, reversible effect on various neuroanatomical loci of the brain using a yet undiscovered psychopharmacological concoction or other interventional procedures.

## Sedation and Pediatric Dentistry

A popular method used today in clinical care of patients who experience fear, anxiety, and/or pain is that of pharmacological interventions. In fact, sedation of children is a common and accepted modality of patient management during potentially painful procedures. Its popularity is due, in part, to its effective and efficient ability to overcome in variable degrees the mental and emotional anguish and behavioral expressions of the patient who otherwise is unable to provide satisfactory personal management of the distressing situation. Parents appear to be more accepting of their children today than in previous years of pharmacological management under certain circumstances, (Patel et al. 2016; White et al. 2016) and evidence suggests its use among some practitioners, including female practitioners, is increasing (Wells et al. 2018a).

The process and need for safety in performing sedation during dental procedures involves several factors that are directed toward positive general outcomes. Some of these factors can be seen in Table 11-1. Clinicians must have a strong cognitive understanding, clinical expertise, and respect of each of these factors often reflected in the concept of professional competency. Unfortunately, little is

*Wright's Behavior Management in Dentistry for Children*, Third Edition. Edited by Ari Kupietzky.
© 2022 John Wiley & Sons, Inc. Published 2022 by John Wiley & Sons, Inc.

**Table 11-1** Major factors and their considerations in performing sedations.

| Major factors | Considerations |
| --- | --- |
| Child characteristics | Age, cognition, temperament, style of coping, parent–child relationship, and caries burden |
| Drug characteristics | Dose and concentration, mechanism of action, effects, pharmacokinetics, pharmacodynamics, adverse events, contraindications, formulations, and combinations of agents |
| Protocol | Standardized process, checks and balances, and quality improvement measures |
| Patient monitoring | Monitors and significance and implications of measures monitored |
| Practitioner training | Breadth and types of experiences, programmatic versus empirical influences, and recognition and response to patient signs and symptoms |
| Clinical staff knowledge | Similar to practitioner training |
| Sedation guidelines | Knowledge and adherence to guidelines |
| State rules and regulations | Knowledge and adherence to state regulations which supersede guidelines |
| Emergency prevention and management | Training, recognition, and interventional abilities, including algorithm efficiencies |

currently known about practitioner competency surrounding the knowledge and adherence to these factors either in the educational or practice communities. Indirect information through surveys over the decades has suggested that many practitioners perform sedations on a regular basis (Houpt 1989, 1993, 2002; Wilson and Houpt 2016), but documented information of the details of the sedations and even their effectiveness are mostly non-existent. Nonetheless, several important factors are discussed briefly in the following sections, which the dentist should have gleaned through formal training and experience.

## The Child

Essential knowledge of the child's age, cognitive development, temperament, and coping styles become key to planning and negotiating interactions aimed at arriving at a safe and successful clinical outcome (see Chapter 2). Usually, children less than three years of age are not easily managed during stressful or painful procedures using behavioral interactive techniques. The likelihood increases that such techniques will become more successful once the youngster has a better comprehension and mastery of speech, symbolic manipulations, and coping strategies. Thus, pharmacological management of the child who is less than three years becomes a more promising and rational approach in managing behavior assuming the depth of the sedation is enough to overcome the child's natural instincts of fight or flight without compromising the child's safety during the procedure. Deep sedation (DS) or GA is needed for these younger children but may carry a greater risk for the children and clinical team.

Children cope with varying degrees of success during challenging clinical situations. There are few studies in dentistry investigating cognitive coping strategies, parental or staff-assisted interventions (e.g., distraction or breathing exercises), or other mechanisms used in coping with acute or chronic pain and perceived stress. However, interventional studies designed to minimize anxiety, stress, and pain during distressful procedures have been investigated by others (Campbell et al. 2017; Flowers and Birnie 2015; Mahoney et al. 2010; McCarthy et al. 2010). Investigations of how children cope with stressful situations potentially involving pain have led to such concepts as information-seeking and information-limiting individuals (Fortier et al. 2009). In other words, some children do better when told about details of a procedure they will undergo, whereas others use different techniques including limiting information about the procedure.

Temperament may be defined as how a child typically responds to a novel environment as well as the child's basic daily expression pattern in a host of solitary and social situations. It was initially described in relationship to the clinical environment in the 1960s by Thomas et al. (1963). As such, temperament has received considerable attention in explaining some behaviors associated with various settings (Fortier et al. 2010; Lee and White-Traut 1996; Lopez et al. 2008). There are several scales or measures of temperament and conceptual domains used to describe conceptual domains and qualities of temperament (Cloninger et al. 2019). The work by Lochary et al. was one of the first to describe characteristics of temperament as it relates to the dental setting (Lochary et al. 1993) and can be seen in Table 11-2. Temperament is thought to have some genetic component (DiLalla and Jamnik 2019; Goldsmith

**Table 11-2** Domains of temperament according to Thomas and Chess.

| Parameter | Characteristic |
| --- | --- |
| Sensitivity | Threshold level for change in environment |
| Approachability | Initial response to new settings |
| Adaptability | Response over time to new settings |
| Mood | Tendency toward happy/unhappy attitude |
| Distractibility | Tendency to be sidetracked |
| Activity | Daily amount of energy expended |
| Regularity | Predictability in daily routine |
| Intensity | Amount of energy in response to setting |
| Persistence | Ability to stick to task |

*Source:* Based on Lochary et al. (1993).

et al. 1997; Plomin and Rowe 1977), and, interestingly, there have been some brain loci associated with temperament characteristics (Cloninger et al. 2019; Helfinstein et al. 2012; Martinos et al. 2012; Morgan 2006). The degree to which sedative agents may modulate these brain areas and affect expressions of temperament is unknown at this time but may be further elucidated by research in the future.

Temperamental characteristics of children are thought to be related to child behavior in clinical situations (Caldwell-Andrews and Kain 2006; Fortier et al. 2010; Koller and Goldman 2012; McCarthy et al. 2010; Tripi et al. 2004; Wolff et al. 2011). Interestingly, there is a significant amount of information concerning the contribution of child temperament to behaviors witnessed in the dental environment (Aminabadi et al. 2015; Arnkup et al. 2003; Arnrup et al. 2007; Klingberg and Broberg 1998, 2007; Gustafsson 2010; Gustafsson et al. 2010; Isik et al. 2010; Jabin and Chaudhary 2014; Krikken et al. 2012; Lane et al. 2015; Nelson 2013; Nelson et al. 2017; Salem et al. 2012; Santos and Quinonez 2014; Tsoi et al. 2018). Clinically and simplistically, children can be divided into three groups: (1) easy—those who are very interactive, friendly, and easily managed; (2) slow-to-warm up—those who generally do well with appropriate guidance but need some time to overcome minor anxieties; and (3) difficult—those who are withdrawn and display overt disruptive behaviors with little provocation (Lochary et al. 1993). The results of some studies suggest that shy children in the dental setting express more distress and negative behaviors in response to dental procedures (Aminabadi et al. 2014; Arnrup et al. 2007; Jensen and Stjernqvist 2002; Quinonez et al. 1997; Tsoi et al. 2018), whereas those who are adaptable and approachable exhibit less disruptive and more appropriate interactive behaviors (Lochary et al. 1993;

Radis et al. 1994). Relationships between sedation and temperament in the dental setting have also been studied (Cohen et al. 2006; Isik et al. 2010; Lane et al. 2015; Nelson et al. 2017). One study concluded that children sedated with midazolam and who exhibit specific temperament characteristics and behavior problems may be more likely to experience sedation failure (Isik et al. 2010). A clinician should always be cognizant of children's behaviors preoperatively in hopes of finding clues that may aid in anticipating interactions with the child once dental procedures begin. For instance, a concerted effort should be made to observe the interaction of the dental staff with children during initial introductions and exchange of pleasantries, patient weighing, and introduction to the office in general and in the clinical operatory. These interactions can be predictive of behavior and help anticipate potential behavior management strategies when one interacts with the child.

A parent's demeanor, body language, concerns, desires, anxieties, and opinions are also important considerations. Parents usually have belief and value systems that tend to fit their generation, lifestyle, and life experiences. It is appropriate for the practitioner to ascertain the parent's opinion in discussing behavior management possibilities.

There is some evidence suggesting that parenting skills have changed over recent decades and that these changes influence how children tend to respond in the dental environment as well as other social settings (Casamassimo et al. 2002; Schor 2003). Practitioners report that children tend to cry and are more difficult to manage than in the past. Furthermore, some view today's parent(s), compared to a generation or two ago, as more liberal in rearing their children. As an extension of that view, many believe this less involved parenting style is a detrimental trend in that parents fail to set limits and are less involved in guiding their children in psychosocial and socialization processes. Even the concept of the family is different than it was when this textbook was initially written (see Chapter 4). Some have shown that parenting styles are an important consideration in the dental setting (Aminabadi, et al. 2015; Howenstein et al. 2015; Miranda-Remijo et al. 2016; Oliver and Manton 2015; Tsoi et al. 2018; Wells et al. 2018b). Aminabadi et al. (2015) have proposed a new perspective involving a dynamic patient–parent–dentist relationship. They found that children of authoritative parents had significantly less anxiety and behavior problems during dental care. Children of authoritarian and permissive parents had significantly high levels of anxiety and behavior problems. As a newer generation of professional transition into providing care, their attitudes, opinions, and orientations toward delivery of care may change reflecting similar sentiments of parents of their age. It will remain speculative as to what management technologies may prevail in the future. But it is possible based on trends today in society that a greater reliance on pharmacological management will predominate in the future in managing children for medical and dental procedures.

## Patient Assessment

One of the most important and comprehensive aspects in the decision to use pharmacological agents in aiding the management of the child is that of patient assessment. Patient assessment includes a detailed review of the patient's medical and social history and major physiological systems (e.g., cardiovascular), performing a physical assessment of the child focusing on auscultation of the chest and heart, viewing the upper airway structures including tonsils, ascertaining an impression of the patient's behavior and temperament, and determining the number of dental needs of the patient. Medical consults following the initial review of the patient's conditions are also a part of this process.

By performing these preliminary procedures, one may determine the physical risk and status of the patient in undergoing the sedation and dental procedure, the drug(s) and dose(s) selected, and possibly an impression of the likelihood of a successful outcome. A similar process occurs when assessing a patient for GA with the outcome being a physical risk category assigned to the patient. The standard physical risk categories used in medical and dental care is that of the American Society of Anesthesiology (i.e., ASA classifications) and can be seen in Table 11-3.

The review of systems and medical history implies asking appropriate questions and if anything, other than "normal" arises, follow-up queries to determine the issue and its impact, medications, hospitalizations, acute or chronic home care, and outcome of any previous intervention. If there is or has been a problem with a system, a consultation with the patient's primary care physician often is advisable.

Auscultation of the chest using a stethoscope is needed to confirm that the intrathoracic airway is clear and not congested or indicative of other abnormalities (e.g., asthmatic wheezing). Typically, placement of the bell on the various fields of the chest and back is done. In preschoolers, another good location to hear breath sounds in under the armpit and lateral border of the chest. Also, the heart sounds should be auscultated with a stethoscope. The primary goal in listening to the heart is determining if there is a regular rate and rhythm (e.g., sinus rhythm). If there is anything unusual or different from a typical "lub-dub" of each cardiac cycle, or any other sound is heard, a consultation with the child's physician is usually indicated. Sites can be found on the Internet allowing one to hear differences between normal and abnormal respiratory and cardiac sounds (e.g., https://www.youtube.com/watch?v=dBwr2GZCmQM). A visit to those websites is highly recommended. Listen to the sounds to gain a basic appreciation of what is normal and abnormal.

**Table 11-3** American Society of Anesthesiology (ASA) physical risk categories.[§]

| ASA Class[§] | Patient status | Comment |
|---|---|---|
| I | A normal healthy patient | Healthy, non-smoking, and no or minimal alcohol use |
| II | A patient with mild systemic disease | Mild diseases only without substantive functional limitations. Examples include (but not limited to): current smoker, social alcohol drinker, pregnancy, obesity (30 < BMI < 40), well-controlled DM/HTN, and mild lung disease |
| III | A patient with severe systemic disease | Substantive functional limitations; one or more moderate to severe diseases. Examples include (but not limited to): poorly controlled DM or HTN, COPD, morbid obesity (BMI ≥40), active hepatitis, alcohol dependence or abuse, implanted pacemaker, moderate reduction of ejection fraction, ESRD undergoing regularly scheduled dialysis, premature infant PCA < 60 weeks, and history (>3 months) of MI, CVA, TIA, or CAD/stents |
| IV | A patient with severe systemic disease that is a constant threat to life | Examples include (but not limited to): recent (< 3 months) MI, CVA, TIA, or CAD/stents; ongoing cardiac ischemia or severe valve dysfunction; severe reduction of ejection fraction; sepsis; and DIC, ARD, or ESRD not undergoing regularly scheduled dialysis |
| V | A moribund patient who is not expected to survive without the operation | Examples include (but not limited to): ruptured abdominal/thoracic aneurysm, massive trauma, intracranial bleed with mass effect, and ischemic bowel in the face of significant cardiac pathology or multiple organ/system dysfunction |

There is an ASA VI but refers to a brain death individual whose organs may be harvested.
[§] See https://www.ncbi.nlm.nih.gov/books/NBK441940/
*Source:* Based on National Center for Biotechnology Information, U.S. National Library of Medicine 8600 Rockville Pike, Bethesda MD, 20894 USA.

Soft tissue (e.g., tonsils and adenoids) and the structural relationships of the upper airway are important considerations in decisions related to the use of sedatives. Tonsil size is important in appreciating the amount of airway space they occupy as they rest between the anterior and posterior pillars separating the oral from the pharyngeal portion of the oropharynx (Figure 11-1). Strong consideration of the risk of large tonsil size is imperative, especially if the likelihood that unconsciousness may occur during sedation. Tonsils greater than 50% of the airway diameter are usually contraindicated with drugs like chloral hydrate because of the increased likelihood of loss of consciousness. Chloral hydrate may increase the probability of airway blockage due to relaxation of the tongue and airway muscles and mandible, which due to gravity in a supine patient tends to fall backward against soft tissue. A very important question that should always be asked of the parent is whether the child routinely snores during sleep. The likelihood of snoring increases as the size of the tonsils increase.

It is rare that one cannot visualize the tonsils and transitional aspects of a portion of the oropharynx. If the child is cooperative, one may ask them to point their chin toward the ceiling while in a supine position, open as wide as possible, and say a soft "ahhh." The clinician sitting directly *behind* the patient with good lighting should be able to judge the size of the tonsils and how much of the patent airway space they occupy. If a child is not cooperative, the following technique can be used to visualize the tonsils. A mouth mirror can be placed on the anterior part of the tongue which naturally causes the child to posture or stiffen the tongue against the mirror and slowly slide the mirror distally until the gag reflex is triggered. The clinician must be prepared to quickly observe the tonsil size during the gag movement wherein the tonsils and soft tissue collectively move into the center of the airway space and rise slightly cephalad. The patient will not vomit, but the clinician must be ready to observe the tissues during this quick reflex. A second gag attempt is not recommended. A courteous apology of the maneuver to the child is appropriate.

Finally, an assessment of the child's dental needs is critical in terms of the number of teeth or quadrants of dentistry requiring treatment, the technical challenge of the procedures, and degree of patient immobility needed for the type of procedures anticipated. These, along with the child's temperament, are important variables in deciding the selection of agent(s) and their doses prior to preparing the sedation "cocktail." For instance, an ultra-short procedure such as extraction of the maxillary primary incisors may only require a low dose of midazolam. Caution is advised for these short invasive procedures in terms of allowing enough time for profound local anesthesia onset before beginning the exodontia procedure. Midazolam has a rapid onset but a short duration of action, whereas two or more quadrants of dental restorations may require a triple combination of drugs such as low-dose chloral hydrate (or benzodiazepine such as midazolam or diazepam), meperidine, and hydroxyzine. This combination affords the dentist a longer working time. Those who do not vary the drug regimen(s) or dose(s) are less likely to have a higher rate of successful sedations than those who do have the training and skills associated with various drug regimens.

## Sedation Protocol

Establishing and adhering to a good sedation protocol will facilitate pharmacological management of the child and minimize the likelihood of making an error within a

(a)

(b)

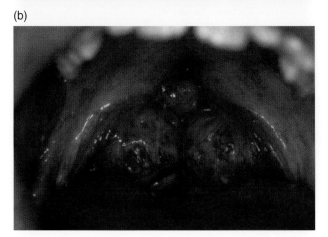

**Figure 11-1** Tonsil size is very important in appreciating the amount of airway space that they occupy between the anterior and posterior pillars separating the oral from the pharyngeal portion of the oropharynx visible tonsils of average size (a) versus enlarged tonsils which may result in airway blockage (b).

sequence of activities associated with the delivery of dental care. Another benefit of relying on a regular and standardized procedural sequence is that it allows incorporating and synchronizing other staff or colleagues in the process as collaborators in the safeguard of patient welfare. As a team, a set of checks or stops (e.g., time-out procedure) throughout the process diminishes errors of omission, overt forgetfulness, and probabilities of sequential flaws. A sense of teamwork will evolve and can be strengthened by regular reviews, application of risk management principles, and practicing emergency patient rescue with the goal of continual quality improvement and safety.

There are key steps within a protocol that should be highlighted for emphasis in guaranteeing the best possible outcome for the patient. They are important because they increase favorable interactions between controlled and uncontrolled factors (e.g., dental procedure versus child temperament, respectively), provide primary and secondary defenses against procedural hazards, and communicate a strong feeling of competency in performing professional duties. An example of a sedation protocol that may reflect these principles is shown in Table 11-4. The following are recommended approaches to increase the likelihood of a good outcome when performing sedations.

**Table 11-4** An example of a sedation protocol.

| Timing | Steps |
| --- | --- |
| Pre-sedation prior to sedation appointment | Behavioral assessment |
| | Dental examination and needs including radiographs if behavior permits |
| | Medical, dental, and social history |
| | Focused physical examination including respiratory, airway, and cardiovascular |
| | Informed consent with risk/benefits and alternatives |
| | Pre-operative counseling and pre-operative written instructions for parents |
| | Consults, as needed |
| | Office policy and requests during sedation visit |
| | Financial considerations |
| | State and professional regulations/guidelines |
| Pre-sedation steps on day of sedation | Review of above for completeness |
| | Matching temperamental factors with selection of drug(s) and dose(s) |
| | Drawing up drug(s) in presence of colleague/staff for confirmation check |
| | Drug administration considerations and method |
| | Clinical monitoring (or affixing monitors, as needed) during latency period between administration of drug and start of operative procedure |
| | Feedback to parents, as needed |
| | Safety interventions, as needed (e.g., emesis and decision to continue) |
| Intra-operative steps | Dental instruments, supplies, medicaments, and assessment of nitrous oxide system functionality |
| | Emergency equipment including positive pressure oxygen delivery system (i.e., bag-valve-mask) checked and readily available |
| | Continued monitoring from last step or affixing monitors and beginning monitoring per AAP/AAPD guidelines |
| | Decision on need for immobilization of patient |
| | Adjusting airway initially and frequently during procedure and use of shoulder roll/device |
| | Administration of topical and local anesthetics never exceeding a minimal and appropriate dose for a child (e.g., no more than 4 mg/kg regardless of ". . .caine"). Sometimes, this dictates how many sedation visits are needed |
| | Use of rubber dam or its equivalency (e.g., Isolite system) |
| | Variable suction (i.e., high/low suction, appropriate tips, and back-up) and lighting |
| | Documentation of vitals, behavior, and incidents with sedation record per guidelines/state regulations |
| Post-operative steps | Appropriate monitoring per guidelines/state regulations |
| | Post-operative counseling and written instructions for parents |
| | Discharge only after criteria are attained per guidelines |
| | Complete and appropriate documentation of procedure per guidelines |
| | Follow-up phone call with parents in evening |

## Clinical Technique During Sedation

### Case 11.1

Jessica, a four-year-old female weighing 18 kg, was scheduled to receive quadrant restorative dentistry under sedation. Her mother was given a plastic syringe filled with the appropriate dose (20 mg/kg) of chloral hydrate syrup and instructed to administer the drug to her daughter. After a couple of minutes, the mother called for assistance. Jessica had refused to swallow the medicine spitting it out and onto her mother, all the time screaming hysterically and kicking.

*Case 11.1, Discussion*: One of the challenging aspects of using oral sedatives is the administration of the drug. Essentially the drug can be administered by the parent or the clinician depending on the latter's practice philosophy. Many patients undergoing minimal sedation are uncooperative and may exhibit defiant behavior. There are essentially three ways to administer the regimen. A first unique way to "encourage" the hesitant child to enthusiastically drink the entire amount of liquid is to play the "race" game. The child and parent are given cups filled with either the sedative regimen (for the child) or the same color of flavored water (for the parent), respectively. The race is to see who can drink the liquid the fastest. A count of "1-2-3" is done and then both parent and child race to see who downs the liquid fastest.

A second approach involves the dentist offering the parent the option of giving the child the drug, explaining the necessity of the child swallowing the entire dose. A good gut feeling on the part of the dentist toward the parent's conviction that they can be successful in administering the regimen is beneficial. A cup or needleless syringe filled with the regimen may be offered. Some children will be willing to drink the liquid from a cup or a syringe depending on their experience in taking over-the-counter medications at home. The parent may be or may not be successful in administering the agent. If successfully administered, then wait for the appropriate time, depending on the agents used, to begin restorative procedures. If unsuccessful, and the dentist is unsure how much of the drug has been consumed, it may be hazardous and therefore not recommended to administer more of the drug(s) in order to continue with the appointment. It is the author's recommendation that the practitioner always observe the parent–child interaction during the attempt to administer the agent, whether in the room or watching outside the doorway. If the interaction was not observed, keep the child in the office to determine if some of the regimen was consumed causing some degree of sedation. It is possible that some restorative work can be done even if the child did not consume all the sedative.

The third option is when the parent initially states they do not wish to or they failed to successfully administer the regimen, then the dentist may intercede. A convenient way to facilitate the consumption of the regimen is using the "knee-to-knee" procedure. Incidentally, this procedure can be used for administering sedatives orally or intranasally. During this procedure, the child sits on the parent's lap facing the parent with his/her legs wrapped around the parent's waist. The dentist sits in a chair facing the parent and slides his/her chair to touch the knees of the parent and dentist together. The child is then reclined into the lap of the dentist and the parent secures the child's hands. A slight alternative to this maneuver is to have the child stand in front of the dentist and the child's head is tilted backward while the parent restrains the hands (Figure 11-2).

In either case, the dentist embraces the child's head and with a needleless syringe slowly dribbles the solution down and off the finger or thumb of the non-dominant hand that is strategically placed on the retromolar pad of the patient (Figure 11-3). This usually stimulates the swallowing reflex and gives the child a chance to coordinate breathing and swallowing. Infrequently, the child refuses to swallow and a pool of solution begins to form; the parent is asked to pinch off the nose briefly causing either swallowing or expectoration (usually the former). Often, the child is crying and struggling. Occasionally, they have a very difficult time between the crying and swallowing resulting in coughing while reclined. Care must be taken not to dispense too large a bolus. Pause and let the child swallow and "catch their

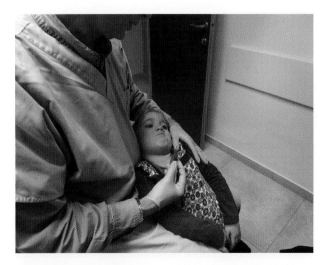

**Figure 11-2** The child's head is embraced by the dentist during administration of the premedication.

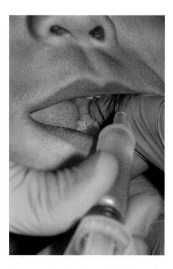

**Figure 11-3** Photograph showing administration to sedative solution using a needleless syringe technique. The tip of the thumb is placed on the retromolar pad just distal to the last mandibular molar. The tip of the syringe is aligned and placed at the first knuckle of the thumb. When the sedative solution is expressed slowly from the syringe, it flows along the thumb, over the retromolar pad, and into the back of oropharyngeal airway for swallowing. This technique minimizes choking and coughing.

breath" before proceeding. Verbally encourage them to swallow. Continue slowly until the liquid is consumed.

The time between administration of the regimen and the beginning of restorative care is known as the latency time. Latency time will vary depending on the regimen (e.g., regimens with chloral hydrate or diazepam take 45 minutes compared to that involving midazolam which only takes 15–25 minutes). During the latency period, the child's behavior is noted to change. Usually, they are more friendly, interactive, and disinhibiting. The disinhibition is exhibited as more talkativeness, exploratory hyperactivity in the environment, social interaction, and general silliness and desire to color or play with an electronic gadget (e.g., iPad), but occasionally the disinhibition can be frank agitation. This phase is usually followed by drowsiness, sleepiness, or sleep itself depending on the regimen. Even if the child appears to be sleeping, separation of the child from the parent to start dental procedures is not recommended until the appropriate latency for the regimen has passed. Otherwise, the drug has not reached enough therapeutic blood levels and if the child is disturbed, they will become uncooperative. Anytime the child is sleeping prior to separation from the parent, careful monitoring clinically and with electronic monitors (e.g., pulse oximetry) must be done. The child is never left alone, even with the parent present, and must be continuously assessed during the latency period. Practitioners may have preferences for

parental presence during the entire sedation procedure. Others prefer the parent to be dismissed before dental procedures are initiated.

Next begins the operative or working time phase. The working time will depend on the regimen used with agents (e.g., diazepam or chloral hydrate lasting nearly an hour and midazolam lasting only 20–30 minutes), the patient's level of natural fatigue, use of nitrous oxide, and child characteristics such as temperament and cognitive development.

The first item to consider during the working time is whether to use nitrous oxide as a means of slightly deepening the level of the sedation or at least controlling the uncooperative behavior of the child. Generally, nitrous oxide is very beneficial. Nitrous oxide administration is ideally used for "settling" a child at the beginning of the working phase. The settling will promote the likelihood of good behavior throughout the procedure. If any procedure is started without settling first, the likelihood of disruptive behavior will increase significantly. Thus, before any topical or local administration occurs, nitrous oxide, if used, must be delivered for a period of not less than 5 minutes to "settle" the child. Usually, the concentration of nitrous oxide for settling the child is between 35% and 50%, but if the child is screaming, crying, and generally disruptive, the concentration of nitrous oxide can be increased to 70% temporarily (not longer than 8–10 minutes) to aid in settling the child. Chapter 12 describes in detail the administration of nitrous oxide. A good method of delivering high concentration nitrous oxide when the child is moving his/her head is to hold the hood slightly off the nose and mouth by grasping the tubing on either side of the hood to steady and move the hood as the child's head moves (see Figure 11-4). If the child fails to settle, continuation of the sedation appointment will be challenging and likely fail. Then an alternative approach for managing the child's behavior at another visit should be considered. However, if successfully implemented with the nasal hood covering the nose, begin with slow but deliberate movements to open the airway. Either ask the child to point the chin of a supine patient toward the ceiling or do a head tilt to point the chin skyward. The clinician can distract the child with chatter using a low voice if the child is awake. Tell–show–do is just as important during sedation appointments as it is for routine restorative appointments. Following proper titration of nitrous oxide concentration and flow, gently open the mouth slightly, insert a mouth prop, and slowly open the mouth wider. After reviewing and confirming the planned treatment, topical and local anesthesia are administered. Chapter 9 describes in detail the administration of local anesthesia. If the child becomes agitated during the

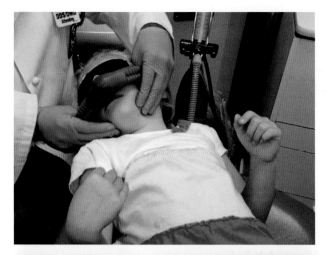

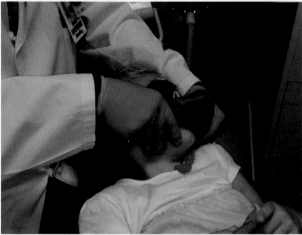

**Figure 11-4** Dentist stabilizing the nitrous oxide hood slightly off the face of patient matching the orientation of the hood with the head movement during "settling" of the patient.

injection, the clinician should "re-settle" the child once local anesthetic is administered.

Isolation of the operative field is extremely important for the safety of the child and facilitates the delivery of quality dental restorations. A rubber dam or a comparable method (e.g., Isolite,) should always be used for sedations. Generally, one can cut teeth dry or use a very light water spray that is rapidly suctioned from the mouth with high-speed suction. Note that the high-speed suction should initially be activated at some distance from the patient and slowly brought closer to the patient's mouth to not startle the patient. The same is true for the overhead lamp. Activate it away from the patient's face and slowly adjust it to illuminate the mouth. Tooth preparation can generally begin once adequate anesthesia is obtained. For pulpal procedures or extractions, the minimum time for profound bony anesthesia is 10–15 minutes—a long but necessary time to

wait before initiating such treatment. The restorative phase, if working efficiently, can be completed quickly. Occasionally, a child may become agitated during the restorative procedures and need to be re-settled with nitrous oxide and pausing the restorative care. If this sequence of events is followed, and the patient begins the procedure in a non-agitated state, it usually results in a good sedation outcome.

## Monitoring and Monitors

Monitoring means to warn or alert. Monitoring implies the possibility that both (1) clinical assessment of the patient is done by a clinician (i.e., observation of skin coloring) and (2) monitoring equipment aid in assisting the clinician in making decisions about the patient's state and need for intervention. Several monitors are used in clinical dentistry, and they can be broadly categorized as *electronic* and *non-electronic* monitors (e.g., pulse oximeter and precordial stethoscope, respectively). Some of the electronic monitors measure the same parameter as non-electronic monitors (e.g., heart rate). Automated blood pressure machines can determine the systolic and diastolic blood pressure as an isolated event or in repeated, regularly timed intervals. Likewise, a manual blood pressure cuff (BPC) can determine the same parameters of blood pressure but usually requires another tool (i.e., stethoscope) and a clinician's sense of hearing and sound discrimination. Although individual monitors are available such as a free-standing pulse oximeter, some monitors of today are referred to as *multifunctional monitors* because they incorporate three or four measured parameters into one unit. For example, blood pressure, pulse oximetry, capnography, EKG, and temperature can be assessed by a single monitor with those built-in capabilities (Figure 11-5).

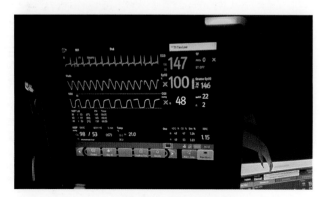

**Figure 11-5** Multifunctional monitor showing multiple physiological parameters being recorded.

## Auscultation

Stethoscopes have been available for decades and can assist in obtaining sounds of heart, respiratory, gastrointestinal, joint, and cardiovascular anomalies (e.g., arteriovenous malformations). They are particularly useful for monitoring airway and heart sounds during sedation. Optimizing and highlighting the specific sound of either the airway or heart is greatly dependent on the site of placement of the stethoscope's bell on the chest wall. In healthy children, the clinician should focus on the airway sounds, as respiratory issues typically occur before cardiac issues.

To facilitate conceptualizing the maximizing of airway versus heart sounds, one can imagine a triangle on the chest of a child with a line connecting the two nipples representing the base of the triangle (see Figure 11-6).

(a)

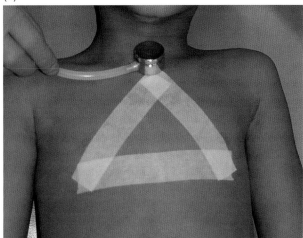

(b)

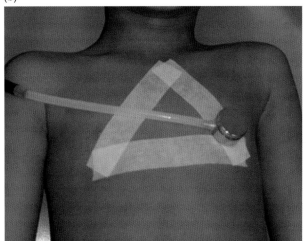

**Figure 11-6** Imaginary triangle on patient's chest. Ideally, to hear maximum upper airway sounds, the stethoscope bell is placed in the fossa just above the manubrium (a); maximum heart sounds heard when the bell overlies the heart area (b).

The right and left sides of the triangle run from the corresponding right and left nipple to the notch or soft depression on the neck just superior to the manubrium bone of the chest cage. In a supine patient, placement of the stethoscope bell at the notch will cause breathing sounds to be loud and dominant compared with the faint sounds of the heart. As the stethoscope bell is moved along the imaginary line connecting the notch to the left nipple, the sounds of breathing become fainter and the heart sounds begin to dominate. Airway sounds are more important during sedation as they transmit information on the function and patency of the upper airway as well as secondary anatomical structures and sounds (e.g., esophagus and vomiting, respectively). Thus, during sedations, the bell should be placed toward the apex of the triangle. It should be gently but well-attached to the body without causing increased pressure against the throat either with adhesive tape or 3M Double-Stick Discs® (3M Medical Device Division, St Paul, MN).

When listening through a stethoscope, competing sounds come from various sources including handpiece noise, a metal rubber dam frame touching the stethoscope bell and conducting sounds when the handpiece contacts the frame, and ambient room noise (e.g., talking or music). Often, these sounds can be comparatively loud and drown out the airway sounds, increasing the need for additional monitoring, typically the capnograph.

## Blood Pressure Cuffs

The use of BPCs has a long history in medicine and dentistry. BPCs can be used manually or electronically. The manual BPC has a cuff in which an inflatable bladder is embedded, a pressure gauge indicating the pressure inside the bladder, and a valve-controlled bulb to inflate/deflate the bladder connected to the cuff via a flexible rubber tube. Manual use of a BPC may be very helpful in emergency situations to gain a quick insight as to the approximate systolic pressure of the patient. For example, a very quick but less precise measure of systolic blood pressure can be obtained by inflating the cuff with a valve-controlled bulb and fairly rapidly decreasing the pressure in the cuff until the needle which had been traveling in a smooth constant rate from higher to lower pressures begins to "bounce" or waiver. This technique gives the clinician a rapid means of determining the general range of systolic pressure.

Automated BPCs indirectly indicate the systolic and diastolic blood pressures, as well as heart rate at discrete but modifiable intervals. The automated BPCs also use a bladder and transducer embedded cuff, a rubber tube connecting the cuff to the frame of the blood pressure apparatus, and inside the apparatus, a pump and micro-chip to control the inflation and deflation of the cuff as well as perform algorithms to determine various blood pressure and heart rate parameters.

With many automated units, a typical cycle of determining blood pressure involves periods of inflation and deflation of the cuff to obtain blood pressure parameters and variable inactive periods of time between blood pressure measurements. A cycle period for sampling blood pressure can be varied over a wide range of time periods (e.g., every 3 up to 90 minutes).

Functionally, the bladder is inflated over a few seconds to a pressure that essentially occludes blood flow in arteries. Normally, this initial pressure is set internally to around 150 mm Hg, but if vibrations are still detected, the pressure is increased until such vibrations cease. The bladder then is deflated in small steps of pressure change during which the transducer monitors oscillatory signals emanating from the arteries through the bladder. When the first increase in the size of oscillatory signals per step of decreasing pressure change is repeatedly detected, the BPC reports this pressure value as the systolic blood pressure. The cuff continues to deflate in pressure steps and the pulse pressure in the limb initially increases, then declines, until finally no further change in oscillatory signals is detected. The bladder pressure at that point represents the diastolic blood pressure. Control of this cycle is done electronically through an algorithm which determines and reports mean arterial pressure in some units which is approximately two-thirds of systolic blood pressure. The pulsating oscillatory signals detected can also be used to calculate heart rate.

There are a few factors that can cause artifact information with manual and BPCs, including (1) different width-sized cuffs with oversized cuffs tending to cause erroneously low pressure readings and too small a cuff erroneously causing high blood pressure readings; (2) air leaks anywhere within the system; and (3) patient movement. The latter is clinically significant. Movements or attempts to dislodge the cuff by an uncooperative child may result in constant recycling at high pressures. Eventually, the inflated, high pressure cuff begins to cause distal pain in the occluded limb on which it is affixed. Under normal circumstances, most automated BPCs require less than 30 seconds to determine blood pressure. However, with a struggling child, the prolonged inflation pressure of the cuff (often greater than a minute or so) causes pain and can aggravate disruptive behaviors. Failure to attend to and terminate the prolonged inflation pressure in the struggling child could conceivably lead to temporary or permanent paresthesia distal to the cuff on the limb.

In dosages designed to produce minimal and moderate sedation, most sedative agents do not cause significant clinical changes in blood pressure in the unprovoked, resting child. And in general, the blood pressure and heart rate vary with age (the younger the child, the lower the resting blood pressure and the higher the heart rate).

### Pulse Oximetry

The principle of pulse oximetry is based on the red and infrared light absorption characteristics of oxygenated and deoxygenated hemoglobin. Oxygenated and deoxygenated hemoglobin absorbs light of different wavelengths. The oxisensor probe that is attached to a vascularized tissue (e.g., toe or finger) alternatively emits red, infrared, and no light in a frequency sequence that cannot be detected by human eyes. In other words, when looking at the activated oxisensor, one only sees the red light as a constant light, but it is flickering and alternating with infrared and a no light phase that cannot be seen by human eyes. The sequencing of lights and no lights is controlled by the microchip in the pulse oximeter and aids in displaying a moving signal across the window of the pulse oximeter. Using the microchip processor, pulse oximetry takes advantage of the principle that there is a difference in light absorption of the two different states of hemoglobin depending on the amount of oxygen being carried on the hemoglobin molecule. Oxygenated hemoglobin absorbs more infrared wavelengths of light allowing more red light to pass through, while deoxygenated hemoglobin absorbs proportionately more red wavelengths with more infrared transmitted through the tissue. Hence, the microchip can discern the ratio of the two wavelengths of light and calculate the percent of oxygen saturation ($SaO_2$) of blood flowing within a tissue bed. Because the tissue bed expands slightly during pulsatile (arterial) periods, the light travels over a slightly longer distance throughout the pulse and the amount of light collected per unit time changes. Simultaneously, the oxisensor determines the change in light transmitted at a very high frequency due to the arterial pulse passing through tissue bed (plethysmography). Thus, pulse oximeters theoretically measure only arterial saturation of hemoglobin. If no blood is flowing or pulsing, no meaningful signal is detected.

The primary disadvantage of pulse oximetry is that it measures oxyhemoglobin saturation rather than arterial oxygen tension ($PaO_2$). The $PaO_2$ and the $SaO_2$ are not linearly related, but rather are related by the oxyhemoglobin dissociation curve (Figure 11-7). The "S" shape of the oxyhemoglobin dissociation curve is important for physiologic uptake and delivery of oxygen in the body. In the lungs, hemoglobin is rapidly and almost totally saturated over a wide range of $PaO_2$ (flat portion of the curve), while at the

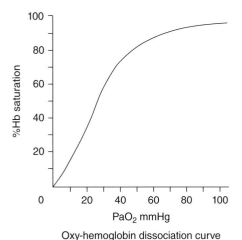

Oxy-hemoglobin dissociation curve

**Figure 11-7** Oxygen hemoglobin desaturation curve. The curve reveals the nonlinear relationship between partial pressure of oxygen in blood and oxyhemoglobin saturation. Note that blood leaving the lungs is well oxygenated under normal circumstances, but venous blood returning to the heart is less oxygenated. If the blood is not appropriately oxygenated as it passes through the lungs, then desaturation in peripheral tissues will occur rapidly (i.e., hypoxia). *Source:* Anderson and Vann (1988). Reproduced with permission from AAPD. © 1998, American Academy of Pediatric Dentistry.

tissues, large amount of oxygen is unloaded as desaturation occurs over a relatively small drop in PaO$_2$ on the steep portion of the curve. An understanding of the relationship between PaO$_2$ and the SaO$_2$ is essential for those using pulse oximetry clinically (Anderson and Vann 1988).

Changes in oxygenation are not detected until the PaO$_2$ falls to the point where oxyhemoglobin desaturation occurs, that is, the 70–80 mm Hg range, where the steep portion of the oxyhemoglobin dissociation curve is rapidly approached. When one is breathing room air, the normal PaO$_2$ is in the 90–100 mm Hg range, which corresponds to a SaO$_2$ of 96–100%. Because a PaO$_2$ of 60 mm Hg corresponds to a SaO$_2$ of approximately 90%, the PaO$_2$ must fall from approximately 100%–90%. Often, patients undergoing dental sedation or GA are receiving supplemental oxygen (with or without nitrous oxide), thus the PaO$_2$ may range from 150 to above 600 mm Hg. The PaO$_2$ must fall drastically before any change will be detected in the SaO$_2$. Large decreases in oxygenation may occur without any change being detected by pulse oximetry. Only when the PaO$_2$ falls to less than 70 mm Hg will a significant desaturation occur and be detected by pulse oximetry. The pulse oximeter will not warn of downward trends in PaO$_2$ over the wide range of oxygen tensions above this level.

To summarize, when oxyhemoglobin desaturation begins to occur, serious respiratory depression may be present. Furthermore, more rapid desaturation may be imminent as the steep portion of the curve is approached.

Therefore, during pediatric sedation, even a small change in saturation (e.g., 99–96%) must be noted quickly and evaluated before further desaturation occurs. If the saturation is trending in a downward state (i.e., less saturation state) and falls into the 95%–90% saturation range, all dental procedures must be stopped and the patient must be rapidly assessed for airway patency and efficiency of ventilation.

Any interference with information processing of the signal can produce an erroneous reading (e.g., patient movement affects tissue bed pressures and signal transmission causing motion artifact, and some fingernail polish wavelength overlaps that of red). The clinician needs to be aware that certain clinical conditions and situations can cause false signals unrelated to hemoglobin saturation. These are motion artifact; crying that may involve a Valsalva's maneuver (airway is momentarily closed while muscular efforts are made to compress air in the lungs—grunting); cold limbs or tissue bed; cessation of a prolonged crying bout; some nail polishes; profound tissue pigmentation in some African Americans; some hemoglobinopathies (e.g., methemoglobinemia); improperly attached oxisensor to tissue bed or re-used oxisensor; or any condition that reduces blood flow into the tissue bed. Pulse oximeters have alarms (both high and low) that are set by the manufacturer but can be reset for heart rate and oxygen saturation. The oxygen saturation alarm sets should not be changed; however, the high heart rate alarm can be raised to values exceeding 200 beats per minute to avoid constantly sounding alarm noise for sedation of two- to four-year-old children who are struggling because of anger and frustration (usually when in a restraint) during minimal sedation.

Clinically, it is important to attach the oxisensor probe to accessible, well-perfused tissue. The toe next to the great toe seems best suited in the young, active toddler. The oxisensor can be wrapped or placed on that toe and the great toe, second (on which the oxisensor is placed), and middle toe secured together as a unit using adhesive tape. It is also wise to tape the oxisensor cable onto the plantar surface of the foot; otherwise, its movement can cause dislodging of either the oxisensor during struggling or electromagnetic (motion) artifacts. Fingers also are useful sensor sites in the older child or adult, but most uncooperative toddlers will tend to remove the oxisensor, especially if they struggle or do not want the probe on their finger. The ear lobe is another convenient site in older children.

Since 1985, almost every article on sedation of the pediatric dental patient published today reports the use of PO (per os). Generally, most reports indicate oxygen saturation to be very stable during sedations with only an occasional desaturation episode. Unfortunately, these desaturation episodes can be erroneously associated with a specific sedative agent, including questionable attribution of the agent's purported effects on airway compromise. Other conditions do and have been shown to account for what appears to be temporary "desaturations" that are of no clinical significance. Nonetheless, vigilance of the patient's ventilation and attending to signals from the pulse oximeter are necessary during any sedation.

## Capnography

Capnography is one of the least understood monitoring techniques in dentistry. When used properly, it is the only electronic monitor on the market that indicates some degree of the airway patency and ventilation. Capnographs measure expired carbon dioxide concentrations. Normal carbon dioxide concentrations in children range from 33 to 40 mm Hg. But usually it is not the absolute carbon dioxide concentration that is important during lighter stages of sedation but the fact that some exchange of air can be "visualized" on the monitor. Capnographs can be classified as either main- or side-stream units. The main-stream is used with intubated patients, whereas the side-stream units are appropriate for sedated, non-intubated patients. For side-stream units, air is vacuumed or sucked through a port that is either inserted into the nostrils or placed in close approximation to the orifice of the nostril or mouth. Sucked air is delivered to a chamber inside the capnograph where the concentration of carbon dioxide can be determined by infrared absorption technology. The amount of infrared absorption in the test chamber is compared to a standardized chamber containing a known amount of carbon dioxide. The microchip processor determines and displays the carbon dioxide concentration. Capnographs can display single excursions representing the concentration of expired carbon dioxide during the expiratory cycle of breathing, and some can display trended data in which each excursion is compressed over time and appears as a single vertical line.

The expired carbon dioxide curve is displayed on a capnograph as is depicted in Figure 11-8. During normal circumstances, the beginning rise in the curve represents the first portion of carbon dioxide gas, just prior to dead space air, exiting the lungs during the initial phases of expiration. As expiratory process continues, gases from deeper portions of the lungs containing greater concentrations of carbon dioxide exit and the height of the curve rises dramatically at first then at a constant rate. As the expiratory process stops and inspiration begins, the concentration of carbon dioxide dramatically drops back to baseline. The expired carbon dioxide concentration displayed on a capnograph represents the greatest concentration (i.e., the final height) achieved during that expiration (end-tidal

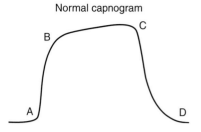

Normal capnogram

A: Exhalation begins
B-C: Plateau = outflow of alveolar gas
C: End-tidal $CO_2$

**Figure 11-8** Typical capnograph waveform showing excursions associated with expired $CO_2$. Capnography produces a waveform by the continuous analysis of respired gas for $CO_2$. The presence of the waveform implies exhalation of gases from the lungs. The end-tidal $CO_2$ (point C) corresponds to alveolar gas which may correlate closely with the $PaCO_2$. *Source:* Anderson and Vann (1988). Reproduced with permission from AAPD. © 1998, American Academy of Pediatric Dentistry.

$CO_2$). It represents gas coming from the alveoli and has been shown to correlate closely with the $PaCO_2$ (partial pressure of $CO_2$ in arterial blood). During normal breathing, that concentration is typically 40 mm Hg pressure. A child who is breathing normally but primarily moving expired gas through the mouth tends to have a waveform that is less square in shape and the height (and displayed concentration value of carbon dioxide) is reduced. Crying results in a waveform with multiple "blips" whose height is small. The height and shape of the waveform will be affected in various ways depending on the condition of the patient during monitoring.

Importantly, most capnographs have an alarm to indicate an obstruction anywhere along the sampling route, including the airway. Mucous blockage is one possible clinical situation causing the alarm mechanism to indicate an obstruction. Crying is a clinical event that causes most of the expired air to exit via the mouth; thus the capnograph will detect, if any, a lower concentration of expired carbon dioxide (i.e., the majority was shunted through the mouth leaving proportionately less to be sucked into the port). This phenomenon is also true of predominant mouth breathers. Also, many capnographs can electronically filter out the wavelength associated with nitrous oxide absorption; hence, the sampling tube can be placed under a nitrous hood without affecting the capnograph's functioning.

## Monitoring on Day of Procedure

Common sense, standard protocol, and sedation guidelines will require patient monitoring on the day of the procedure. Vital signs before administration of a sedative agent(s) should be routinely obtained unless behavior interferes with their acquisition. If behavior does prevent obtaining vital signs, a note indicating such should be placed in the patient's chart.

Monitoring should occur pre-operatively after the administration of the sedative(s) but may only involve clinical assessment of the patient (i.e., continual observation of the patient). However, if the patient becomes noticeably sedated (e.g., more quiet, peaceful, or even closes eyes), then more monitors need to be used depending on the level of sedation noted (e.g., pulse oximeter). The patient should be closely monitored until the intra-operative phase begins.

The patient needs to be monitored intra-operatively as indicated by sedation guidelines. The type and number of monitors required intra-operatively should be dependent on the patient's depth of sedation and could include a stethoscope, pulse oximeter, BPC, capnograph, EKG, or more. Table 11-5 indicates the monitors that may be recommended according to the behaviors of the patient. Importantly, the American Academy of Pediatrics and American Academy of Pediatric Dentistry sedation guidelines have changed recently including the monitors and monitoring of the patient for different depths of sedation (Cote et al. 2019). The language for moderate depths of sedation has significantly changed and reads as follows:

> There shall be continuous monitoring of oxygen saturation and heart rate; when bidirectional verbal communication between the provider and patient is appropriate and possible (i.e., patient is developmentally able and purposefully communicates), monitoring of ventilation by (1) capnography (preferred) or (2) amplified, audible pretracheal stethoscope (e.g., Bluetooth technology) or precordial stethoscope is strongly recommended. If bidirectional verbal communication is not appropriate or not possible, monitoring of ventilation by capnography (preferred), amplified, audible pretracheal stethoscope, or precordial stethoscope is required.

**Table 11-5** Patient behavior intra-operatively and recommended monitors.[§]

| Behavior | Clinical signs | Pre-cordial stethoscope | Pulse oximetry | Blood pressure cuff | Capnograph |
|---|---|---|---|---|---|
| Peaceful and content Screaming or yelling with movement | Little tears Controlled breathing Struggling against wrap | Take earpiece out of ear Replace it when patient becomes less noisy | Keep it stabilized on foot Set upper heart rate limits to > 230 bpm | Place on limb but do not inflate if child is uncooperative | Not needed at this time but can place if anticipating patient may attain deeper levels of sedation |
| Mild crying | Tearing variable; eyelids open/some ptosis Sobbing, but controlled Little or no struggling | Same as above, but be ready to insert earpiece if child becomes quiet | Same as above | Place on limb (upper arm or lower leg above ankle); obtain blood pressure occasionally (10-15 minutes) | Same as above |
| Quiet, but responsive | Eyes closed; opens when requested or mildly stimulated Breathing within normal limits Occasional sobbing | Earpiece in and listening Attentive to gurgling (fluids in airway) or snoring (partially blocked airway adjust with head tilt–jaw thrust) | Same as above Heightened awareness for incidence of desaturation (pitch) | Place on limb (upper arm or lower leg above ankle); obtain blood pressure every 5 minutes unless its function upsets patient (then obtain occasionally) | Place probe Monitor ventilation and record respiratory rate |
| Quiet | Eyes closed or partial ptosis with possible divergent eyes; does not open upon command Breathing shallow, subtle super-inspiration may occur and intermittent or infrequent in rate | Same as above Maximal focus on airway sounds | Same as above Critically important Heightened awareness for incidence of desaturation (pitch) | Place on limb (upper arm or lower leg above ankle); obtain blood pressure every 5 minutes | Critically important Be aware of frequency of breathing, expired [conc], and apnea |

[§] Behavior and physiological parameters must be recorded on sedation record.

Also important is the change in personnel required during DS. For DS, an independent observer in addition to the clinician providing the dental care must be present whose sole purpose is to monitor the patient. This independent observer must have anesthesia training and be certified and able to perform patient rescue procedures (e.g., intubation). The guidelines specifically identify the independent observer as either a physician with sedation training and advanced airway skills (e.g., medical anesthesiologist), dentist anesthesiologist, oral surgeon, or other medical specialists with requisite licensure, training, and competencies (e.g., certified registered nurse anesthetist).

The frequency of recording of the monitored parameters will also depend on the depth of sedation attained.

Monitoring of the patient should continue after the procedure is completed and during the post-operative phase until the patient meets discharge criteria and is released from the dentist's care. Again, the type of monitoring required will depend on the patient's behavior and depth of sedation during this phase. A child should never leave the office until discharge criteria are met as per sedation guidelines.

Detailed record keeping before, during, and after sedation procedures are extremely important and carry significant medico-legal implications for the practitioner. Information on the type of documentation that is needed can be found in sedation guidelines (Cote et al. 2019). For example, written and signed informed consent documents should be a part of the patient's record. Also important are consultation documents, pre- and post-operative instructions for parents, detailed progress notes of the procedure, and a time-based record of the sedation. The American Academy of Pediatric Dentistry's website (www.aapd.org) has a sedation record that is detailed and consistent with all requirements of the sedation guidelines. It is advisable to visit the website and download a copy of the sedation record as a template for sedations performed by the practitioner.

## Practitioner and Staff Training

Practitioner competency and staff training are essential to safe sedation practices. Unfortunately, there are few regulations or processes that guarantee practitioner competency and staff training specifically related to sedation procedures. The Commission on Dental Accreditation (CODA) has language related to sedation for advanced programs of some dental specialties in the United States, but the accreditation process allows institutions liberty in interpreting and instituting such training (http://www.ada.org/115.aspx). Hence, there is considerable variability among training programs despite advocacy for improving and somewhat standardizing sedation training (Wilson and Nathan 2011). Likewise, although state boards of dentistry regulate sedation practices, the degree of consistency among the state rules and regulations is variable. Recent changes in CODA standards for advanced programs in Pediatric Dentistry have gone into effect in July 2013 with language changes reflecting requirements for increased sedation experiences for trainees but not necessarily the scope and quality of such experiences. The current CODA standard indicates that students/residents (1) must complete 20 nitrous oxide analgesia patient encounters as the primary operator and (2) must complete a minimum of 50 patient encounters in which sedative agents other than nitrous oxide are used (although nitrous oxide can be a part of the sedation regimen). Each student/resident must act as the sole primary operator in a minimum of 25 sedation cases of the 50 encounters. Of the remaining 25 cases, each student/resident must gain clinical experience in a variety of settings including human simulation. CODA does not address training of individuals once they graduate from a program. However, other options are available to the practicing dentist, including continuing education courses involving sedation as well as human simulation of sedation emergencies (e.g., see website of AAPD).

The American Dental Association (ADA) has guidelines on the teaching of pharmacological management of patients, including dentists seeking continuing education (http://www.ada.org/sections/about/pdfs/anesthesia_guidelines.pdf). These guidelines are currently under review and likely will be modified soon. Practitioners should be aware of such guidelines and take precautions not to provide sedation in their practices unless their training meets or exceeds these guidelines. Practitioners also should have training in advanced cardiac life support or its equivalency before sedating patients, especially those in the pediatric age group (e.g., pediatric advanced life support).

Practitioners who provide sedation services to pediatric patients should train or provide options for training for their staff. The training should meet minimum objectives and criteria not unlike that offered via ADA guidelines to practitioners. The American Academy of Pediatric Dentistry currently offers a didactic course on sedation for office staff.

Finally, dentists and their staff should enroll in emergency management courses on a regular basis to obtain a review of and recognition of emergencies and basic skill sets associated with lifesaving procedures such as airway management. Basic and advanced life support knowledge and skills tend to dissipate quickly following courses, and hence, emergency drills and practice should occur on a frequent basis (Wik et al. 2002). Interestingly, high-fidelity human simulation training has become very popular and is highly recommended for those in performing emergency procedures (Tipa and Bobirnac 2010). Teamwork, including communication, decision-making, and role responsibilities, is critical to effectively manage emergencies. Evidence suggests that higher frequency of errors in team is associated with lower-rated teamwork scores (Herzberg et al. 2019). It is the opinion of the author that emphasis on teamwork training in sedation protocols in the office should be conducted quarterly, and human simulation of sedation emergencies performed on an annual basis. Currently, the greatest barriers for human simulation are access and cost.

### Sedation Guidelines

The history for the development of sedation guidelines for children sedated for dental procedures has been published (Creedon 1986; Wilson et al. 1996). Since the first publication of sedation guidelines for children and dentistry in 1985, there have been several revisions. The latest revision of the sedation guidelines, entitled "Guidelines for Monitoring and Management of Pediatric Patients During and After Sedation for Diagnostic and Therapeutic Procedures," was published jointly by the American Academy of Pediatrics and the American Academy of Pediatric Dentistry (Cote et al. 2019).

The current guidelines are designed for any medical or dental procedures involving sedation and children regardless of the setting. The well-referenced guidelines address prominent issues surrounding sedation of children and can best be summarized in the abstract of the guidelines which states:

> *The safe sedation of children for procedures requires a systematic approach that includes the following: no administration of sedating medication without the safety net of medical/dental supervision, careful presedation evaluation for underlying medical or surgical conditions that would place the child at increased risk from sedating medications, appropriate fasting for elective procedures and a balance between the depth of sedation and risk for those who are unable to fast because of the urgent nature of the procedure, a focused airway examination for large (kissing) tonsils or anatomic airway abnormalities that might increase the potential for airway obstruction, a clear understanding of the medication's pharmacokinetic and pharmacodynamic effects and drug interactions, appropriate training and skills in airway management to allow rescue of the patient, age- and size-appropriate equipment for airway management and*

> *venous access, appropriate medications and reversal agents, sufficient numbers of appropriately trained staff to both carry out the procedure and monitor the patient, appropriate physiologic monitoring during and after the procedure, a properly equipped and staffed recovery area, recovery to the presedation level of consciousness before discharge from medical/dental supervision, and appropriate discharge instructions. This report was developed through a collaborative effort of the American Academy of Pediatrics and the American Academy of Pediatric Dentistry to offer pediatric providers updated information and guidance in delivering safe sedation to children.*

One of the key concepts of safety in the guidelines is that of "rescue." Rescue is defined as the necessary skills of a practitioner to (1) recognize various levels of sedation and (2) possess the skills to provide appropriate cardiopulmonary support. Furthermore, rescue interventions require specific training and skills. The current guidelines state that the practitioner must be sufficiently skilled to rescue a child with apnea, laryngospasm, and/or airway obstruction, including the ability to open the airway, suction secretions, provide CPAP, and perform successful bag-valve-mask ventilation should the child progress to a level of DS. Training in, and maintenance of, advanced pediatric airway skills is required.

Indirect evidence suggests that the impact of guidelines is favorable in terms of outcomes and that adverse events are rare, especially in hospitals (Cravero et al. 2006; Langhan et al. 2012). Adverse events, including death, have occurred in dental offices and at a higher rate than other venues such as hospitals (Cote et al. 2000a; Cote et al. 2000b), but when cases are available for review, it seems obvious that most of the adverse events occurred when general tenets of guidelines were not followed (Chicka et al. 2012; Krippaehne and Montgomery 1992; Lee et al. 2013). Sedation guidelines do not assure that adverse events will not occur if faithfully followed. However, it is highly recommended that dentists who sedate patients, especially children, should be intimately familiar with sedation guidelines and incorporate the guideline recommendations into their practice and protocols to maximize favorable outcomes and safety for children.

## Emergency Management

Any discussion of sedation and its safety must include the topic of emergency management (see Chapter 16). Not only do sedation guidelines stress the importance of recognition of emergencies and the knowledge and skills in performing emergency management interventions, but common sense also dictates a strong respect for factors contributing to the likelihood that emergencies will occur as the depth of sedation increases or as therapeutic management boundaries are violated.

Enough data are available to understand that the respiratory system is most likely the first system that will fail during a sedation mishap (Cote el al. 2000a). Once this system has been significantly compromised and not adequately addressed, the natural progression of events that rapidly follows involves the cardiovascular system and collapse of the CNS and autonomic nervous system. This fact points to the need for appreciating and adhering to some very basic tenets of patient management, including, among others, knowledge of pharmacokinetics and pharmacodynamics of drugs, not exceeding recommended therapeutic doses of drugs, focusing on patient monitoring and airway competency, and intimate knowledge of and skill sets in managing a compromised airway.

## Summary

Sedation can be a valuable and effective aid in the management of children's behaviors during dental procedures. However, the risks for adverse outcomes, including death and brain damage associated with sedation, are daunting and carry profound and significant implications for any clinician who performs sedations. Thus, any consideration for implementing sedation as part of the possibilities in behavior management armamentaria must include both competency in training and in-depth knowledge in the fields of pharmacology, behavior, emotional and physiological functioning, monitoring, and emergency management principles and skills. An equally strong familiarity with and adherence to sedation guidelines and state rules and regulations is essential for promoting safety during sedation.

## References

Aminabadi, N.A., Deljavan, A.S., Jamali, Z. et al. (2015). The influence of parenting style and child temperament on child–parent–dentist interactions. *Pediatric Dentistry*, 37, 342–347.

Aminabadi, N.A., Ghoreishizadeh, A., Ghoreishizadeh, M. et al. (2014). Can child temperament be related to early childhood caries? *Caries Research*, 48, 3–12.

Anderson, J.A. and Vann, W.F. Jr. (1988). Respiratory monitoring during pediatric sedation: pulse oximetry and capnography. *Pediatric Dentistry*, 10, 94–101.

Arnrup, K., Broberg, A.G., Berggren, U. et al. (2007). Temperamental reactivity and negative emotionality in uncooperative children referred to specialized paediatric dentistry compared to children in ordinary dental care. *International Journal of Paediatric Dentistry*, 17, 419–429.

Arnrup, K., Broberg, A.G., Berggren, U. et al. (2003). Treatment outcome in subgroups of uncooperative child dental patients: an exploratory study. *International Journal of Paediatric Dentistry*, 13, 304–319.

Caldwell-Andrews, A.A. and Kain, Z.N. (2006). Psychological predictors of postoperative sleep in children undergoing outpatient surgery. *Paediatric Anaesthesia*, 16, 144–151.

Campbell, L., DiLorenzo, M., Atkinson, N. et al. (2017). Systematic review: A systematic review of the interrelationships among children's coping responses, children's coping outcomes, and parent cognitive–affective, behavioral, and contextual variables in the needle-related procedures context. *Journal of Pediatric Psychology*, 42, 611–621.

Casamassimo, P.S., Wilson, S., and Gross, L. (2002). Effects of changing U.S. parenting styles on dental practice: Perceptions of diplomates of the American Board of Pediatric Dentistry presented to the College of Diplomates of the American Board of Pediatric Dentistry 16th Annual Session, Atlanta, GA, Saturday, May 26, 2001. *Pediatric Dentistry*, 24, 18–22.

Chicka, M.C., Dembo, J.B., Mathu-Muju, K.R. et al. (2012). Adverse events during pediatric dental anesthesia and sedation: A review of closed malpractice insurance claims. *Pediatric Dentistry*, 34, 231–238.

Cloninger, C.R., Cloninger, K.M., Zwir, I. et al. (2019). The complex genetics and biology of human temperament: A review of traditional concepts in relation to new molecular findings. *Transl Psychiatry*, 9, 290.

Cohen, L.L., Francher, A., MacLaren, J.E. et al. (2006). Correlates of pediatric behavior and distress during intramuscular injections for invasive dental procedures. *Journal of Clinical Pediatric Dentistry*, 31, 44–47.

Cote, C.J., Karl, H.W., Notterman, D.A. et al. (2000a). Adverse sedation events in pediatrics: analysis of medications used for sedation. *Pediatrics*, 106, 633–644.

Cote, C.J., Notterman, D.A., Karl, H.W. et al. (2000b). Adverse sedation events in pediatrics: a critical incident analysis of contributing factors. *Pediatrics*, 105, 805–814.

Cote, C.J., Wilson, S., American Academy of Pediatrics and American Academy of Pediatric Dentistry. (2019). Guidelines for monitoring and management of pediatric patients before, during, and after sedation for diagnostic and therapeutic procedures. *Pediatrics*, 143.

Cravero, J.P., Blike, G.T., Beach, M. et al. (2006). Incidence and nature of adverse events during pediatric sedation/anesthesia for procedures outside the operating room: Report from the Pediatric Sedation Research Consortium. *Pediatrics*, 118, 1087–1096.

Creedon, R.L. (1986) Guidelines for the elective use of conscious sedation, deep sedation, and general anesthesia in pediatric patients. *Anesthesia Progress*, 33, 189–190.

DiLalla, L.F. and Jamnik, M.R. (2019). The Southern Illinois Twins/Triplets and Siblings Study (SITSS): A longitudinal study of early child development. *Twin Res Hum Genet*, 1–4.

Flowers, S.R. and Birnie, K.A. (2015). Procedural preparation and support as a standard of care in pediatric oncology. *Pediatric Blood & Cancer*, 62(Suppl. 5), S694–723.

Fortier, M.A., Chorney, J.M., Rony, R.Y. et al. (2009). Children's desire for perioperative information. *Anesthesia and Analgesia*, 109, 1085–1090.

Fortier, M.A., Del Rosario, A.M., Rosenbaum, A. et al. (2010). Beyond pain: Predictors of postoperative maladaptive behavior change in children. *Paediatric Anaesthesia*, 20, 445–453.

Goldsmith, H.H., Buss, K.A., and Lemery, K.S. (1997). Toddler and childhood temperament: Expanded content, stronger genetic evidence, new evidence for the importance of environment. *Developmental Psychology*, 33, 891–905.

Gustafsson, A. (2010). Dental behaviour management problems among children and adolescents–a matter of understanding? Studies on dental fear, personal characteristics and psychosocial concomitants. *Swedish Dental Journal Supplement*, 2 p preceding 1–46.

Gustafsson, A., Broberg, A., Bodin, L. et al. (2010). Dental behaviour management problems: The role of child personal characteristics. *International Journal of Paediatric Dentistry*, 20, 242–253.

Helfinstein, S.M., Fox, N.A., and Pine, D.S. (2012). Approach-withdrawal and the role of the striatum in the temperament of behavioral inhibition. *Developmental Psychology*, 48, 815–826.

Herzberg, S., Hansen, M., Schoonover, A. et al. (2019). Association between measured teamwork and medical errors: an observational study of prehospital care in the USA. *BMJ Open*, 9, e025314.

Houpt, M. (2002). Project USAP 2000–use of sedative agents by pediatric dentists: A 15-year follow-up survey. *Pediatric Dentistry*, 24, 289–294.

Houpt, M. (1993). Project USAP the use of sedative agents in pediatric dentistry: 1991 update. *Pediatric Dentistry*, 15, 36–40.

Houpt, M. (1989). Report of Project USAP–the use of sedative agents in pediatric dentistry. *Journal of Dentistry for Children*, 56, 302–309.

Howenstein, J., Kumar, A., Casamassimo, P.S. et al. (2015). Correlating parenting styles with child behavior and caries. *Pediatric Dentistry*, 37, 59–64.

Isik, B., Baygin, O., Kapci, E.G. et al. (2010). The effects of temperament and behaviour problems on sedation failure in anxious children after midazolam premedication. *European Journal of Anaesthesiology*, 27, 336–340.

Jabin, Z. and Chaudhary, S. (2014). Association of child temperament with early childhood caries. *Journal of Clinical and Diagnostic Research*, 8, ZC21-4.

Jensen, B. and Stjernqvist, K. (2002). Temperament and acceptance of dental treatment under sedation in preschool children. *Acta Odontologica Scandinavica*, 60, 231–236.

Klingberg, G. and Broberg, A.G. (2007). Dental fear/anxiety and dental behaviour management problems in children and adolescents: A review of prevalence and concomitant psychological factors. *International Journal of Paediatric Dentistry*, 17, 391–406.

Klingberg, G. and Broberg, A.G. (1998). Temperament and child dental fear. *Pediatric Dentistry*, 20, 237–243.

Koller, D. and Goldman, R.D. (2012). Distraction techniques for children undergoing procedures: A critical review of pediatric research. *Journal of Pediatric Nursing*, 27, 652–681.

Krikken, J.B., van Wijk, A.J., ten Cate, J.M. et al. (2012). Child dental anxiety, parental rearing style and referral status of children. *Community Dental Health*, 29, 289–292.

Krippaehne, J.A. and Montgomery, M.T. (1992). Morbidity and mortality from pharmacosedation and general anesthesia in the dental office. *Journal of Oral and Maxillofacial Surgery*, 50, 691–698; discussion 698-9.

Lane, K.J., Nelson, T.M., Thikkurissy, S. et al. (2015). Assessing temperament as a predictor of oral sedation success using the children's behavior questionnaire short form. *Pediatric Dentistry*, 37, 429–435.

Langhan, M.L., Mallory, M., Hertzog, J. et al. (2012). Physiologic monitoring practices during pediatric procedural sedation: A report from the Pediatric Sedation Research Consortium. *Archives of Pediatrics and Adolescent Medicine*, 166, 990–998.

Lee, H.H., Milgrom, P., Starks, H. et al. (2013). Trends in death associated with pediatric dental sedation and general anesthesia. *Paediatric Anaesthesia*, 23, 741–746.

Lee, L.W. and White-Traut, R.C. (1996). The role of temperament in pediatric pain response. *Issues in Comprehensive Pediatric Nursing*, 19, 49–63.

Lochary, M.E., Wilson, S., Griffen, A.L. et al. (1993). Temperament as a predictor of behavior for conscious sedation in dentistry. *Pediatric Dentistry*, 15, 348–352.

Lopez, U., Habre, W., Van der Linden, M. et al. (2008). Intra-operative awareness in children and post-traumatic stress disorder. *Anaesthesia*, 63, 474–481.

Mahoney, L., Ayers, S., and Seddon, P. (2010). The association between parent's and healthcare professional's behavior and children's coping and distress during venepuncture. *Journal of Pediatric Psychology*, 35, 985–995.

Martinos, M., Matheson, A., and de Haan, M. (2012). Links between infant temperament and neurophysiological measures of attention to happy and fearful faces. *Journal of Child Psychology and Psychiatry and Allied Disciplines*, 53, 1118–1127.

McCarthy, A.M., Kleiber, C., Hanrahan, K. et al. (2010). Factors explaining children's responses to intravenous needle insertions. *Nursing Research*, 59, 407–416.

Miranda-Remijo, D., Orsini, M.R., Correa-Faria, P. et al. (2016). Mother–child interactions and young child behavior during procedural conscious sedation. *BMC Pediatrics*, 16, 201.

Morgan, B.E. (2006). Behavioral inhibition: A neurobiological perspective. *Current Psychiatry Reports*, 8, 270–278.

Morin, A., Ocanto, R., Drukteinis, L. et al. (2016). Survey of current clinical and curriculum practices of postgraduate pediatric dentistry programs in nonintravenous conscious sedation in the United States. *Pediatric Dentistry*, 38, 398–405.

Nelson, T. (2013) The continuum of behavior guidance. *Dental Clinics of North America*, 57, 129–143.

Nelson, T.M., Griffith, T.M., Lane, K.J. et al. (2017). Temperament as a predictor of nitrous oxide inhalation sedation success. *Anesthesia Progress*, 64, 17–21.

Oliver, K. and Manton, D.J. (2015). Contemporary behavior management techniques in clinical pediatric dentistry: Out with the old and in with the new? *Journal of Dentistry for Children (Chic)*, 82, 22–28.

Patel, M., McTigue, D.J., Thikkurissy, S. et al. (2016). Parental attitudes toward advanced behavior guidance techniques used in pediatric dentistry. *Pediatric Dentistry*, 38, 30–36.

Plomin, R. and Rowe, D.C. (1977). A twin study of temperament in young children. *Journal of Psychology*, 97, 107–113.

Quinonez, R., Santos, R.G., Boyar, R. et al. (1997). Temperament and trait anxiety as predictors of child behavior prior to general anesthesia for dental surgery. *Pediatric Dentistry*, 19, 427–431.

Radis, F.G., Wilson, S., Griffen, A.L. et al. (1994). Temperament as a predictor of behavior during initial dental examination in children. *Pediatric Dentistry*, 16, 121–127.

Salem, K., Kousha, M., Anissian, A. et al. (2012). Dental fear and concomitant factors in 3–6-year-old children. *Journal of Dental Research Dental Clinics Dental Prospects*, 6, 70–74.

Santos, R.G. and Quinonez, R. (2014). Child temperament is as strongly associated with early childhood caries (ECC) as poor feeding practices: Positive temperament appears protective, negative temperament may increase ECC risk. *Journal of Evidence-Based Dental Practice*, 14, 85–88.

Schor, E.L. (2003). Family pediatrics: Report of the Task Force on the Family. *Pediatrics*, 111, 1541–1571.

Thomas, A., Chess, S., Birch, H.G. et al. (1963). Behavior Individuality in Early Childhood. Brunner-Mazel, New York, NY.

Tipa, R.O. and Bobirnac, G. (2010). Importance of basic life support training for first and second year medical students—a personal statement. *Journal of Medicine and Life*, 3, 465–467.

Tripi, P.A., Palermo, T.M., Thomas, S. et al. (2004). Assessment of risk factors for emergence distress and postoperative behavioural changes in children following general anaesthesia. *Paediatric Anaesthesia*, 14, 235–240.

Tsoi, A.K., Wilson, S., and Thikkurissy, S. (2018). A study of the relationship of parenting styles, child temperament, and operatory behavior in healthy children. *Journal of Clinical Pediatric Dentistry*, 42, 273–278.

Wells, M.H., Dormois, L.D., and Townsend, J.A. (2018a). Behavior guidance: That was then but this is now. *General Dentistry*, 66, 39–45.

Wells, M.H., McCarthy, B.A., Tseng, C.H. et al. (2018b). Usage of behavior guidance techniques differs by provider and practice characteristics. *Pediatric Dentistry*, 40, 201–208.

White, J., Wells, M., Arheart, K.L. et al. (2016). A questionnaire of parental perceptions of conscious sedation in pediatric dentistry. *Pediatric Dentistry*, 38, 116–121.

Wik, L., Myklebust, H., Auestad, B.H. et al. (2002). Retention of basic life support skills 6 months after training with an automated voice advisory manikin system without instructor involvement. *Resuscitation*, 52, 273–279.

Wilson, S., Creedon, R.L., George, M. et al. (1996). A history of sedation guidelines: Where we are headed in the future. *Pediatric Dentistry*, 18, 194–199.

Wilson, S. and Houpt, M. (2016). Project USAP 2010: Use of sedative agents in pediatric dentistry–a 25-year follow-up survey. *Pediatric Dentistry*, 38, 127–133.

Wilson, S. and Nathan, J.E. (2011). A survey study of sedation training in advanced pediatric dentistry programs: Thoughts of program directors and students. *Pediatric Dentistry*, 33, 353–360.

Wolff, N.J., Darlington, A.S., Hunfeld, J.A. et al. (2011). The influence of attachment and temperament on venipuncture distress in 14-month-old infants: The Generation R Study. *Infant Behavior & Development*, 34, 293–302.

## 12

# Nitrous Oxide/Oxygen Inhalation Sedation in Children

*Ari Kupietzky and Dimitris Emmanouil*

## Introduction

Nitrous oxide ($N_2O$) is an invaluable tool for managing the mild to moderately anxious child. Its ease of administration, wide margin of safety, analgesic and anxiolytic effects, and, most of all, its rapid reversibility make it an ideal drug for use in children (Houpt et al. 2004; Paterson-Tahmassebi 2003). The American Academy of Pediatric Dentistry (AAPD), among other organizations, recognizes $N_2O$/oxygen inhalation sedation as a safe and effective technique to reduce anxiety, produce analgesia, and enhance effective communication between a patient and healthcare provider (AAPD 2020). However, clinicians though should not make the mistake of thinking that $N_2O$ sedation, by itself, controls behavior. $N_2O$ serves as an adjunct to behavior management.

$N_2O$ is widely accepted as a behavior management technique in pediatric dentistry. Wilson and Alcaino's (2011) international survey revealed that at least 56% of the respondents used $N_2O$ in their practices. A survey of AAPD members by Wilson in 1996 and then repeated in 2016 found an increase in the use of $N_2O$ from 66.3% to 97%. Wilson found that practitioners have the perception that more pediatric patients require $N_2O$ than before. Adair et al. (2004), who surveyed behavior management teaching techniques in USA pediatric dentistry advanced education programs, reported that all programs taught $N_2O$ sedation. Its use is not limited to pediatric specialists. The results from a survey conducted by the Academy of General Dentistry demonstrated that about 74% of American dentists used $N_2O$–oxygen sedation (Lynch 2007). Thus, in contrast to earlier studies, $N_2O$ is used by more practitioners and used more frequently than before. Its utilization is likely to continue, and it will probably increase.

## $N_2O$ Historic Milestones

$N_2O$ has an interesting history of use and abuse after it was first synthesized by Joseph Priestley in 1772 nearly 250 years ago. Sir Humphrey Davy was the first to report on the pleasurable and unusual sensations following the inhalation of $N_2O$ and coined the term "laughing gas." In the early 1840s, a dentist named Horace Wells made the first practical use of $N_2O$ having his own tooth extracted while inhaling $N_2O$ (Archer 1944).

Although the analgesic properties of $N_2O$ were recognized for some time, the risk of asphyxia when using it as the sole anesthetic agent prevented its use for lengthy operations. However, in 1868, Chicago surgeon Edmund W. Andrews published the results of a large survey which suggested that the anesthetic use of ether and chloroform would be safer by combining these agents with 70% $N_2O$ and 30% oxygen. This extended the anesthetic time for longer operations, and the notion of balanced anesthesia was born. At about the same time, gas machines were introduced, making anesthesia more convenient. Dentistry took advantage of this progress. Before the turn of the century, a limited number of dentists were beginning to use $N_2O$ and oxygen for cavity preparations.

Throughout the first half of the twentieth century, the primary interest in $N_2O$ was in its analgesic properties (Langa 1968). Most discussions concerning $N_2O$ stressed the analgesic and anesthetic properties for extractions. Dental offices remained dependent upon $N_2O$ for pain control until the introduction of local anesthesia. The feeling of euphoria caused by $N_2O$, which was so sought-after during the "laughing gas parties" 100 years earlier, were either ignored or considered a minor benefit during dental procedures.

Since the prevalent attitude among dentists in the early twentieth century was that young children were not suitable patients, few references have suggested using $N_2O$ for the child patient. However, in 1925, physician John S. Lundy specifically described the use of $N_2O$ as an induction agent to prepare children for extractions. Sorenson and Roth (1973) emphasized the value of inhalation sedation to reduce children's fears, particularly fear of injections. They de-emphasized the analgesic effect of $N_2O$–oxygen, which is associated with concentrations of $N_2O$ exceeding 40%, and emphasized the sedative–tranquilizing–euphoric benefits of dilute concentrations, that is, less than 40% of $N_2O$.

It may be because of the history, but, for many years, there has been some confusion regarding the terms *$N_2O$ inhalation sedation* and *anesthetic $N_2O$*. As a consequence, anesthesiologists were opposed to the use of $N_2O$ by dentists. This is unfortunate because it delayed the widespread use of the agent by dentists. Although $N_2O$ now is routinely used in dentistry and considered a safe drug, in medicine, $N_2O$ is frequently combined with other general anesthetic agents to produce a balanced anesthesia. Lately, it has also found its way into managing pain and distress in children undergoing emergency or brief diagnostic and therapeutic procedures in hospitals (Trottier et al. 2019).

## Physiology and Pharmacology

$N_2O$ is a non-irritating, colorless gas with a faint sweet taste and odor. It is a true general anesthetic, but the least potent of all anesthetic gases in use today. It is an effective analgesic/anxiolytic agent which causes central nervous system (CNS) depression and euphoria with little effect on the respiratory system. $N_2O$ has rapid uptake, as it is absorbed quickly from the alveoli and held in a simple solution in the serum. It is dissolved and transported in blood; it does not combine with hemoglobin, and it does not undergo biotransformation.

It is relatively insoluble, passing down a gradient into other tissues and cells in the body, such as the CNS. It is excreted quickly from the lungs. Elimination of $N_2O$ occurs by means of expiration in a manner that is precisely the reverse of uptake and distribution, and $N_2O$'s low solubility allows it to be removed rapidly (Emmanouil and Quock 2007).

### Cardiovascular Effects

$N_2O$ causes minor depression in cardiac output while peripheral resistance is slightly increased, thereby maintaining normal blood pressure. This is of particular advantage in treating patients with cerebrovascular system disorders. There are no changes in the heart rate (pulse) or blood pressure. $N_2O$ is transported through the blood stream in a free gaseous state. Total saturation in the blood occurs within 3–5 minutes. Total circulation time for one breath of $N_2O$/oxygen is 3–5 minutes. Any noted changes in respiratory rate are related more to the relaxation of the patient than to the $N_2O$ itself.

### CNS Effects

$N_2O$ has multiple mechanisms of action that underlie its varied pharmacological properties. $N_2O$ and nitric oxide are now what in pharmacology is considered a new class of neurotransmitters. Their interactions affect a host of neuronal activities like cognition, emotion, and behavior (Emmanouil 2020).

### Analgesia and Anxiolysis

Analgesic $N_2O$ has a long history of use in obstetrics for labor-pain relief (Likis et al. 2014). $N_2O$ is also used for self-administered analgesia in cancer patients (Parlow et al. 2005) to alleviate pain and discomfort associated with a number of medical procedures, and in emergency medicine departments for procedures such as treatment of lacerations and orthopedic procedures (Baskett 1970). It is essential to make a clear distinction between the high anesthetic concentrations of $N_2O$ producing unconsciousness and the much lower doses that are associated with consciousness and its psychotropic actions (i.e., analgesia, anxiolysis, and euphoria). Subanesthetic concentrations of $N_2O$ produce only analgesic and anxiolytic effects without unconsciousness (Dundee and Moore 1960). The main difference between the analgesic and anesthetic actions of $N_2O$ as far as the mechanisms of action are considered is the lack of opioid system involvement in the anesthetic actions, whereas opioid mediation is required for the analgesic properties of $N_2O$ (Sanders et al. 2008). There is also now evidence that the relief from anxiety during inhalation of $N_2O$ is a specific anxiolytic effect that is independent of its analgesic action. Emmanouil and Quock (2007) proposed a possible mechanism for $N_2O$ anxiolytic actions at a cellular level where $N_2O$ activates the benzodiazepine binding site of the $GABA_A$ receptor.

### Anesthesia

$N_2O$ has a well-known role in medical history because it was the first drug used for surgical anesthesia. Despite its limited anesthetic potency, $N_2O$ is the most widely used general anesthetic agent. With a minimum alveolar concentration of 104% at 1 atm in humans, $N_2O$ by itself would require high volume percentage and hyperbaric conditions to achieve anesthesia (Hornbein et al. 1982). Therefore, due to its low potency, in clinical practice, $N_2O$ is generally used to reduce the minimum alveolar concentration of a second inhalation agent for anesthesia and increase the rate of induction (i.e., the second gas effect) and to provide or augment the analgesic component of general anesthesia. It is suggested that a common property of NMDA receptor antagonism may underlie the similar pharmacological profiles of $N_2O$ and ketamine, an intravenous dissociative anesthetic. The two drugs, in fact, produce synergistic neurotoxicity when used together (Jevtovic-Todorovic et al. 2000).

*Amnesia:* In addition to analgesia, anxiolysis, and anesthesia, $N_2O$ can also cause amnesia or memory loss (Ramsay et al. 1992) by possibly again affecting the $GABA_A$ receptor complex (Emmanouil et al. 2020).

## Nitrous Oxide in Pediatric Dentistry: Rationale and Objectives

Dentistry generates more stress than most other professions, primarily because of the working conditions of the dental practice (Bodner 2008). In particular, the specialty of pediatric dentistry can feature crying children, clashes with parents, and children's small mouths and teeth, which contribute to a stressful environment. The use of $N_2O$ sedation can reduce some of these stresses in the dental office—it helps produce a relaxed atmosphere and can benefit everyone in the pediatric dental treatment triangle.

The administration of $N_2O$ has major advantages not common to other sedation agents used in dentistry for children. These include rapid onset, rapid withdrawal, and convenient dosage adjustment to maintain a tranquil and sedated state.

In modern dentistry, children do not often experience real physical pain. Although many procedures are less than pleasurable, children usually fail to recognize shades of gray—only the polarity of black or white, pain or no pain. However, pain, with its physiological and psychological components, can be somewhat difficult to define in the clinical setting. As a result, minor discomforts can be magnified and interpreted as pain. $N_2O$ can modify these discomforts by the diminution or elimination of pain and anxiety in a conscious patient. It is well recognized for these analgesia/anxiolysis properties.

Like children, adults have fears and anxieties, but they are contained by previous experiences. A child lacking the experiences of an adult has an emotional overflow when placed in an anxious or stressful situation. Due to a lack of experience, the child acts out primary feelings. This reaction or emotional outburst to stress or anxiety is usually in the form of fight-or-flight behavior. Children reacting this way may need assistance in controlling their emotions. $N_2O$, as an adjunct to behavior management, can help many children learn to cope with the stressful environment.

Emotions and pain thresholds are interwoven. When a child patient is fearful, anxious, or apprehensive, there is a lower pain threshold. Minor things may irritate and upset the patient. If minimizing pain during treatment is one of the objectives, then reducing the child patient's level of anxiety is critical. There is a positive association between anticipatory anxiety and procedural pain. Interventions designed to reduce task-specific anticipatory anxiety may help reduce pain responses in children and adolescents (Tsao et al. 2004). When $N_2O$ sedation eliminates or reduces fear or anxiety, it raises the pain reaction threshold and reduces fatigue (Weinstein et al. 1986). Both pain sensitivity and pain reaction are altered. Additionally, the pain threshold can be raised with attention and distraction tasks. When the placebo effect of distraction is combined with the sedative properties of $N_2O$, the injection experience is much more easily accomplished.

Studies have reported on the effects of $N_2O$ from children's perspective. Children described dreaming or being on a "space-ride" (Hogue et al. 1971). Berger et al. (1972) reported that some children described a "floating, warm, and tingling sensation" with $N_2O$. In yet another study, children indicated a preference for music in conjunction with $N_2O$ during dental treatment (Anderson 1980). Langa (1968) described the child under $N_2O$ sedation as being in "suspended animation"—that is, the child's body does not move, head and extremities remain relaxed, and sudden movements commonly associated with children are eliminated. With the child in a relaxed state, a dentist can provide optimum treatment for a child with minimum trauma for both dentist and patient. Following the foregoing rationale for the use of $N_2O$/oxygen sedation, many pediatric dentists adopted the technique for managing their child patients. The objectives for $N_2O$ usage are shown in Table 12-1.

**Table 12-1** Objectives of nitrous oxide/oxygen inhalation sedation.

---

1. Reduce or eliminate anxiety.
2. Reduce untoward movement and negative reaction to dental treatment.
3. Enhance communication and patient cooperation.
4. Raise the pain reaction threshold.
5. Increase tolerance for longer appointments.
6. Reduce gagging.

---

## Stages of Anesthesia

Four stages of general anesthesia were recognized in Guedel's classification: (1) induction (also referred to as *analgesia*), (2) excitement, (3) surgical anesthesia, and (4) overdose (Guedel 1937). The first stage begins with the induction of anesthesia and ends with a patient's loss of consciousness. Patients still feel pain in this stage. In 1968, Langa introduced a term to represent $N_2O$ inhalation sedation: *relative analgesia (RA).* Langa (1968) proposed that there were three planes of analgesia in the first stage. The planes vary from moderate to total analgesia and are dependent on the concentration of $N_2O$ in the mixture and the signs and symptoms shown by patients (Table 12-2). During $N_2O$ inhalation sedation, the patient always remains at the first stage of anesthesia.

In Plane One (5–25% $N_2O$) the patient appears normal, relaxed, and awake and may feel slight tingling in toes, fingers, tongue, or lips, and may giggle. Vital signs remain normal. There are no definite clinical manifestations.

In Plane Two, or RA (20–55% $N_2O$), the patient may have a dreamy look, eyes appearing "glassy" (occasionally with tears), reactions are slowed, and the voice may sound "throaty." The patient will feel warm and drowsy, may drift in and out of the surrounding environment, and may hear pleasant ringing in the ears. Partial amnesia may occur. Vital signs remain normal. Pain is reduced or eliminated, but touch and pressure are still perceived. The patient is less aware of surroundings; sounds and smells are dulled. The term *psychotropic analgesic $N_2O$* (PAN) was introduced by Gillman and Lichtigfeld (1994) to describe Plane Two of analgesia. This term clearly distinguishes the concentrations of $N_2O$ used for anxiolysis/analgesia from the much higher doses used for anesthesia, wherein the patient is totally unconscious.

In Plane Three (55–70% $N_2O$), the patient becomes angry, with a hard stare; the pupils usually are centrally fixed and dilated, the mouth tends to close frequently, and the patient is unaware of his surroundings and may hallucinate. When patients are in Plane Three, Roberts (1990) reported that they may experience sensations of flying, falling, or uncontrolled spinning, or the chest may feel heavy, and the patient will no longer cooperate.

Plane Two provides adequate $N_2O$ sedation and allows dentist–child communication, although some clinicians prefer the dream period, usually characterized by closed eyes and difficulty with speech. Figure 12-1 portrays a patient's appearance in Plane Two. Plane One is usually of short duration, while Plane Two can be maintained for several hours. Children in Plane Two usually respond to questions by moving the head rather than speaking.

**Table 12-2**   Effects of $N_2O$ in relation to its concentration.

| |
|---|
| 100% will produce anoxia. |
| 80% will produce hypoxia with hallucinations and bizarre dreams; may cause respiratory, cardiovascular, kidney or liver damage. |
| 65% can cause patients to enter the excitement stage. |
| 35% usually provides maximum analgesia with maintenance and cooperation of the patient. |
| 25% is an analgesic equipotent to 10 mg morphine sulphate. |

Facial features are relaxed, and the jaw usually sags, remaining open without mouth props. The eyes are usually closed but will open in response to questions. The arms are heavy and will stay where placed, and the hands are open. The legs often slide off the side of the chair. All vital signs are stable. There is no significant risk of losing protective reflexes, and the child is able to return to pre-procedure mobility. The objective of the sedation should be to reach, but not pass, this plane. This is the desirable sedation level when performing $N_2O$ sedation.

For some patients, the feeling of "losing control" may be troubling. Others may be claustrophobic and unable to tolerate the nasal hood, finding it confining and unpleasant (Stach 1995). A patient's experience after $N_2O$ is believed to be similar to a posthypnotic state. During $N_2O$, there is an enhancement of suggestibility and imaginative ability that may be utilized while managing the child's behavior and dental experience. This can be advantageous. Suggestions, such as "fixing teeth is fun," made while a patient is experiencing $N_2O$ sedation might make subsequent visits easier and more readily accepted (Whalley and Brooks 2009). Another beneficial suggestion is to instruct ways to improve oral hygiene.

Individual biovariability accounts for different reactions to various concentrations of $N_2O$. Some individuals experience several symptoms, while others experience only a few. Symptoms are intense for some and insignificant for others. Sometimes, signs are obvious; at other times, they are subtle. Titration allows for the biovariablility of any patient that may be associated with the administration of the substance. Titrating $N_2O$ /oxygen and careful observation of patient responses are keys to successful administration.

Clinicians must know what signs and symptoms to look for when administering and monitoring $N_2O$ sedation (Table 12-3). Keeping a constant vigil is imperative because pleasant sensations may quickly change and become unpleasant. Knowledge of the appropriate technique and associated physical, physiologic, and psychological changes minimizes negative patient experiences.

(a)          (b)          (c)

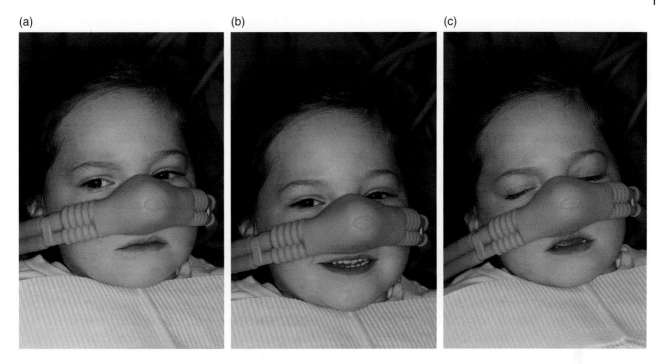

**Figure 12-1** A patient's appearance in Plane Two. Facial features are relaxed, and the jaw usually sags, remaining open without mouth props. The eyes are usually closed but will open in response to questions. *Source:* Courtesy of Dr. Ari Kupietzky.

**Table 12-3** Clinical tips to evaluate level of $N_2O$ inhalation sedation.

Eyes are very indicative of the sedation level.

Reduced activity of the eyes indicative of desirable level of sedation.

Increased activity of the eyes may indicate that sedation is too light.

Fixed, hard stare of the eyes: sedation is too deep, $N_2O$ % needs to be decreased.

Arms and legs crossed: the patient is not relaxed yet, increase $N_2O$ %.

Patient talks too much: sedation is too light due to mouth breathing. Do not increase; just try to get patient to stop talking. Use of a rubber dam will prevent this situation.

Patient answers rapidly: sedation is too light.

Patient answers slowly and deliberately: good sedation.

Patient does not answer: may be tired and asleep. If used in combination with another sedative agent, stimulate patient and check verbally.

Perspiration appears on the face: reassure patient that this is expected and will pass.

Paraesthesia of extremities: reassure patient that this is normal and will dissipate after treatment.

Paraesthesia of lips, tongue, or oral tissues: profound depth; time for injection of local anesthetic.

### Case 12.1

Donna, aged five years, was a healthy child requiring four quadrants of restorative dentistry. At the initial examination, the child appeared cooperative, but the dentist recognized her apprehension. Despite this observation, the dentist elected to treat Donna through behavior shaping, a non-pharmacological approach. Performing dentistry quadrant by quadrant, the dentist achieved good patient cooperation at the first and second restorative dentistry appointments. At the third visit, the child cried during the injection but eventually calmed down. When the time arrived for the fourth and final restorative treatment, Donna's parent forcibly brought her to the office. The child cried continuously and hysterically refused the injection.

*Case 12.1, Discussion:* While the ultimate goal is to increase patient comfort through relaxation (Clark and Brunick 2007), another important goal is for $N_2O$/oxygen to serve as an adjunct to behavior management. It is not for all patients, and before selecting a management method for any pediatric patient, careful behavior observation is needed. After observing the child during the examination visit, the dentist has to anticipate future cooperation and balance this evaluation against treatment requirements. In Donna's case, where minor apprehension was observed at the examination visit, one or two restorative appointments likely would not have created a problem. However, sitting for four restorative visits is a different matter, and the child failed to tolerate the protracted series of appointments. There is no formula for precisely predicting such problems, and the ability to detect them in advance is usually gained by experience. Choosing the proper behavioral strategy in this type of case can be difficult. Nonetheless, whenever a dentist begins treating an apprehensive but cooperative and likeable child who becomes a behavior problem, the behavior management approach is open to question.

In hindsight, the negative outcome of Donna's case should not have occurred. If her perceived apprehension had been addressed, it likely would have created an improved end result. A pharmacological adjunct would benefit the child, helping her with a difficult initiation to dentistry. Donna is the ideal candidate for $N_2O$/oxygen inhalation sedation. She was communicative and in control of herself. $N_2O$ offers a reasonable adjunctive therapy for Donna's behavior management. This is the type of situation that Musselman and McClure referred to as a "preventive medication" (1975) in the original behavior management book. It is given to a child who is unnecessarily strained by the dental situation and who could become a more difficult management problem. Providing comfort with $N_2O$ at an initial dental visit impacts children's later experiences, resulting in improved behaviors and less anxiety at subsequent visits. This effect can be seen even if $N_2O$ is not administered at later visits (Collado et al. 2006; Nathan et al. 1988).

## Administration Technique

Before the first operative appointment, an introductory explanation must be given to the parent. It is important to state that the child's feelings of anxiety or fear are not unique, but are observed in many children coming for the first operative visit. A brief explanation, such as the one following, assures a parent that the drug has no lingering effects and is routinely used safely.

> Dentist: Mrs. Jones, Donna is such a nice girl. I have noticed that most children feel nervous at the first few visits. As we explained earlier, our goal is to help Donna become a good dental patient without fears. To make the visit more acceptable to her, we are going to use nitrous oxide, which is commonly known as "laughing gas." As she breathes in the gas,

she will feel less nervous. The nitrous oxide will make the injection of local anesthesia easier. Donna will have the feeling of a relatively shorter session. When it is used with proper technique, it helps children enjoy dentistry. Its effects will be gone at the end of the appointment, so you shouldn't worry after the appointment.

Additionally, parents may be given a $N_2O$ parent information pamphlet and the opportunity to ask questions regarding the procedure. Informed consent for the procedure and for the $N_2O$ sedation must be obtained and filed in the patient's chart. The patient's record should also include the indication for use of $N_2O$ sedation. Indeed, as for other pharmacologic agents, documentation is very important. A written record detailing the concentration of $N_2O$ administered, monitored patient variables, the duration of the procedure, post-treatment oxygenation procedure, and any complications encountered (or lack thereof) should be entered in the patient chart.

Critical to beginning the $N_2O$–oxygen procedure is the acceptance of the nasal mask by the child; hence, this treatment is not advised for the resistant pediatric patient. At the outset, it is important to check that the child does not have a cold and can breathe through the nose. There are many techniques to introduce the nasal mask. In all instances, however, clinicians must use child management techniques with explanations adjusted for the child's level of comprehension. The introduction should be brief and presented in a matter-of-fact manner. Elaborating unnecessarily may build apprehension and create undesirable responses. Usually, tell-show-do (TSD) is employed. The child must be told in advance what is being done and why.

### Tell

- Plant positive suggestions.
- "Donna, because you have so many teeth to fix and I want it to be easy for you", I am going to use my magic air. It is something special. It will make you feel funny. Some children even laugh at it."
- Thus, the suggestion of an extraordinary and pleasant experience is established.
- Explain the nasal mask.
- "To do this, I use a little, funny nose."
- The dentist places a nasal mask on herself and says,
- "See? I look like an airplane pilot!" or "I look funny with my funny nose!" (Figure 12-2).
- Explain the immediate effect of the mask.
- "Through the special nose, you will be able to smell yummy flavors."

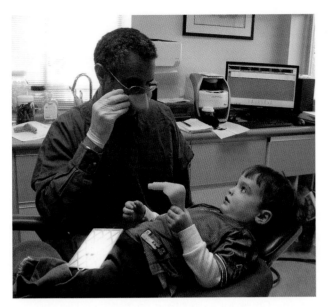

**Figure 12-2** "See? I look like an airplane pilot!" or "I look funny with my funny nose!" *Source:* Courtesy of Dr. Ari Kupietzky.

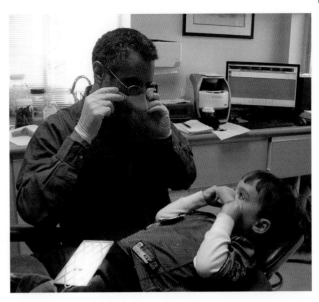

**Figure 12-3** The next move is to have the apprehensive child place a nasal mask over the nose. *Source:* Courtesy of Dr. Ari Kupietzky.

## Show

The child is shown the nasal mask. At this point, the child should not be offered a choice. Avoid asking, "Would you like to wear this nose?"

The next move is to have the apprehensive child place a nasal mask over her nose (Figure 12-3). ("Let me show you how funny it looks." "Donna, I have another funny nose for you. It is smaller because your nose isn't as big as mine." "To do this, I need you to wear this clown nose." Let the child hold the nasal mask on the nose.)

## Do

- Begin by repeating the plan.
- "Since you have so many teeth to fix and I want it to be easy for you, I am going to use my magic air. It is something special. It will make you feel funny. Some children even laugh at it."
- Place the mask on the child. There should be a gas flow through the mask before it is placed.
- "Try it on, it smells nice."
- The child is given a mirror and the nasal mask is gently placed on her nose. Since the child is holding the mirror with both hands, she is less likely to remove the mask (Figure 12-4).
- "Hold this mirror in your hands so you can see how funny you look."

Some dentists prefer to have the child begin by breathing through the mouth. In their preferred method, the child is told not to breathe through his nose and to keep

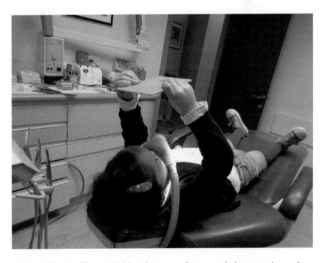

**Figure 12-4** The child is given a mirror and the nasal mask is gently placed on her nose. *Source:* Courtesy of Dr. Ari Kupietzky.

his mouth open (Figure 12-5). "Don't close your mouth. Keep it open. And don't breathe from your nose yet. Wait until I tell you." "I can make it smell like chocolate chip cookies or strawberries. Which smell do you like?"

Some dentists prefer to use scented nasal masks or a little dab of flavoring that can be placed on the mask beforehand to provide a more pleasant smell. However, with power of suggestion, many children will attest that the funny gas smelled like chocolates or strawberries, according to their choice. The child breathes through the mouth and looks at herself through the mirror.

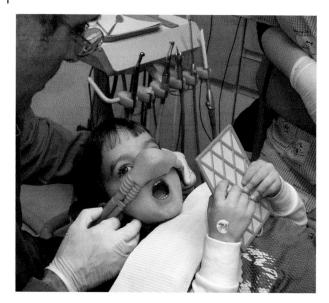

**Figure 12-5** Some dentists prefer to have the child begin by breathing through the mouth. The child is told not to breathe through the nose and to keep the mouth opened. *Source:* Courtesy of Dr. Ari Kupietzky.

## Determining the Tidal Volume and Gas Flow

Tidal volume is the amount of air moved into or out of the lungs during quiet breathing. The goal is to match the gas flow with the tidal volume. For a four-year-old child, approximately 20 kg (40 lbs.), the tidal volume will be near 4 liters. To verify this, the sedation procedure begins with a flow of 4 liters of oxygen through the system. Total liters flow per minute (L/min) is adjusted depending on the size and age of the child. The reservoir bag should be approximately 2/3 full. When the patient breathes in, the bag moves and collapses slightly, but not fully. When expiration occurs, the bag distends, but not fully. Tidal volumes have to be tailored to individual patients. To assist in determining the starting point, Table 12-4 provides data for children up to age 10 years. Note that as children get older, the respiration rate decreases. Conversely, as children get older and larger, the tidal volume increases.

**Table 12-4** Respiratory data for children.

| Weight (Kg) | Age (Yrs) | Respiration Rate/Minute | Minute Volume (ml) |
|---|---|---|---|
| 13.6 | 2–3 | 30 | 2700 |
| 20.0 | 4 | 30 | 4000 |
| 28.0 26.0 43.0 | 6 8 10 | 27 22 20 | 5000 5300 5700 |

*Source:* Adapted from Stephen et al. (1970).

## Titrating Gases for Sedation

Children need to be instructed to breathe properly. After three or four breaths, the child is instructed to close the mouth once and breathe once through the nose. Afterward, the child is told to breathe twice, and then three times. Increasingly, the child will switch over to breathing exclusively through the nose—a gradual introduction of the gas has occurred.

Observing the movement of the reservoir bag is essential for monitoring breathing. A fully distended bag hampers monitoring. Therefore, if the bag is distended, the clinician needs to start by checking the child's breathing. Instruct the child to breathe deeply and demonstrate what is meant. "I would like you to breathe more: breathe in as hard as you can."

If the bag does not move, lower the volume of gas inflowing. Check for a snug fit of the nasal mask to ensure a closed circuit. An improper fit allows gas leakage to contaminate the clinician's immediate environment (breathing zone). Escaping gas influences the movement of the reservoir bag and can irritate a child's eyes. A further check should be made for any kinks in the gas lines that might obstruct the gas flow. Once the volume of gas flow has been established (about 2–3 minutes of oxygen), titration of gases for sedation commences.

Young children often have to be instructed to breathe properly. Rapid, shallow breathing (tachypnea) may not provide the alveolar ventilation required for uptake of a gas mixture. In these cases, the dentist can demonstrate the breathing technique. Most children imitate the modeling. Repeated instructions are made to keep the mouth closed, thus encouraging nasal breathing. It may be necessary to place a finger on the lips of very young children to teach them to breathe properly through the nasal mask. The use of the rubber dam also helps with proper breathing. Once the dam is in place, mouth breathing is difficult and nasal breathing is easier.

There are two methods to initially administer $N_2O$ to children: the standard titration technique and the rapid induction technique.

### Standard Titration Technique

The standard titration technique (also known as *slow titration technique* or *slow induction technique*) is used by many dentists for adults and older children. The technique begins slowly with 100% oxygen. After 2–3 minutes, gases are adjusted to approximately 20% $N_2O$ and 80% oxygen. Every 1–2 minutes, the gas ratio is altered. The nitrous level is increased about 10%, and the oxygen flow is lowered concomitantly. The total gas flow, which was established at the outset, is maintained. Often, gas is titrated close to a 1:1 ratio for the injection and rubber dam procedures and then decreased to about a 30% N₂O level during restorative procedures. Success with the standard titration technique is dependent, to a large degree, on the patient properly describing the effects of the gas. If used for younger children, they have to be guided throughout the process. The child is told, "Soon the magic air will make you feel funny, and you will probably laugh, too. Don't forget to breathe through your nose and not through your toes!"

After about a half minute, the child is asked, "Are your arms getting tired? You sure hold that well." Following the usual affirmative response, the child is told to lower her arms and the assistant is instructed to secure the nasal mask. "Soon you will feel funny. You remember why I am doing this—so it doesn't hurt you when I fix your teeth. You know, you are doing this better than most four-year-old children. We all like you here (positive verbal reinforcement). Pretty soon you are going to start to feel funny. Your legs and feet might tickle or feel heavy. You might feel as if you are flying in an airplane. You will feel really good (elements of hypnosis, see Chapter 7)."

Maintaining a constant and almost monotonous voice contact lulls the patient into a state of security. Try not to use specific terms about how the patient will feel, especially with older children. The power of suggestion can lead them to respond positively and create a false perception of the N₂O effectiveness. On the other hand, if a child makes noncoherent comments or show signs of loss of control or agitation, this could be indicative of an overdose. Lower the concentration: do not increase it under this circumstance.

At the end of the procedure, 100% oxygen should be delivered for at least 3–5 minutes. This is specifically important while treating children (AAPD guideline), as they de-saturate rapidly. As N₂O is 34 times more soluble than nitrogen in blood, diffusion hypoxia may occur. The patient may be discharged when he/she has returned to normal (pre-sedation) levels of consciousness and has regained normal speech and gait (Jastak and Orendruff 1975).

With removal of the nasal mask from a patient, particularly following a lengthy one, a depression may appear over the child's nose and along the cheek (Figure 12-6). These facial signs are caused by a firm fitting nasal mask and will fade away within minutes. However, if the parent is not told about the phenomenon at the outset or right before the mask is removed, much ado could be made about nothing.

### Rapid Induction Technique

An alternative method for N₂O administration is the rapid induction technique. This technique can be divided into four phases and is described in Table 12-5 (Simon and

(a)
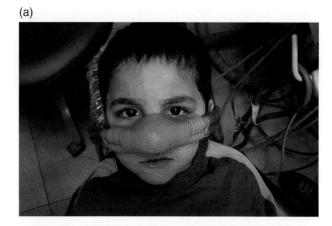
(b)
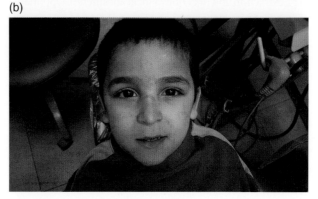

**Figure 12-6** A firm fitting mask (a) may leave transient signs on the child's face (b).

**Table 12-5** Phases of inhalation sedation with dosages.

| Phase | Dosage |
| --- | --- |
| Introduction | 3–5 liters oxygen |
| Injection | 2 liters nitrous oxide: 2 liters oxygen (50%) |
| Maintenance | 1–2 liters nitrous oxide: 3 liters oxygen (25–40%)* |
| Withdrawal | 3–5 liters oxygen |

*Some clinicians maintain a level of 50% nitrous throughout the entire treatment.

Vogelsberg 1975). Similar to the standard titration technique, rapid induction begins for our four-year-old patient with about 4 l of oxygen. However, after 1–2 minutes, the gas is delivered in a 1:1 ratio: half N₂O and half oxygen. It is maintained at this level for 5–10 minutes, and once injections have been given and a rubber dam has been placed, the N₂O level is decreased and the oxygen is increased. The patient is maintained on a 25–35% nitrous level using the pre-established volume of gas, however, some clinicians maintain 50% nitrous throughout the entire treatment. Similar to the slow titration, 100% oxygen is administered at the end of the procedure for about 3–5 minutes. Because the administration is much more rapid, the patient's signs are watched closely. These can involve body movements, eye signs, or even slurring of speech. If there is concern that the sedation is too deep, the $N_2O$ is lowered. This technique is most appropriate for the very young child or the highly anxious patient, as it allows the clinician to deal with the behavior much more quickly.

Regardless of the technique that is used, two opinions are found regarding changes in $N_2O$ concentration during treatment. One approach (which is part of the AAPD guidelines) is that it may be decreased during easier procedures (e.g., restorations) and increased during more stimulating ones (e.g., extraction and injection of local anesthetic). Opponents of this technique opine that frequent changes in $N_2O$ concentrations may cause unnecessary nausea and result in vomiting; the sensation is likened to a roller coaster ride. These clinicians keep the $N_2O$ concentration steady throughout all types of dental procedures.

Generally, during $N_2O$/oxygen analgesia/ anxiolysis, the concentration of $N_2O$ should not routinely exceed 50%. At concentrations greater than 50%, $N_2O$ may cause deep sedation, which generally has been found to be associated with an increased risk of adverse events (Babl et al. 2008; Hoffman et al. 2002). In addition, during $N_2O$ sedation without any additional sedative agent, the AAPD guideline requires that only continual clinical observation of the patient's responsiveness, color, and respiratory rate and rhythm be performed. However, if higher concentrations are used, the patient may experience minimal or moderate sedation, which requires monitoring with pulse oximetry, blood pressure cuff, and precordial stethoscope or capnography (Coté and Wilson 2019).

For safety reasons, the dentist should always be accompanied by assisting personnel. At least one staff member must be present in the treatment room at all times during the administration of $N_2O$, and the patient should never be left unattended.

Generally, the $N_2O$ should not be used without local anesthesia. However, to avoid any local anesthesia discomfort, some clinicians take advantage of $N_2O$ analgesic properties and perform minor procedures, like class I cavity restorations, without local anesthesia (Hammond and Full 1984). The downside of avoiding local anesthesia is that the operative procedure may or may not be pain-free. As with other pharmacotherapeutic and nonpharmacotherapeutic techniques, the key to success is the avoidance of pain. Some dentists will try to avoid the injection of local anesthesia when confronted with a resistant child or parent. However, with $N_2O$ sedation and good injection technique, the small amount of discomfort from the injection becomes subclinical and the use of local anesthetic is highly recommended.

## Adverse Effects

When administered by trained personnel on carefully selected patients with appropriate equipment and technique, $N_2O$ is a safe and effective agent for providing pharmacological guidance of behavior in children with relatively few adverse effects. This was documented in a large French survey series of 7,571 children receiving demand valve 50% $N_2O$ in which a low rate of major adverse events was reported (0.3%). All adverse events were resolved within minutes, and none of the patients needed any airway intervention (Gall et al. 2001). The safety of 50% $N_2O$ for procedural sedation also has been demonstrated in studies encompassing thousands of patients (Hennequin et al. 2004; Onody et al. 2006).

Headache and disorientation can occur occasionally. They result from acute hypoxia, a rapid release of $N_2O$ from the blood stream into the alveoli. These adverse effects can be avoided by administering 100% oxygen after discontinuing the $N_2O$ at the end of treatment.

The most common, though infrequent, complication found to occur with the administration of $N_2O$ to children is vomiting. For this reason, some practitioners instruct patients to refrain from eating prior to the dental appointment. There are conflicting views on the need for this and also on the length of fasting time prior to a procedure. Although the frequency of vomiting during $N_2O$ is very low, there are dentists who require fasting for all children undergoing $N_2O$ sedation. They argue that since the foremost adverse reaction associated with $N_2O$ sedation is vomiting, a complete fast should be enforced. Dentists who oppose fasting for the use of $N_2O$ sedation may reason that the incidence of vomiting is very low and, in the event of such an occurrence, no life-threatening risks exist since the patient is not deeply sedated and remains in control of all reflexes, unlike the deeply sedated child. Aspiration of vomitus is unlikely when the protective airway reflexes are intact. Consequently, pulmonary aspiration is highly unlikely to occur.

Several studies have looked at this issue. Babl et al. (2005) examined the relationship between fasting status and adverse events during procedural sedation with $N_2O$ in the emergency department (ED). Pre-procedural fasting is difficult to obtain in the ED, since procedures are unscheduled and non-elective. Although in this study 71.1% of patients did not meet fasting guidelines for solids, no serious adverse events and no episodes of aspiration were found. The study concluded that $N_2O$ is a safe agent for procedural analgesia and sedation, without serious adverse events and with a low rate of temporary, mild adverse events. No association between pre-procedural fasting and emesis was found.

In earlier investigations, there were mixed opinions on the frequency of vomiting. Hogue et al. (1971) reported no ill effects administering between 5% and 40% $N_2O$; however, Houck and Ripa (1971) found that 10% of the children vomited while receiving maintenance concentrations between 30%–60% $N_2O$. These latter investigators recommended that dentists ask the following in health questionnaires to screen for patients who might be potentially high-risk candidates for vomiting:

- Has your child vomited during previous dental treatments?
- Does your child experience motion sickness—car or airplane?
- Does your child have influenza or any gastrointestinal infections?

For patients with a history of vomiting or car sickness, an antiemetic may be prescribed.

More recently, a cross-over design by Kupietzky et al. (2008) assessed the relationship between fasting status and vomiting with $N_2O$ sedation. The average time between eating and treatment in the fasting sessions was 6 hours and 1 hour in the non-fasting group. A rapid induction method of constant, non-fluctuating concentration/flow of 50% $N_2O$ was used. Vomiting occurred in only one subject, immediately after cessation of treatment resulting in a frequency of 1% of subjects or 0.5% of sessions. No other differences were found between fasting and non-fasting subjects.

In addition to the low frequency of vomiting occurring during nitrous administration, there are other reasons not to require preprocedural fasting. A child fasting may be agitated and will be less cooperative during dental treatment, thus defeating the purpose of $N_2O$ sedation use. Unfed children are often cranky, sometimes combative, and occasionally dehydrated (Gleghorn 1997). Parents accompanying a fasting child will also be less cooperative. A hungry child is irritable and therefore more difficult to sedate. Consequently, the dentist may decide to use a higher $N_2O$ sedation concentration to overcome this child's disruptive behavior. The higher dose may result in over-sedation, which in itself can cause of vomiting. Another paradox to be considered is that patients treated on an empty stomach are more susceptible to nausea and vomiting.

Clinical Tip: There are times when a child has been undergoing a lengthy procedure and becomes fidgety. This could be a signal that nausea and vomiting is an impending problem. It also could mean that the patient is slipping into the excitement stage. Because the child is fidgeting, the clinician may consider increasing the $N_2O$ level. This is not an uncommon response. But the correct thing *is to lower the $N_2O$ level.*

Nausea and vomiting that occur during $N_2O$ sedation are usually associated with the following causes: over-sedation ($N_2O$ concentration too high for patient, Malamed 2009); the "roller coaster" effect of sharp increases and decreases in concentrations of $N_2O$ administered (Clark and Brunick 2007); sedation length—the longer the patient has $N_2O$, the greater the incidence of nausea and vomiting (Zier and Liu 2011); and a prior history of nausea and vomiting.

The AAPD guideline on use of $N_2O$ for pediatric dental patients states that "Fasting is not required for patients undergoing nitrous oxide analgesia/anxiolysis. The practitioner, however, may recommend that only a light meal be consumed in the 2 hours prior to the administration of nitrous oxide."

## Contraindications

$N_2O$/oxygen sedation cannot be used to control all forms of child behavior, especially those that are hysterical or defiant. No positive effect will be obtained treating the crying, hysterical child with whom the dentist cannot communicate. Forcing a nasal mask on a child in this circumstance only escalates the torment. Truly defiant children will not accept a nasal hood gracefully or cooperate adequately for nasal inhalation of $N_2O$.

$N_2O$ sedation should not be used in any condition which might lead to nasal blockage and prevents a child from sufficiently inhaling the nitrous administered: the common cold, upper respiratory infections (URI) or bronchitis, allergies, and hay fever. Patients with blocked Eustachian tubes can experience ear pain due to distention of the tympanic membrane. Administering $N_2O$ to a child with a middle ear infection may result in a ruptured eardrum. $N_2O$ is 40 times more soluble in blood than nitrogen. This allows it to rapidly diffuse into closed gas spaces within the body, exerting pressure effects locally. Related to this cavity-expanding phenomenon, $N_2O$ can prove problematic in those patients with bowel obstruction since it may lead to expansion of gas with readily apparent adverse consequences. Other areas of trapped gas may not be so clinically apparent; patients who have undergone recent retinal surgery may have intraocular gas that may expand during $N_2O$ administration, leading to intraocular hypertension and irreversible loss of vision (Lockwood and Yang 2008).

Although $N_2O$ can be safely administered to most asthmatics and those with other forms of chronic obstructive pulmonary disease (COPD); there is a small subset of these patients in whom its use is not prudent. Those patients with severe pulmonary disease who utilize hypoxic drive (lack of oxygen) to stimulate breathing, rather than the normal mechanisms mediated by carbon dioxide accumulation, reflect a relative contraindication to the use of $N_2O$. This is due to (1) the patients usually being more sensitive to the sedative effects of $N_2O$ and (2) supplemental oxygen being also administered with $N_2O$, increasing the patient's oxygen uptake, thereby removing the stimulus to breathe. Generally, those patients with bronchial asthma can receive $N_2O$ because it is nonirritating to the bronchial and pulmonary tissues. Increased stress can lead to an asthmatic attack; therefore, nitrous sedation can be helpful.

$N_2O$ also can have a disproportionately stronger effect on special patients taking tranquilizers, analgesics, antidepressants, antipsychotic drugs, or who have a depressed level of consciousness. $N_2O$ may cause neurological and hematological signs and symptoms, as it inhibits vitamin B12 (cobalamin) by irreversibly oxidizing the cobalt atom of cobalamin (Lindstedt 1999). Inhibition of vitamin B12 lasts several days because of the irreversible nature of the reaction. Exposure of $N_2O$ to patients with methylenetetrahydrofolate reductase (MTHFR) gene polymorphisms, which are operant in the folate cycle, is associated with neurological symptoms, which were reversed after supplementary therapy with folic acid and vitamin B12 (Lacassie et al. 2006). Recent studies have revealed that the genes involved in the folate pathway may be risk factors for autism spectrum disorders (ASDs), and at the same time, ASD syndromes are associated with single nucleotide mutations of the MTHFR gene (Arab and Elhawary 2019). The AAPD guidelines state that MTHFR is a contraindication for use of $N_2O$ based only on one extreme case (Selzer et al. 2003).

*UpToDate*, an anesthesiology peer-reviewed online "textbook" though, states that chronic elevated homocysteine levels are the primary concern with this gene, and therefore, intermittent increases from $N_2O$ use would be negligible. Finally, treatment with bleomycin sulfate is contraindicated for use of $N_2O$ (Fleming et al. 1988).

The increased risk of spontaneous abortions and malformations in humans is controversial although animal studies show various risk potentials (fetotoxicity at 450–1,000 ppm in rats). No association has been found between trace levels of waste $N_2O$ in *scavenged* locations and adverse health effects to personnel. Reduced fertility has been reported for those not using scavenging equipment and exposed to $N_2O$ for more than 3 hours per week (Rowland et al. 1995). Still, it is advised that females should not administer $N_2O$ during the first trimester of pregnancy.

In an effort to reduce occupational health hazards associated with $N_2O$, the AAPD recommends exposure to ambient $N_2O$ be minimized through the use of effective scavenging systems and periodic evaluation and maintenance of the delivery and scavenging systems (AAPD 2020). Scavenging significantly reduces ambient $N_2O$ levels in the dentist's breathing zone but not to the level (25 ppm) recommended by The National Institute for Occupational Safety and Health. Supplemental oral evacuation should be employed in conjunction with the scavenging system during dental procedures or when patient behaviors such as increased talking or crying can result in increased environmental $N_2O$ exposure to staff (Henry et al. 1992).

## Safety

The most important safety consideration is the prevention of hypoxia. Safety features have been designed to prevent hypoxia by ensuring a minimal oxygen flow, thus limiting the amount of $N_2O$ that can be administered. Donaldson et al. (2012) reviewed the 12 safety features used to ensure the safety and efficacy of $N_2O$ sedation. The authors discussed examples of safety feature failures, as well as steps to follow to help prevent negative outcomes.

$N_2O$–oxygen delivery systems for dental use typically are limited to a maximum of 70% $N_2O$ and 30% oxygen delivery, which ensures that the patient is receiving at least 9% more oxygen than found in ambient air. Other safety features stop the delivery of $N_2O$ if oxygen flow stops. The pin-index safety system prevents the accidental attachment of a non-oxygen tank to the oxygen attachment portal, and diameter index systems help ensure that the appropriate gas flows through the appropriate tubing. Although these safety features are in place, dentists have reported incidents of hypoxia involving incorrect equipment installation or equipment damage. If a safety feature failure is suspected during administration of $N_2O$ sedation, the clinician should remove the face mask from the patient immediately.

Scavenging of waste gas ideally should be with the aid of an ejector run by compressed air and not through the vacuum system of the dental unit. This ejector should have a capacity of scavenging 25 liters per minute.

## Summary

N$_2$O may be considered to be the most popular form of sedation among pediatric dentists. It has earned this place due to its excellent safety record and ease of use. It provides rapid onset and offset of sedation. Because of its unique inhalation application, it has been allocated to this chapter, separate from other pharmacologic agents. The mechanisms of its action have been discussed and its practical administration described in detail.

## References

Adair, S.M., Rockman, R.A., Schaefer, T.E. et al. (2004). Survey of behavior management techniques in advanced education programs. *Pediatric Dentistry*, 26, 151–158.

American Academy of Pediatric Dentistry (AAPD). (2020). *Use of nitrous oxide for pediatric dental patients. The Reference Manual of Pediatric Dentistry*. Chicago, Ill.: American Academy of Pediatric Dentistry, pp. 324–329.

Arab, A.H. and Elhawary, N.A. (2019). Methylenetetrahydrofolate reductase gene variants confer potential vulnerability to autism spectrum disorder in a Saudi community. *Neuropsychiatric Disease and Treatment*, 27, 3569–3581.

Anderson, W. (1980). The effectiveness of audio-nitrous oxide- oxygen psychosedation on dental behavior of a child. *Journal of Pedodontics*, 5, 3–21.

Archer, W.H. (1944). Life and letters of Horace Wells: Discoverer of anesthesia. *Journal of the American College of Dentistry*, 11, 81.

Babl, F.E., Puspitadewi, A., Barnett, P. et al. (2005). Preprocedural fasting state and adverse events in children receiving nitrous oxide for procedural sedation and analgesia. *Pediatric Emergency Care*, 21, 736–743.

Babl, F.E., Oakley, E., Seaman, C., Barnett, P. et al. (2008). High-concentration nitrous oxide for procedural sedation in children: Adverse events and depth of sedation. *Pediatrics*, 121, 528–532.

Berger, D., Allen, G., and Everett, G. (1972). An assessment of the analgesic effects of nitrous oxide on the primary dentition. *Journal of Dentistry for Children*, 39, 265–268.

Bodner, S. (2008). Stress management in the difficult patient encounter. *Dental Clinics of North America*, 52, 579–603.

Clark, M.J. and Brunick, A. (2007). Handbook of Nitrous Oxide and Oxygen Sedation, 3rd ed. CV Mosby Co, St. Louis, MO, USA.

Collado, V., Hennequin, M., Faulks, D. et al. (2006) Modification of behavior with 50% nitrous oxide/oxygen conscious sedation over repeated visits for dental treatment: A 3-year prospective study. *Journal Clinical Psychopharmacology*, 26, 474–481.

Coté, C.J. and Wilson, S. (2019). Guidelines for monitoring and management of pediatric patients before, during, and after sedation for diagnostic and therapeutic procedures. *Pediatric Dentistry*, 41(4), 26E–52E.

Donaldson, M., Donaldson, D., and Quarnstrom, F.C. (2012). Nitrous oxide-oxygen administration: When safety features no longer are safe. *Journal of the American Dental Association*, 143, 134–143.

Dundee, J.W. and Moore, J. (1960). Alterations in response to somatic pain associated with anaesthesia. *IV. The effect of subanaesthetic concentrations of inhalation agents. British Journal of Anaesthesiology*, 32, 453–459.

Emmanouil, D. (2020). Mechanism of action of nitrous oxide (Chapter 3). In: K. Gupta, D. Emmanouil, A. Sethi (Eds.), Nitrous Oxide in Pediatric Dentistry (pp. 77–94). Springer, Switzerland.

Emmanouil, D.E. and Quock, R.M. (2007). Advances in understanding the actions of nitrous oxide. *Anesthesia Progress*, 54, 9–18.

Emmanouil, D., Klein, E.D., Chen, K. et al. (2020). Nitrous oxide-induced impairment of spatial working memory requires activation of GABAergic pathways. *Current Psychopharmacology*, 9, 68–78.

Fleming, P., Walker, P.O., and Priest, J.R. (1988). Bleomycin therapy: A contraindication to the use of nitrous oxide-oxygen psychosedation in the dental office. *Pediatric Dentistry*, 10, 345–346.

Gall, O., Annequin, D., and Benoit, G. et al. (2001). Adverse events of premixed nitrous oxide and oxygen for procedural sedation in children. *Lancet*, 358, 1514–1515.

Gillman, M.A. and Lichtigfeld, F.J. (1994). Opioid properties of psychotropic analgesic nitrous oxide (laughing gas). *Perspectives in Biology and Medicine*, 38, 125–138.

Gleghorn, E. (1997). Preoperative fasting: You don't have to be cruel to be kind. *Journal of Pediatrics*, 131, 12–13.

Guedel, A.E. (1937). Inhalation Anesthesia. McMillan Co, New York, NY, USA.

Hammond, N.I. and Full, C.A. (1984). Nitrous oxide analgesia and children's perception of pain. *Pediatric Dentistry*, 6, 238–242.

Hennequin, M., Maniere, M.C., Albecker-Grappe, S. et al. (2004). A prospective multicentric trial for effectiveness and tolerance of a N2O/O2 premix as a sedative drug. *Journal Clinical Psychopharmacology*, 24, 552–554.

Henry, R.J., Primosch, R.E., and Courts, F.J. (1992). The effects of various dental procedures and patient behaviors upon nitrous oxide scavenger effectiveness. *Pediatric Dentistry*, 14, 19–25.

Hoffman, G.M., Nowakowski, R., Troshynski, T.J. et al. (2002). Risk reduction in pediatric procedural sedation by application of an American Academy of Pediatrics/American Society of Anesthesiologists process model. *Pediatrics*, 109, 236–243.

Hornbein, T.F., Eger, E.I. 2nd, Winter, P.M. et al. (1982). The minimum alveolar concentration of nitrous oxide in man. *Anesthesia Analgesia*, 61, 553–556.

Hogue, D., Ternisky, M., and Iranpour, B. (1971). The response of nitrous oxide analgesia in children. *Journal of Dentistry for Children*, 38, 129–135.

Houpt, M.I., Limb, R., and Livingston, R.L. (2004). Clinical effects of nitrous oxide conscious sedation in children. *Pediatric Dentistry*, 26, 29–36.

Jastak, J.T. and Orendruff, D. (1975). Recovery from nitrous sedation. *Anesthesia Progress*, 22, 113–116.

Jevtovic-Todorovic, V., Benshoff, N., and Olney, J.W. (2000). Ketamine potentiates cerebrocortical damage induced by the common anaesthetic agent nitrous oxide in adult rats. *British Journal of Pharmacology*, 130, 1692–1698.

Kupietzky, A., Tal, E., Shapira, J. et al. (2008). Fasting state and episodes of vomiting in children receiving nitrous oxide for dental treatment. *Pediatric Dentistry*, 30, 414–419.

Lacassie, H.J., Nazar, C., Yonish, B. et al. (2006). Reversible nitrous oxide myelopathy and a polymorphism in the gene encoding 5,10 methylenetetrahydrofolate reductase. *British Journal of Anaesthesia*, 96, 222–225.

Langa, H. (1968). Relative Analgesia in Dental Practice: Inhalation Analgesia with Nitrous Oxide. W B Saunders, Philadelphia, PA, USA.

Likis, F., Andrews, J.C., Collins, M.R. et al. (2014). Nitrous oxide for the management of labor pain: A systematic review. *Anesthesia & Analgesia*, 118, 153–167.

Lindstedt, G. (1999). Nitrous oxide can cause cobalamin deficiency. Vitamin B12 is a simple and cheap remedy. *Lakartidningen*, 96(44), 4801–4805.

Lockwood, A.J. and Yang, Y.F. (2008). Nitrous oxide inhalation anaesthesia in the presence of intraocular gas can cause irreversible blindness. *British Dental Journal*, 204, 247–248.

Lundy, J.S. (1925). Anesthesia by nitrous oxide, ethylene, carbon dioxide and oxygen for dental operations on children. *Dental Cosmos*, 67, 906–909.

Lynch, K. (2007). Sedation modifications: How will the proposed guidelines affect your practice? *AGD Impact*, 35, 48–54.

Malamed, S.F. (2009). Sedation: A Guide to Patient Management, 5e. CV Mosby Co, St. Louis, MO, USA.

Musselman, R.J. and McClure, D.B. (1975). Pharmacotheraputic approaches to behavior management (Chapter 8). In: G.Z. Wright (Ed.), Behavior Management in Dentistry for Children (pp. 146–177). W.B. Saunders Co., Philadelphia.

Nathan, J.E., Venham, L.L., West, M.S. et al. (1988). The effects of nitrous oxide on anxious young pediatric patients across sequential visits: A double-blind study. *Journal of Dentistry for Children*, 53, 220–230.

Onody, P., Gil, P., and Hennequin, M. (2006). Safety of inhalation of a 50% nitrous oxide/oxygen premix: A prospective survey of 35 828 administrations. *Drug Safety*, 29, 633–640.

Paterson, S.A. and Tahmassebi, J.F. (2003). Pediatric dentistry in the new millennium: 3. *Use of inhalation sedation in pediatric dentistry. Dental Update*, 30, 350–356, 358.

Ramsay, D.S., Leonesio, R.J., Whitney, C.W. et al. (1992). Paradoxical effects of nitrous oxide on human memory. *Psychopharmacology*, 106, 370–374.

Rowland, A.S., Baird, D.D., Shore, D.L. et al. (1995). Nitrous oxide and spontaneous abortion in female dental assistants. *American Journal of Epidemiology*, 141, 531–537.

Roberts, G.J. (1990). Inhalation sedation (relative analgesia) with oxygen/nitrous oxide gas mixture: 1. Principles. *Dental Update*, 17, 139–146.

Sanders, R.D., Weimann, J., and Maze, M. (2008). Biologic effects of nitrous oxide: A mechanistic and toxicologic review. *Anesthesiology*, 109, 707–722.

Selzer, R.R., Rosenblatt, D.S., Laxova, R. et al. (2003). Adverse effect of nitrous oxide in a child with 5,10-methylenetetrahydrofolate reductase deficiency. *New England Journal of Medicine*, 349, 45–50.

Simon, J.F. Jr., and Vogelsberg, G.M. (1975). Use of nitrous-oxide-oxygen inhalation sedation for children (Chapter 9). In: G.Z. Wright (Ed.), Behavior Management in Dentistry for Children (pp. 177–196). W.B. Saunders Co., Philadelphia.

Sorenson, H.W. and Roth, G.I. (1973). A case for N2O/oxygen inhalation sedation: An aid in the elimination of the child's fear of the needle. *Dental Clinics of North America*, 17, 51–66.

Stach, D.J. (1995). Nitrous oxide sedation: Understanding the benefit and risks. *American Journal of Dentistry*, 8, 47–50.

Trottier, E.D., Doré-Bergeron, M., Chauvin-Kimoff, L. et al. (2019). Managing pain and distress in children undergoing brief diagnostic and therapeutic procedures. *Paediatrics and Child Health*, 24, 509–535.

Tsao, J.C., Myers, C.D., Craske, M.G. et al. (2004). Role of anticipatory anxiety and anxiety sensitivity in children's and adolescents' laboratory pain responses. *Journal of Pediatric Psychology*, 29, 379–388.

UpToDate, https://www.uptodate.com/contents/overview-of-homocysteine.

Weinstein, P., Domoto, P.K., and Holleman, E. (1986). The use of nitrous oxide in the treatment of children: results of a controlled study. *Journal of the American Dental Association*, 112, 325–331.

Whalley, M.G. and Brooks, G.B. (2009). Enhancement of suggestibility and imaginative ability with nitrous oxide. *Psychopharmacology (Berl)*, 203, 745–752.

Wilson, S. and Alcaino, E.A. (2011). Survey on sedation in paediatric dentistry: A global perspective. *International Journal of Paediatric Dentistry*, 21, 321–332.

Wilson, S. (1996). A survey of the American Academy membership: Nitrous oxide sedation. *Pediatric Dentistry*, 18, 287–293.

Wilson, S. and Gosnell, S.E. (2016). Survey of American Academy of Pediatric Dentistry on nitrous oxide and sedation: 20 years later. *Pediatric Dentistry*, 38, 385–392.

Zier, J.L. and Liu, M. (2011). Safety of high-concentration nitrous oxide by nasal mask for pediatric procedural sedation: experience with 7802 cases. *Pediatric Emergency Care*, 27, 1107–1112.

# 13

# Minimal and Moderate Sedation Agents

*Stephen Wilson*

## Introduction

Sedation usually implies a modification of the level of consciousness of an individual resulting ideally in a state of lessened anxiety or fear, relaxation, and sometimes favorable mood enhancement. The change in consciousness can be induced through non-pharmacological or pharmacological intervention (see Figure 1-2). This chapter will focus solely on pharmacologically mediated changes in consciousness.

Sedative medications alter the level of consciousness of an individual. Consciousness is represented as a continuum ranging from full wakefulness to complete coma and is dependent, to a degree, on the number and dose of pharmacological agents administered to the individual (Figure 13-1). Hence, the level or depth of sedation often is referred to as an *indirect, continuous index* of the patient's level of consciousness at any given point in time.

There are many ways to define levels or depths of sedation. Nonetheless, definitions of sedation are found in sedation guidelines offered by various professional organizations (American Dental Association, see https://www.ada.org/~/media/ADA/Member%20Center/FIles/anesthesia_guidelines.pdf?la=en; American Academy of Pediatrics and American Academy of Pediatric Dentistry (Cote et al. 2019); American Society of Anesthesiology (see https://www.asahq.org/standards-and-guidelines/continuum-of-depth-of-sedation-definition-of-general-anesthesia-and-levels-of-sedationanalgesia)). The most frequently used guidelines for sedation of the pediatric patient in any setting including dentistry is that of the current American Academy of Pediatrics/American Academy of Pediatric Dentistry (AAP/AAPD) (Cote et al. 2019).

Three different levels of sedation are defined in those guidelines:

*Minimal* (old terminology of "anxiolysis"): A drug-induced state during which patients respond normally to verbal commands. Although cognitive function and coordination may be impaired, ventilatory and cardiovascular functions are unaffected.

*Moderate* (old terminology "conscious sedation" or "sedation/analgesia"): A drug-induced depression of consciousness during which patients respond purposefully to verbal commands or after light tactile stimulation. No interventions are required to maintain a patent airway, and spontaneous ventilation is adequate. Cardiovascular function is usually maintained. However, in the case of procedures that may themselves cause airway obstruction (e.g., dental or endoscopic), the practitioner must recognize an obstruction and assist the patient in opening the airway. If the patient is not making spontaneous efforts to open his/her airway to relieve the obstruction, then the patient should be considered to be deeply sedated. For older patients, this level of sedation implies an interactive state; for younger patients, age-appropriate behaviors (e.g., crying) occur and are expected. Reflex withdrawal, although a normal response to a painful stimulus, is not considered as the only age-appropriate purposeful response (e.g., it must be accompanied by another response, such as pushing away the painful stimulus to confirm a higher cognitive function).

*Deep*: A drug-induced depression of consciousness during which patients cannot be easily aroused but

*Wright's Behavior Management in Dentistry for Children*, Third Edition. Edited by Ari Kupietzky.
© 2022 John Wiley & Sons, Inc. Published 2022 by John Wiley & Sons, Inc.

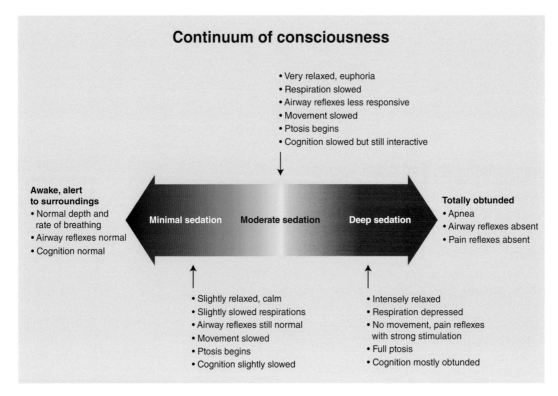

**Figure 13-1** Continuum of consciousness.

respond purposefully (see discussion of reflex withdrawal above) after repeated verbal or painful stimulation (e.g., purposefully pushing away the noxious stimuli). The ability to independently maintain ventilator function may be impaired. Patients may require assistance in maintaining a patent airway, and spontaneous ventilation may be inadequate. Cardiovascular function is usually maintained. A state of deep sedation may be accompanied by partial or complete loss of protective airway reflexes.

In this chapter, the focus is on minimal and moderate sedation. However, it is important to remember that any sedative drug and its dose can produce variable depths of sedation in individuals. Hence, it is impossible and inappropriate to refer to any one drug or a combination of drugs as a "drug(s) that produces minimal, moderate, or deep sedation." Indeed, a drug and its therapeutic dose may produce a given depth of sedation in most children, but others may respond either in a less (hypo-responder) or a more exaggerated fashion (hyper-responder) than expected.

A major theme and important concept in the AAP/AAPD sedation guidelines is that of rescue (Cote et al. 2019). Rescue as used in the guidelines refers to a practitioner's knowledge, training, and skills in providing competent management for the patient who is in the process of or potentially could drift into a compromised condition. Ultimately, any practitioner who sedates a child for the

purposes of undergoing a procedure must be able to recognize any compromised state of the child and act immediately to stabilize the patient until help arrives (e.g., paramedics) and prevent a disastrous adverse outcome. The most frequently occurring compromising states resulting from sedation involves the respiratory system. Therefore, practitioners must be efficient and effective in basic airway management skills including the use of positive pressure oxygen with a bag-valve-mask or other advanced airway adjuncts (e.g., oral airway). It is, therefore, essential that specialty training programs provide appropriate didactic and clinical experiences for trainees before they sedate children. Training may best be obtained via dedicated anesthesiology rotations in which trainees are frequently and directly exposed to compromised respiratory conditions and mentored by highly trained, skilled professionals. Training, especially in emergency management situations involving sedation, may be supplemented by frequent human simulation settings.

## Drugs

Drugs have been used to sedate children for dental procedures for well over a century. Isolated reports reviewing drugs as "premedications" for children during dental procedures can be found in the older literature, that of the 1950s and 1960s, for example, see Aduss et al. 1961; Album 1955;

Buckman 1956; Kracke 1962; and Lampshire 1950. The same drugs, besides alcohol, paralleling that era were also used in medicine for various conditions with barbiturates dominating for almost the first half of the twentieth century (Lopez-Munoz et al. 2005). Other notable drugs of that time were chloral hydrate, narcotics (primarily morphine), and bromides.

A classic review of agents of that era was done in 1952 by Ruble (Ruble 1952). He described the current literature of the primary and popular drugs of that era including barbiturates, bromides, and morphine. Interestingly, as described in his review, the issues and challenges during that day remain consistent with those of today. The premedication was indicated for the "nervous and highly apprehensive child." Concern revolved around the depth of sedation and dose and route of administration. The occurrence of family guidance at home, school, and in the dental office, or its lack resulted in the "happy" versus "maladjusted" individual. It was noted that a "screaming, violent child" made relatively simple procedures difficult and time-consuming for the dental team, and that sedation was "helpful to the child and the dentist." Other studies and written opinions of the day addressed these issues as well (Aduss et al. 1961; Album 1955; Buckman 1956; Lampshire 1950).

There have been several surveys over the past four decades identifying several agents used to sedate children for dental procedures (Adair et al. 2004; Badner et al. 1994; Davis 1988; Houpt 2002; Houpt 1989; Morin et al. 2016; Tilliss 1993; Wilson 1996; Wilson and Alcaino 2011; Wilson and Gosnell 2016; Wilson and Houpt 2016; Wilson and McTigue 1989; Wilson and Nathan 2011). The more common agents identified were nitrous oxide, chloral hydrate, meperidine, midazolam (and other benzodiazepines), and hydroxyzine (and other antihistamines). Agents such as morphine, alphaprodine, barbiturates, and chlorpromazine have been mentioned as well (Brandt and Bugg 1984; Doring 1985; Lambert et al. 1988; Myers and Shoaf 1977; Riekman and Ross 1981; Roberts et al. 1992). And more recently Ketamine and other agents (e.g., dexmedetomidine) have been reported in the literature (Gomes et al. 2017; Hitt et al. 2014; Malhotra et al. 2016; Pandey et al. 2011; Sado-Filho et al. 2019). The more common agents fall into five categories of agents: inhalation agents, hypnotics, analgesics, benzodiazepines, and antihistamines. The focus in this chapter will be on the oral route.

## Hypnotics

Hypnotics are drugs that promote drowsiness and sleep. Hypnotic agents are generally classified as barbiturates and non-barbiturate types. Barbiturates such as pentobarbital were popular decades ago. However, because of their potential to create paradoxical reactions, they are no longer favored as sedating agents for children.

### Chloral Hydrate

The most common hypnotic agent used in pediatric dentistry for decades has been chloral hydrate. Although chloral hydrate has and can be used as a single agent (Anderson 1960; Czaarnecki and Binns 1963), most recent studies have investigated chloral hydrate in combination with one or more other agents (Badalaty et al. 1990; Campbell et al. 1998; Chowdhury and Vargas 2005; da Costa et al. 2007; Hasty et al. 1991; Houpt, Weiss et al. 1985; Iwasaki et al. 1989; Leelataweewud et al. 2000; Meyer et al. 1990; Needleman et al. 1995; Poorman et al. 1990; Reeves et al. 1996; Sams et al. 1993; Sams and Russell 1993; Sheroan et al. 2006; Tafaro et al. 1991; Torres-Perez et al. 2007; Wilson et al. 2000; Wilson et al. 1998).

*Characteristics* Chloral hydrate was discovered in 1832 by Justus Liebig. It was introduced in medicine as an anesthetic and hypnotic drug in 1869 (Stetson and Jessup 1962). It acts by depressing the central nervous system. Its mechanism of action is not well understood but thought to involve the GABA receptor complex (Lu and Greco 2006). As a hypnotic, therapeutic doses of chloral hydrate can cause sleepiness, drowsiness, or in some cases, hyperactivity. Care must be exercised whenever using chloral hydrate in combination with other agents, including nitrous oxide, as the depth of sedation may increase and respiratory depression can occur (Leelataweewud et al. 2000). A unique effect of chloral hydrate is that of potential inhibition of the genioglossal muscle of the tongue (Hershenson et al. 1984). Children with large tonsils and adenoid tissue may not be appropriate recipients of chloral hydrate, especially higher doses (e.g., >25 mg/kg) because of the increased likelihood of upper airway blockage, especially when the patient is in the prone position.

Chloral hydrate is an oily substance and a noted irritant to mucosal tissue. Hence, it should not be used in patients who have conditions involving gastritis, esophagitis, or oral lesions. Care must also be taken to avoid contact of chloral hydrate with the conjunctiva of eyes, which may occur in the patient or person orally administering chloral hydrate when the patient coughs or spits. Rapid administration of chloral hydrate in children using a needleless syringe with splashing against the posterior portion of the mouth should also be avoided. Chloral hydrate in higher doses has also been associated with cardiac dysrhythmias, and thus its use should be avoided in patients with certain cardiac conditions (Table 13-1).

Chloral hydrate has no analgesic properties. Chloral hydrate has an unpleasant taste and usually requires a flavoring vehicle when orally administered. The formulation

**Table 13-1** Chloral Hydrate.

| Drug | Dose (Oral) | Characteristics | Warnings[§] | Sedation considerations (timing) | Reversible |
|---|---|---|---|---|---|
| Chloral hydrate (Sedative-hypnotic) | 20–50 mg/kg | Oily Not palatable | *Airway blockage* | Onset: 20–45 min | No |
| | Max: 1 g | Irritability Sleep/drowsiness | *Mucosal irritant* | Separation time: 45 min | |
| *Contraindications\*:* | | | | | |
| Hypersensitivity | | | *Laryngospasms* | Work: 1–1.5 hr | |
| Hepatic or renal impairment | | | Respiratory depressant | | |
| Severe cardiac disease | | | *Cardiac arrhythmias* | | |
| Gastritis | | | | | |
| Esophagitis | | | | | |
| Gastric ulcers | | | | | |

*Note:* Usually, one's sedation goals are the first two depths of sedation of the American Academy of Pediatric Dentistry guidelines (i.e., minimal and moderate sedation). However, in small uncooperative children, the optimal level of sedation is that of very light sleep from which one can be easily aroused with minimal verbal or tactile stimulation. The therapeutic dose range that usually produces this type of effect, when used alone, in most children is 30–50 mg/kg of body weight. If used with any other sedative, the author recommends a dose range of 10–25 mg/kg for minimal to moderate levels of sedation. Chloral hydrate can cause hypotonicity of the muscles of the tongue causing it to fall backward against the posterior oro-pharyngeal structures. Appropriate patient monitoring (pulse oximetry and capnography) is necessary because of the possibility that airway compromise may occur due to hypotonicity of glossal muscles, deep sleep, exhaustion, and/ or some respiratory depression.
[§] The listed warnings are incomplete, and the reader is strongly advised to view more warnings from a reliable source (e.g., Lexi-Comp)
[*] The listed contraindications are incomplete, and the reader is strongly advised to review more contraindications from a reliable source (e.g., Lexi-Comp)

and production of the oral solution of chloral hydrate in the United States was ceased as of April 2012. It remains available, however, in other countries. However, other formulations of chloral hydrate (e.g., capsules) are still available, and oral solutions of chloral hydrate can be formulated on an individual prescription basis by registered compound pharmacists should they elect to do so.

The typical sequence of behavioral events following the oral administration to a child of chloral hydrate or a combination of agents dominated by chloral hydrate is slight disinhibition or excitement within the first 15–25 minutes. Sometimes, the disinhibition is exhibited as more talkativeness, exploratory hyperactivity in the environment, social interaction, and general silliness, but occasionally can be frank agitation. This phase is usually followed by drowsiness or sleepiness and can result in sleep within 45–60 minutes depending on the dose. The working time, depending on whether other drugs are "on-board," the patient's level of natural fatigue, and the child characteristics such as temperament and cognitive development, is usually 60 or more minutes.

One of the earlier chloral hydrate studies was that of Anderson in 1960. He used chloral hydrate alone when providing dental care to children. Anderson advocated the use of chloral hydrate to "make a difficult, emotional patient easy to work on" and to help with patient tolerance of the procedure. He indicated that up to five teaspoons (1,200 mg)

was necessary for some 3–4-year-olds one-half hour before dental treatment. He reported on 300 patient sedations indicating that often local anesthesia was unnecessary, and all dental treatment could be accomplished in one appointment. Other studies using chloral hydrate as the single agent or with nitrous oxide have also been reported (Barr et al. 1977; Czaarnecki and Binns 1963; Houpt, Sheskin et al. 1985; Moore et al. 1984). Most of the studies indicate that chloral hydrate produces good to excellent sedations. However, chloral hydrate currently is rarely used as a single agent for children during dental procedures.

The dosage range used in these studies for chloral hydrate and hydroxyzine is 40–75 mg/kg and 15 mg to 2 mg/kg, respectively. There is some support to the expectation that the addition of hydroxyzine to chloral hydrate improves patient behavior compared to chloral hydrate alone (Avalos-Arenas et al. 1998); on the contrary, others have found no improvement in this comparison (Needleman et al. 1995).

Promethazine has also been a popular agent as a sedative with antihistaminic properties that has been used with chloral hydrate (Dallman et al. 2001; Houpt, Weiss et al. 1985; Lu and Lu 2006; Robbins 1967; Sams et al. 1993; Sams and Russell 1993; Wright and McAulay 1973). Its dose has been reported in these studies by body weight (1 mg/kg) and as a single bolus (12.5 mg). Blood pressure may be slightly lower in this combination compared to midazolam or chloral hydrate and meperidine (Dallman et al. 2001; Sams and Russell 1993), but the effect is not perceived as clinically significant.

Hydroxyzine, an antihistaminic, is most popular in recent times. Chloral hydrate has also been used in combination with meperidine and hydroxyzine. This combination has been anecdotally known as a "triple" combination. It is a combination that is still taught in advanced pediatric dentistry training programs and is fairly popular (Wilson and Nathan 2011). Generally, this combination when compared to other sedatives or drug combinations tends to cause improved behavior interpreted as increased quiet and decreased crying behaviors (Chowdhury and Vargas 2005; Hasty et al. 1991; Nathan and West 1987; Wilson et al. 2000). However, this is not always the case as dose differences or other similar "triple" combinations have shown no improvement in behavior or equivalent outcomes (Poorman et al. 1990; Sheroan et al. 2006). It is possible that the dose of chloral hydrate used may make a significant difference in the behavioral outcomes with a higher dose mediating a greater likelihood of quiet/sleep behaviors. Nonetheless, with a greater likelihood of quiet/sleep behaviors comes a higher risk of airway or respiratory compromise.

There may be an increased risk of respiratory compromise manifested as apnea and/or oxygen desaturation when the triple combination involves chloral hydrate at a dose of 50 mg/kg (Croswell et al. 1995; Leelataweedwud and Vann 2001; Leelataweewud et al. 2000; Rohlfing et al. 1998; Sheroan et al. 2006). It is possible that less respiratory compromise may result by lowering the dose of chloral hydrate and increasing that of meperidine or substituting midazolam for chloral hydrate in the triple combination (Chowdhury and Vargas 2005; Sheroan et al. 2006). It is the author's experience that chloral hydrate used in low doses (i.e., 10–20 mg/kg) in combination with meperidine (1–2 mg/kg) and hydroxyzine (0.5 mg/kg) is one of the most reliable sedative combinations aimed at moderate levels of sedation in healthy, young children.

## Narcotics

### Meperidine

Some analgesics administered with other classes of sedative agents may enhance the effectiveness of the sedation visit. Meperidine has been the most commonly used narcotic in pediatric dentistry. It is a synthetic analgesic, sedative, euphoric, and antispasmodic agent (Hasty et al. 1991; Toomarian et al. 2013). The liquid can be administered parenterally or orally. For the child, the oral route is easily accepted (Song and Webb 2003); however, the liquid is bitter leaving a strong unpleasant after-taste. For palatability and like most sedative agents, it should be flavored (Wilson 2000). It apparently is used infrequently alone (Cathers et al. 2005; McKee et al. 1990; Song and Webb 2003). One of the primary reasons to use meperidine in combination with another sedative agent is its analgesic properties, as most other agents with which it is combined usually lack analgesic properties (e.g., midazolam). Additionally, meperidine can slightly potentiate the sedative effect of another agent (Chowdhury and Vargas 2005; Nathan and Vargas, 2002; Wilson et al. 2000) deepening the level of sedation and increasing working time and in many cases gives the impression of altering the mood of the patient (i.e., euphoric response).

Meperidine is often administered orally but due to its bitter taste typical of narcotics, it requires some masking with a flavoring agent. It has an onset time of approximately 30 minutes (see Table 13-2). The submucosal route is another popular means of administering meperidine (Cathers et al. 2005; Chen et al. 2006; Lochary et al. 1993; Roberts et al. 1992; Song and Webb 2003). One study evaluated the behavior of children receiving dental care under sedation with meperidine administered orally versus submucosally. There were no differences in behavior based on the route of administration (Song and Webb 2003).

Generally, the onset of meperidine effects when administered submucosally is faster (i.e., approximately 15 minutes) compared to oral administrations. One drawback of the submucosal administration of meperidine is that it can elicit a hyperemic effect often resulting in a "wheal" and itching over the facial area where the injection was given. These effects are caused by the histamine release from mast cells and even direct vascular effects when exposed to meperidine (Flacke et al. 1985; Flacke et al. 1987; Levy et al. 1989). Another possible side-effect of administering meperidine submucosally is that injection into the large pterygoid venous complex, just distal to the maxillary tuberosity, can potentially cause rapid onset of hypotension. Considering these cautions, it seems more prudent to administer meperidine in therapeutic doses via the oral route which tends to eliminate the occurrence of the submucosal effects. Another serious concern is potential interaction between local anesthetics and some narcotics, including meperidine, when either or both used in excessive amounts can result in seizures and/or death (Moore and Goodson 1985).

Morphine is another narcotic that can be used for sedation. It is quite popular in medicine, but there is very little literature on its use in pediatric dentistry (Chen and Tanbonliong 2018; Huang and Tanbonliong 2015; Roberts

**Table 13-2**  Meperidine.

| Drug | Dose (Oral) | Characteristics | Warnings[§] | Sedation considerations (timing) | Reversible |
|---|---|---|---|---|---|
| Meperidine (Narcotic) | 1–2 mg/kg | Clear | Respiratory depression | Onset: 30 min | Yes (Narcan) |
| | Max: 50 mg | Non-palatable | Hypotension | Separation time: 30 min | |
| *Contraindications\*:* | | | | | |
| Hypersensitivity MAO inhibitors used within 14 days | | Analgesia | | Work: 1 hr | |
| | | Euphoria | | | |
| | | Dysphoria | | | |

*Note:* A major drawback to this agent is its likelihood of causing respiratory depression and hypotension. This is particularly true when administered parenterally with a slightly lessened risk anticipated when delivered in therapeutic doses via the oral route. Its use in combination with other sedatives should be carefully assessed because of the additive or synergistic properties of sedative agents. Narcotics, including meperidine, should be used with caution with local anesthetics. The threshold level for seizures is lowered when both are used in combination.
[§] The listed warnings are incomplete, and the reader is strongly advised to view more warnings from a reliable source (e.g., Lexi-Comp)
[*] The listed contraindications are incomplete, and the reader is strongly advised to review more contraindications from a reliable source (e.g., Lexi-Comp)

**Table 13-3**  Morphine.

| Drug | Dose (Oral) | Characteristics | Warnings[§] | Sedation considerations (timing) | Reversible |
|---|---|---|---|---|---|
| Morphine | 0.08–0.5 mg/kg | Analgesic | CNS depression | Onset: 30 min | Yes (Naloxone) |
| *Contraindications\*:* Hypersensitivity to morphine | | Sedative | Constipation | Separation time: 45 min | |
| | | Sleepiness | Hypotension and cardiac arrhythmias | Work: 1 hr | |
| Respiratory depression | | Euphoria | | | |
| Asthma | | | | | |
| Concomitant use of MAO inhibitors | | | | | |

[§] The listed warnings are incomplete, and the reader is strongly advised to view more warnings from a reliable source (e.g., Lexi-Comp)
[*] The listed contraindications are incomplete, and the reader is strongly advised to review more contraindications from a reliable source (e.g., Lexi-Comp)

et al. 1992; Schneider 1986). When given orally, it has an onset of approximately 45 minutes and lasts another 1–2 hours (Table 13-3).

In one study, morphine was compared to meperidine with similar outcomes (Roberts et al. 1992). In another study, morphine was used in two regimens that also involved benzodiazepines (either midazolam or diazepam) and hydroxyzine in young children undergoing dental treatment. Both regimens reportedly had an overall rate of effectiveness greater than 80%, and increased effectiveness was significantly associated with willingness to take the medication (Chen and Tanbonliong 2018). Seizures have been reported with morphine in children undergoing dental treatment (Schneider 1986). Other reported side effects include nausea, emesis, fever, transient oxygen desaturation, asthma, wheezing, prolonged sleep, and paradoxical child reaction (Chen and Tanbonliong 2018; Huang and Tanbonliong 2015; Schneider 1986). Morphine and meperidine can cause histamine release and should not be administered to children who are asthmatic or have seizure disorders.

## Benzodiazepines

Benzodiazepines are a large class of drugs that tend to have a wide margin of safety when used alone and in therapeutic doses. They have several properties which are beneficial to many conditions and generally cause, to relative degrees, anti-anxiety, sedative-hypnotic, anticonvulsant activity, skeletal muscle relaxation, and amnestic effects. Their mechanism of action is associated with activation of the GABA receptor complex which when activated has a generalized inhibitory effect. Thus, indirectly benzodiazepines tend to increase the inhibitory action of GABA. Although there are many benzodiazepines on the market, the most frequently reported benzodiazepines used for sedating children for dental procedures are midazolam, diazepam, and triazolam.

### Midazolam

Midazolam is purportedly the most popular sedative agent and benzodiazepine for children undergoing dental and medical procedures (Bhatnagar et al. 2012; Isik et al. 2008; Wilson and Nathan 2011). It was first used as a sedative for dental treatment in the early 1990s (Roelofse and de 1990) and in medicine since the early 1980s (Haas et al. 1996). When its popularity rose in dentistry, midazolam was reviewed noting its development, characteristics, metabolism, use in studies, and adverse events (Kupietzky and Houpt 1993).

When midazolam is administered orally, slight but perceptible changes in attitude and even activity can be seen within 5 minutes (Table 13-4). In 10–15 minutes, significant relaxation occurs, and increased socialization is noticeable. Sometimes, the child is overcome by a quieter state, but characteristically a more friendly mood is noted especially if they were initially shy or withdrawn. Somewhere between 15 and 20 minutes after the child has received midazolam, separation of the child from the parent can take place. Unfortunately, the working time for midazolam is only 20–40 minutes. So, midazolam, when used alone, can be used only for short dental procedures. Occasionally, frank agitation and paradoxical excitement will occur in a small fraction of patients resulting in an inconsolable, unmanageable child even in the arms of the parent. This response usually occurs immediately following or during a painful procedure (e.g., local anesthetic administration). Anecdotally, this type of response has been referred to as the "angry child syndrome."

Midazolam has been used alone during dental procedures with approximately two-thirds of the patients reportedly having successful acceptance of dental treatment (Erlandsson et al. 2001). Others have demonstrated midazolam's improvement in patient attitude, behavior, and general procedural outcome compared to a placebo or presedation behavior (Gallardo et al. 1994; Mazaheri et al. 2008; Wan et al. 2006).

Midazolam has been used in combination with meperidine, hydroxyzine, ketamine, chloral hydrate, tramadol, fentanyl, sufentanil, nalbuphine, droperidol, and acetaminophen (Cagiran et al. 2010; Heard et al. 2010; Milnes et al. 2000; Myers et al. 2004; Nathan and Vargas 2002; Padmanabhan et al. 2009; Reeves et al. 1996). Few of these studies are alike in protocol or study design; thus, it is almost impossible to determine what combination is consistently superior, if any. Nonetheless, when another agent is added to midazolam, the combination usually results in a slight improvement of behaviors compared to midazolam alone (Al-Zahrani et al. 2009; Cagiran et al. 2010; Nathan and Vargas 2002; Shapira et al. 2004) but not always and may be a function of doses (Musial et al. 2003).

Midazolam is typically administered orally to small children for dental procedures. However, the intranasal route

**Table 13-4** Midazolam.

| Drug | Dose (Oral) | Characteristics | Warnings[§] | Sedation considerations (timing) | Reversible |
|---|---|---|---|---|---|
| Midazolam (Anticonvulsant hypnotic sedative) | 0.3–1.0 mg/kg | Clear | *Angry child syndrome* (AC/Sxd) | Onset: 10 min | Yes (Flumazenil) |
| | Max: 15 mg (2–5 y/o) | Non-palatable | Respiratory depression | Separation time: 10 min | |
| *Contraindications\*:* Hypersensitivity | 20 mg (older child) | Relaxation | | Work: 20 min | |
| | | Anterograde amnesia | Loss of head righting reflex | | |

*Note:* The major risks associated with high doses are hypoventilation and associated hypoxemia. There are interactive effects when used in patients who are on other types of drugs such as erythromycin and thus should be used with caution under such circumstances. In therapeutic doses, its effect on the cardiovascular system is negligible; however, higher doses produce decreased blood pressure and cardiac output. Occasionally, in children, a paradoxical hyperactivity occurs and is called the "angry response."

[§] The listed warnings are incomplete, and the reader is strongly advised to view more warnings from a reliable source (e.g., Lexi-Comp)

\* The listed contraindications are incomplete, and the reader is strongly advised to review more contraindications from a reliable source (e.g., Lexi-Comp)

of administration also has received attention from researchers (AlSarheed 2016). It has a slightly more rapid onset and is easier to administer to a combative, uncooperative patient. The most recent investigations reported are those of Greaves (2016), Eskandarian et al. (2015), Musani and Chandan (2015), Bahetwar et al. (2011), Heard et al. (2010), Johnson et al. (2010), and Wood (2010). Other routes of administration include intramuscular (Capp et al. 2010; Lam et al. 2005), submucosal (Myers et al. 2004), and intravenous (Arya and Damle 2002). The dose range for midazolam given parenterally (i.e., via any route other than oral and rectal) is less compared to that of the oral route (e.g., 0.2–0.3 mg/kg versus 0.5–1.0 mg/kg, respectively). As with other agents including midazolam, a child's temperament has been shown to be associated with pharmacological outcomes. Shy or withdrawn children tend to have less favorable outcomes (Arnrup et al. 2003; Isik et al. 2010; Jensen and Stjernqvist 2002; Lochary et al. 1993; Primosch and Guelmann 2005). Interestingly, some aspects of temperament has been associated with brain activity in the limbic system, especially the amygdala which by coincidence is populated by GABA complex receptors (Carvalho et al. 2012; Clauss et al. 2011; Helfinstein et al. 2012; Martinos et al. 2012; Sehlmeyer et al. 2011). Usually, a quiet, favorable, and interactive mood occurs soon after midazolam administration, but a dramatic change can occur, manifested as a higher heart rate and disruptive behaviors, when the patient is strongly stimulated (e.g., local anesthetic administration). Midazolam lacks analgesic properties, and hence, when analgesics are used in combination with midazolam, the behavioral outcomes generally improve (Nathan and Vargas 2002).

### Other Benzodiazepines

Diazepam is a commonly used agent in pediatric dentistry, and it is likely that triazolam is used more frequently than is reported. Diazepam produces good skeletal muscle relaxation and anti-anxiety effects. It has a long onset time usually approaching one hour after its administration before a patient is ready for dental procedures (Table 13-5). It also has a good hour of working time, and even longer time is required before it is fully metabolized and eliminated from the body. Hence, discharge time may be prolonged with diazepam, and it may not be very useful in small children in a busy office setting.

Several studies have evaluated the effects of diazepam administered rectally in children for dental procedures (Flaitz et al. 1985; Jensen and Schroder 1998; Jensen et al. 1999; Lowey and Halfpenny 1993; Roelofse and van der Bijl 1993). Most of the studies are older suggesting rectal administration is not as popular as it has been in the past. Also, some of the studies indicated that midazolam was better than diazepam when administered rectally. One interesting study evaluated the amnestic effect of diazepam administered orally (Jensen and Schroder 1998). Apparently, the amount of amnesia was significantly reduced in the subset of patients who exhibited behavior management problems. Others have had similar results (Sullivan et al. 2001). Further study needs to determine if there is an association between disruptive behaviors in young children and amnesia with diazepam and other benzodiazepines.

Diazepam also has been used in combination with ketamine (Okamoto et al. 1992; Reinemer et al. 1996; Sullivan et al. 2001). In these studies, the dose of ketamine was

**Table 13-5** Diazepam.

| Drug | Dose (Oral) | Characteristics | Warnings[§] | Sedation considerations (timing) | Reversible |
|---|---|---|---|---|---|
| Diazepam (Anticonvulsant hypnotic Sedative) | 0.25 mg/kg | Non-palatable | Respiratory depression | Onset: 1 hr | Yes (Flumazenil) |
| | 1 mg per year of age up to 10 mg | Relaxation | | Separation time: 1 hr | |
| | | Anterograde amnesia | Possible hypotension | Work: >1 hr | |
| *Contraindications*[*]: Hypersensitivity Glaucoma Sleep apnea | Max: 10 mg (varies with age) | Sedation | Avoid grapefruit juice | | |

*Note:* In therapeutic doses, its effect on the cardiovascular system is negligible; however, higher doses produce decreases in blood pressure and cardiac output. Respiratory depression occurs with increased dosages (or repeated doses) or when diazepam is used in combination with other sedative agents (e.g., opioids); otherwise, respiratory effect is minimal. Occasionally, in children, the expected sedation does not occur, but rather, a paradoxical hyperactivity occurs. This may be accompanied with rage, hostility, and nightmares.

[§] The listed warnings are incomplete, and the reader is strongly advised to view more warnings from a reliable source (e.g., Lexi-Comp)

[*] The listed contraindications are incomplete, and the reader is strongly advised to review more contraindications from a reliable source (e.g., Lexi-Comp)

varied between 4 and 10 mg/kg given orally. The lower dose was the least successful, and the higher doses were not significantly different from one another; however, a high rate of vomiting was frequently associated with ketamine (Reinemer et al. 1996; Sullivan et al. 2001).

Several studies involved children for dental procedures using triazolam (Table 13-6). These were done in the late 1990s or early 2000s. One study evaluated triazolam versus chloral hydrate and hydroxyzine primarily in preschoolers. The doses were 0.2 mg/kg for triazolam and 40 mg/kg and 25 mg for chloral hydrate and hydroxyzine, respectively. There were no significant differences in behavior or physiology between the two regimens, and the authors suggested triazolam was just as effective as the more traditional regimen of chloral hydrate and hydroxyzine (Meyer et al. 1990). Interestingly, a report comparing triazolam (0.3 mg/kg) to a placebo in a well-controlled study showed little improvement with triazolam over the placebo (Raadal et al. 1999). Also noteworthy is that triazolam potentially can produce ataxia and visual disturbances in young children as the dose of triazolam increases from 0.005 to 0.03 mg/kg (Coldwell et al. 1999). Similar findings were reported in slightly older children when triazolam was administered sublingually (Tweedy et al. 2001).

Other non-benzodiazepine like sedative agents have been used for dental procedures in children, such as zolpidem (Ambien®) which is a sleeping aid for adults (Bhatnagar et al. 2012; Koirala et al. 2006). Zolpidem activates a portion of the GABA complex to aid in initiating sleep and can be reversed by flumazenil. At least two articles have indicated that zolpidem is not a preferred agent in children when compared to other more commonly used agents (e.g., midazolam).

## Antihistamines

Antihistamines (e.g., hydroxyzine [Vistaril and Atarax], promethazine [Phenergan], and diphenhydramine [Benadryl]) are some of the most frequently used adjuncts, second to nitrous oxide, when combined with other sedative agents during sedations for pediatric patients undergoing dental procedures. They also are very popular for mild sedation when used alone and tend to be relatively safe for children (Faytrouny et al. 2007; Shapira et al. 1992). They are also noted for potentiating the effects of other sedative/analgesics such as meperidine. Caution is advised in prescribing hydroxyzine during pregnancy, especially in the first trimester (Table 13-7). Antihistamines are noted to have antiemetic, drying, and mild sedative properties. Many studies indicate that the addition of hydroxyzine to another sedative may or may not always improve behavior (Avalos-Arenas et al. 1998; Cathers et al. 2005; da Costa et al. 2007; Lima et al. 2003; Shapira et al. 2004). This inconsistency in showing a beneficial effect associated with the mix of hydroxyzine with other agents may be due to differences in methodology (e.g., dose). Nonetheless, it remains a popular methodology for sedating children most likely because of its antiemetic properties and slight sedative effects whether truly beneficial or not. Promethazine is also a very popular agent used in combination with other agents (Bui et al. 2002; Campbell et al. 1998; Houpt, Weiss et al. 1985; Myers and Shoaf 1977; Sams et al. 1993; Singh et al. 2002; Song and Webb 2003) but has not been shown definitively to be more or less effective than hydroxyzine. Furthermore, promethazine has been associated with respiratory depression in children less than two years of age resulting

**Table 13-6** Triazolam.

| Drug | Dose (Oral) | Characteristics | Warnings[§] | Sedation considerations (timing) | Reversible |
|---|---|---|---|---|---|
| Triazolam (Benzodiazepine) | Investigational Dose of 0.02 mg/kg has been used | Relaxation | Insomnia issues | Onset: 10–30 min | Yes (Flumazenil) |
| | | Sleep | Serious drug interactions | Separation time: 30 min | |
| *Contraindications\*:* | | | | Work: 1 hr | |
| Hypersensitivity to triazolam or any component; cross-sensitivity with other benzodiazepines may occur | | | Hypersensitivity interactions | | |
| Narrow-angle glaucoma | | | Pre-existing depression | | |
| Pregnancy | | | | | |

*Note:* Dosage has not been stabled for children less than 18 years of age. It may be useful for children aged 8–12 years.

[§] The listed warnings are incomplete, and the reader is strongly advised to view more warnings from a reliable source (e.g., Lexi-Comp)

[*] The listed contraindications are incomplete, and the reader is strongly advised to review more contraindications from a reliable source (e.g., Lexi-Comp)

**Table 13-7** Hydroxyzine.

| Drug | Dose (Oral) | Characteristics | Warnings[§] | Sedation considerations (timing) | Reversible |
|---|---|---|---|---|---|
| Hydroxyzine (Antianxiety | 1–2 mg/kg | Palatable | *Pregnancy* | Onset: 30 min | No |
| Antiemetic Antihistamine | Max: 50 mg/day | Sleep/drowsiness | Hypotension | Separation time: 30 min | |
| Sedative) | | Antihistamine | Potentiates other CNS depressants | Work: 30–45 min | |
| *Contraindication\*:* Hypersensitivity | | Bronchodilator | | | |
| Early pregnancy | | Anti-emetic | | | |
| | | Dry mouth | | | |

[§] The listed warnings are incomplete, and the reader is strongly advised to view more warnings from a reliable source (e.g., Lexi-Comp)
[*] *The listed contraindications are incomplete, and the reader is strongly advised to review more contraindications from a reliable source (e.g., Lexi-Comp)*

**Table 13-8** Promethazine.

| Drug | Dose (Oral) | Characteristics | Warnings[§] | Sedation considerations (timing) | Reversible |
|---|---|---|---|---|---|
| Promethazine (Antiemetic | 0.5–1.0 mg/kg | Palatable | Black box: not recommended in children less than two years of age | Onset: 20–30 min | No |
| sedative) | Max: 50 mg | Sleep/drowsiness | | Separation time: 30 min | |
| *Contraindications\*:* Hypersensitivity | | Antihistamine | Lowers seizure threshold | Work: 30–45 min | |
| > 2 years of age Asthma | | Anti-emetic | Hypotension | | |
| | | Dry mouth | | | |

*Note:* Black box warning: ***Should not be used in children less than two years of age due to the possibility of respiratory depression.***
[§] The listed warnings are incomplete, and the reader is strongly advised to view more warnings from a reliable source (e.g., Lexi-Comp)
[*] The listed contraindications are incomplete, and the reader is strongly advised to review more contraindications from a reliable source (e.g., Lexi-Comp)

in the FDA issuing a black box warning against its use in very young children (Table 13-8).

Diphenhydramine administered orally has had limited study as a sedative agent for children undergoing dental procedures (Davila et al. 1994). It has been used as an adjunct to other agents in medical settings (Cengiz et al. 2006; Roach et al. 2010). There has been some controversy over whether diphenhydramine may affect child performance (Kay 2000); however, some evidence suggests that it does not (Bender et al. 2001).

## Other Sedative Agents

### Ketamine

Ketamine is classified as a dissociative anesthetic and in lower doses as a dissociative sedative. It acts as an antagonist to the N-methyl-D-aspartate receptor and affects other receptors producing anesthesia and produces a state that is characterized by profound analgesia and amnesia, retained protective airway reflexes, spontaneous respiration, and cardiopulmonary stability (Gao et al. 2016; Poonai et al. 2017). Ketamine may cause nausea and vomiting and occasionally some emergence agitation (Poonai et al. 2017). It can be administered orally with an onset of 15–30 minutes or intranasally with a slightly faster onset (Table 13-9).

Ketamine has been used clinically for several decades but has recently had a re-emergence as an alternative to other sedative agents used in dental procedures in children. Ketamine may be administered orally in the pediatric patient for dental procedures in doses ranging from 3 to 6 mg/kg). It can also be administered through the intranasal route by drops or atomizer spray. The spray with the intranasal administration purportedly is associated with less aversive reaction, more rapid onset and recovery compared to drops (Pandey et al. 2011). Ketamine given orally

**Table 13-9** Ketamine.

| Drug | Dose (Oral) | Characteristics | Warnings[§] | Sedation considerations (timing) | Reversible |
|---|---|---|---|---|---|
| Ketamine | 2–6 mg/kg | Water and lipid soluble | Nausea and vomiting | Onset: 10–15 minutes | No |
| *Contraindications\*:* Conditions with significantly elevated blood pressure | | Analgesic | Increased salivary secretions | Separation time: 15 minutes | |
| | | Hypnotic | Laryngospasms | Work: 20–30 minutes | |
| | | Amnesic | Potential hallucinations and delirium | | |
| Elevated intracranial pressure | | | | | |

[§] The listed warnings are incomplete, and the reader is strongly advised to view more warnings from a reliable source (e.g., Lexi-Comp)
[*] The listed contraindications are incomplete, and the reader is strongly advised to review more contraindications from a reliable source (e.g., Lexi-Comp)

was shown to produce better behavior, shorter onset, and less post-operative sleep than a meperidine/promethazine combination; however, there was significantly more vomiting with ketamine (Alfonzo-Echeverri et al. 1993). The addition of benzodiazepines or promethazine seems to lessen the nausea and vomiting effects of ketamine, although higher doses of ketamine given with diazepam apparently doesn't decrease the incidence of vomiting (Sullivan et al. 2001). Evidence suggests that combining ketamine with midazolam results in better behaviors than midazolam alone when the latter is given in higher doses (0.75 mg/kg or greater) (Cagiran et al. 2010; Moreira et al. 2013).

### Dexmedetomidine (Precedex®)

Dexmedetomidine is a selective alpha₂-adrenoceptor agonist with anesthetic and sedative properties. Its action is thought to involve activation of G-proteins by alpha₂-adrenoceptors in the brainstem, at other locations in the brain, and peripherally resulting in inhibition of norepinephrine release. Hypertension, bradycardia, and hypotension can result depending on plasma concentrations. It produces sedation, anxiolysis, sympatholytic effects, and analgesia with minimal depression of respiratory function. Sleep can be induced, but the patient apparently is easily rousable (Weerink et al. 2017). Studies of dexmedetomidine in the pediatric population for dental sedation are limited. One randomized triple blinded study, involving 84 pediatric patients aged 4–14 years and evenly distributed by gender, compared two different doses of dexmedetomidine (1.0 microgram and 1.5 microgram/kg) to midazolam (0.2 mg/kg) and ketamine (5 mg/kg), each delivered intranasally. Sedation level, behavior, analgesia, and physiological variables were recorded. The results showed a significant reduction in systolic blood pressure and heart rate of both

doses of dexmedetomidine compared to midazolam and ketamine (but apparently not clinically significant), better analgesia with dexmedetomidine and ketamine compared to midazolam, faster onset and recovery from midazolam with the highest dose of dexmedetomidine causing the slowest recovery, and finally the "satisfactory behavior" was best for the high dose of dexmedetomidine and least for midazolam. The only adverse effect was vomiting seen in the low dose of both dexmedetomidine and ketamine (Surendar et al. 2014).

Another study compared dexmedetomidine to a combination of midazolam and ketamine with a placebo as a control group. The dose of midazolam was greater in this study (0.5 mg/kg) and the midazolam–ketamine solution was given orally rather than intranasally like the dexmedetomidine. There were other differences in methodology. They found no significant difference between the two drug groups in cardiovascular parameters, similar to Surendar et al. (2014) However, the success rate, satisfactory behavior, and ease of treatment were better with the midazolam–ketamine regimen (Malhotra et al. 2016).

### Summary

Clinicians want to know and understand the best evidenced-based information in delivering oral health care to their patients. This orientation applies not only to a plethora of practice issues such as restorative materials and techniques, special treatments (e.g., Endodontics), dental equipment, practice management, but also to patient management and the management of challenging groups of patients such as the geriatric and pediatric categories. The clinician's desires and goals for maximizing the delivery of efficient, quality of care in a friendly and supportive fashion often require the use of pharmacological techniques to successfully manage challenging patients. Thus, clinicians strive to find compelling evidence for the "best" pharmacological agents in aiding them to meet their goals.

Unfortunately, the amount of sound, scientifically derived data suggesting a ranking of agents to meet patient needs and challenges is woefully less. Issues such as study design with blinding and randomization, allocation of patients to groups, dose-response effects, and even the selection of a common outcome metric become exceedingly difficult to control in clinical situations. Even though many decades of clinical studies have occurred investigating sedative agents and their effects on the behavior and physiology of patients, we remain at the front end of a deep, poorly appreciated cavern of knowledge into which we daily enter seeking the answer to the question of "what is the best and safest sedative agent(s) for my patient and his/her specific needs."

Delving into the obscure body of knowledge on sedative agents, a recent study utilizing a meta-analysis attempted to determine which sedative agents are effective for behavior management in children who are receiving dental care (Lourenco-Matharu et al. 2012). The investigators utilized multiple electronic databases as well as hand-searched many journals. They looked for blinded, randomized, and well-controlled sedation studies involving 0–16-year-old children. Study designs using crossover procedures were excluded due to the possibility of differential patient responses at future visits depending on prior experiences in an initial visit. Only 36 studies involving a total of slightly more than 2,000 patients met their criteria. Many of the studies had the potential for high risk of bias and at least 28 different sedatives were used with or without nitrous oxide. The doses, administration mode, and timing factors varied widely. They found weak evidence for midazolam as an effective agent when sedating children for dental treatment and that nitrous oxide may improve patient behavior when used with other sedatives. They concluded that there is a need for further study using tightly controlled study designs and possible comparison to a standard which they interpreted at this point to be midazolam and nitrous oxide.

It is the impression of this author that such inquiry will require a major paradigm shift. Essential to any shift would be better use of electronic technology; agreement on effective, interactive behavior management principles; and support of pooled data development. Greater use of multiple site modalities such as private practice, teaching programs, and hospital collaborates also is critical to effecting change. Otherwise, for now, the "magic bullet" will continue to be general anesthesia.

# References

Adair, S.M., Rockman, R.A., Schafer, T.E. et al. (2004). Survey of behavior management teaching in pediatric dentistry advanced education programs. *Pediatric Dentistry*, 26, 151–158.

Aduss, H., Bane, R., and Lang, L. (1961). Pedodontic psychology and premedication. *Journal of Dentistry for Children*, 28, 73–83.

Al-Zahrani, A.M., Wyne, A.H., and Sheta, S.A. (2009). Comparison of oral midazolam with a combination of oral midazolam and nitrous oxide-oxygen inhalation in the effectiveness of dental sedation for young children. *Journal of the Indian Society of Pedodontics and Preventive Dentistry*, 27, 9–16.

Album, M.M. (1955). Premedication for difficult children. *Journal of Dentistry for Children*, 22, 48–56.

Alfonzo-Echeverri, E.C., Berg, J.H., Wild, T.W. et al. (1993). Oral ketamine for pediatric outpatient dental surgery sedation. *Pediatric Dentistry*, 15, 182–185.

AlSarheed, M.A. (2016). Intranasal sedatives in pediatric dentistry. *Saudi Medical Journal*, 37, 948–956.

Anderson, J.L. (1960). Use of chloral hydrate in dentistry. *North-West Dentistry*, 89, 33–35.

Arnrup, K., Broberg, A.G., Berggren, U. et al. (2003). Treatment outcome in subgroups of uncooperative child dental patients: an exploratory study. *International Journal of Paediatric Dentistry*, 13, 304–319.

Arya, V.S. and Damle, S.G. (2002). Comparative evaluation of Midazolam and Propofol as intravenous sedative agents in the management of uncooperative children. *Journal of the Indian Society of Pedodontics and Preventive Dentistry*, 20, 6–8.

Avalos-Arenas, V., Moyao-Garcia, D., Nava-Ocampo, A.A.et al. (1998). Is chloral hydrate/hydroxyzine a good option for paediatric dental outpatient sedation? *Current Medical Research and Opinion*, 14, 219–226.

Badalaty, M.M., Houpt, M.I., Koenigsberg, S.R. et al. (1990). A comparison of chloral hydrate and diazepam sedation in young children. *Pediatric Dentistry*, 12, 33–37.

Badner, V.M., Lockhart, P.B., and Hicks, J.L. (1994). The program directors' perspective on the goals and objectives of advanced general dentistry training. *Journal of Dental Education*, 58, 12–18.

Bahetwar, S.K., Pandey, R.K., Saksena, A.K. et al. (2011). A comparative evaluation of intranasal midazolam, ketamine and their combination for sedation of young uncooperative pediatric dental patients: A triple blind randomized crossover trial. *Journal of Clinical Pediatric Dentistry*, 35, 415–420.

Barr, E.S., Wynn, R.L., and Spedding, R.H. (1977). Oral premedication for the problem child: placebo and chloral hydrate. *Journal of Pedodontics*, 1, 272–280.

Bender, B.G., McCormick, D.R., and Milgrom, H. (2001). Children's school performance is not impaired by short-term administration of diphenhydramine or loratadine. *Journal of Pediatrics*, 138, 656–660.

Bhatnagar, S., Das, U.M., and Bhatnagar, G. (2012). Comparison of oral midazolam with oral tramadol, triclofos and zolpidem in the sedation of pediatric dental patients: An in vivo study. *Journal of the Indian Society of Pedodontics and Preventive Dentistry*, 30, 109–114.

Brandt, S.K. and J.L. Bugg, Jr. (1984). Problems of medication with the pediatric patient. *Dental Clinics of North America*, 28, 563–579.

Buckman, N. (1956). Balanced premedication in pedodontics. *Journal of Dentistry for Children*, 23, 111–153.

Bui, T., Redden, R.J., and Murphy, S. (2002). A comparison study between ketamine and ketamine-promethazine combination for oral sedation in pediatric dental patients. *Anesthesia Progress*, 49, 14–18.

Cagiran, E., Eyigor, C., Sipahi, A. et al. (2010). Comparison of oral Midazolam and Midazolam-Ketamine as sedative agents in paediatric dentistry. *European Journal of Paediatric Dentistry*, 11, 19–22.

Campbell, R.L., Ross, G.A., Campbell, J.R. et al. (1998). Comparison of oral chloral hydrate with intramuscular ketamine, meperidine, and promethazine for pediatric sedation–preliminary report. *Anesthesia Progress*, 45, 46–50.

Capp, P.L., de Faria, M.E., Siqueira, S.R.et al. (2010). Special care dentistry: Midazolam conscious sedation for patients with neurological diseases. *European Journal of Paediatric Dentistry*, 11, 162–164.

Carvalho, M.C., Moreira, C.M., Zanoveli, J.M. et al. (2012). Central, but not basolateral, amygdala involvement in the anxiolytic-like effects of midazolam in rats in the elevated plus maze. *Journal of Psychopharmacology*, 26, 543–554.

Cathers, J.W., Wilson, C.F., Webb, M.D. et al. (2005). A comparison of two meperidine/hydroxyzine sedation regimens for the uncooperative pediatric dental patient. *Pediatric Dentistry*, 27, 395–400.

Cengiz, M., Baysal, Z., and Ganidagli, S. (2006). Oral sedation with midazolam and diphenhydramine compared with midazolam alone in children undergoing magnetic resonance imaging. *Paediatric Anaesthesia*, 16, 621–626.

Chen, J.W., Seybold, S.V., and Yazdi, H. (2006). Assessment of the effects of 2 sedation regimens on cardiopulmonary parameters in pediatric dental patients: A retrospective study. *Pediatric Dentistry*, 28, 350–356.

Chen, N. and Tanbonliong, T. (2018). Comparison of two morphine-benzodiazepine-hydroxyzine combinations for the oral sedation of pediatric dental patients: A retrospective study. *Pediatric Dentistry*, 40, 43–48.

Chowdhury, J. and Vargas, K.G. (2005). Comparison of chloral hydrate, meperidine, and hydroxyzine to midazolam regimens for oral sedation of pediatric dental patients. *Pediatric Dentistry*, 27, 191–197.

Clauss, J.A., Cowan, R.L., and Blackford, J.U. (2011). Expectation and temperament moderate amygdala and dorsal anterior cingulate cortex responses to fear faces. *Cognitive, Affective & Behavioral Neuroscience*, 11, 13–21.

Coldwell, S.E., Awamura, K., Milgrom, P. et al. (1999). Side effects of triazolam in children. *Pediatric Dentistry*, 21, 18–25.

Cote, C.J., Wilson, S., American Academy of Pediatrics and American Academy of Pediatric Dentistry. (2019). Guidelines for monitoring and management of pediatric patients before, during, and after sedation for diagnostic and therapeutic procedures. *Pediatrics*, 143(6), e20191000. https://doi.org/10.1542/peds.2019-1000

Croswell, R.J., Dilley, D.C., Lucas, W.J. et al. (1995). A comparison of conventional versus electronic monitoring of sedated pediatric dental patients. *Pediatric Dentistry*, 17, 332–339.

Czaarnecki, E.S. and Binns, W.H. (1963). The use of chloral hydrate for the apprehensive child. *Pennsylvania Dental Journal*, 30, 40–42.

da Costa, L.R., da Costa, P.S., and Lima, A.R. (2007). A randomized double-blinded trial of chloral hydrate with or without hydroxyzine versus placebo for pediatric dental sedation. *Brazilian Dental Journal*, 18, 334–340.

Dallman, J.A., Ignelzi, M.A., Jr., and Briskie, D.M. (2001). Comparing the safety, efficacy and recovery of intranasal midazolam vs. oral chloral hydrate and promethazine. *Pediatric Dentistry*, 23, 424–430.

Davila, J.M., Herman, A.E., Proskin, H.M. et al. (1994). Comparison of the sedative effectiveness of two pharmacological regimens. *ASDC Journal of Dentistry for Children*, 61, 276–281.

Davis, M.J. (1988). Conscious sedation practices in pediatric dentistry: A survey of members of the American Board of Pediatric Dentistry College of Diplomates. *Pediatric Dentistry*, 10, 328–329.

Doring, K.R. (1985). Evaluation of an alphaprodine-hydroxyzine combination as a sedative agent in the treatment of the pediatric dental patient. *Journal of the American Dental Association*, 111, 567–576.

Erlandsson, A.L., Backman, B., Stenstrom, A. et al. (2001). Conscious sedation by oral administration of midazolam in paediatric dental treatment. *Swedish Dental Journal*, 25, 97–104.

Eskandarian, T., Arabzade Moghadam, S., Reza Ghaemi, S. et al. (2015). The effect of nasal midazolam premedication on parents-child separation and recovery time in dental procedures under general anaesthesia. *European Journal of Paediatric Dentistry*, 16, 135–138.

Faytrouny, M., Okte, Z., and Kucukyavuz, Z. (2007). Comparison of two different dosages of hydroxyzine for sedation in the paediatric dental patient. *International Journal of Paediatric Dentistry*, 17, 378–382.

Flacke, J.W., Bloor, B.C., Kripke, B.J. et al. (1985). Comparison of morphine, meperidine, fentanyl, and sufentanil in balanced anesthesia: A double-blind study. *Anesthesia and Analgesia*, 64, 897–910.

Flacke, J.W., Flacke, W.E., Bloor, B.C. et al. (1987). Histamine release by four narcotics: A double-blind study in humans. *Anesthesia and Analgesia*, 66, 723–730.

Flaitz, C.M., Nowak, A.J., and Hicks, M.J. (1985). Double-blind comparison of rectally administered diazepam to placebo for pediatric sedation: The cardiovascular response. *Anesthesia Progress*, 32, 232–236.

Gallardo, F., Cornejo, G., and Borie, R. (1994). Oral midazolam as premedication for the apprehensive child before dental treatment. *Journal of Clinical Pediatric Dentistry*, 18, 123–127.

Gao, M., Rejaei, D., and Liu, H. (2016). Ketamine use in current clinical practice. *Acta Pharmacologica Sinica*, 37, 865–872.

Gomes, H.S., Miranda, A.R., Viana, K.A. et al. (2017). Intranasal sedation using ketamine and midazolam for pediatric dental treatment (NASO): Study protocol for a randomized controlled trial. *Trials*, 18, 172.

Greaves, A. (2016). The use of Midazolam as an Intranasal Sedative in Dentistry. *SAAD Digest*, 32, 46–49.

Haas, D.A., Nenniger, S.A., Yacobi, R. et al. (1996). A pilot study of the efficacy of oral midazolam for sedation in pediatric dental patients. *Anesthesia Progress*, 43, 1–8.

Hasty, M.F., Vann, W.F., Jr., Dilley, D.C. et al. (1991). Conscious sedation of pediatric dental patients: an investigation of chloral hydrate, hydroxyzine pamoate, and meperidine vs. chloral hydrate and hydroxyzine pamoate. *Pediatric Dentistry*, 13, 10–19.

Heard, C., Smith, J., Creighton, P. et al. (2010). A comparison of four sedation techniques for pediatric dental surgery. *Paediatric Anaesthesia*, 20, 924–930.

Helfinstein, S.M., Fox, N.A., and Pine, D.S. (2012). Approach-withdrawal and the role of the striatum in the temperament of behavioral inhibition. *Developmental Psychology*, 48, 815–826.

Hershenson, M., Brouillette, R.T., Olsen, E. et al. (1984). The effect of chloral hydrate on genioglossus and diaphragmatic activity. *Pediatric Research*, 18, 516–519.

Hitt, J.M., Corcoran, T., Michienzi, K. et al. (2014). An evaluation of intranasal sufentanil and dexmedetomidine for pediatric dental sedation. *Pharmaceutics*, 6, 175–184.

Houpt, M. (2002). Project USAP 2000—use of sedative agents by pediatric dentists: A 15-year follow-up survey. *Pediatric Dentistry*, 24, 289–294.

Houpt, M. (1989). Report of Project USAP—the use of sedative agents in pediatric dentistry. *Journal of Dentistry for Children*, 56, 302–309.

Houpt, M.I., Sheskin, R.B., Koenigsberg, S.R. et al. (1985). Assessing chloral hydrate dosage for young children. *ASDC Journal of Dentistry for Children*, 52, 364–369.

Houpt, M.I., Weiss, N.J., Koenigsberg, S.R. et al. (1985). Comparison of chloral hydrate with and without promethazine in the sedation of young children. *Pediatric Dentistry*, 7, 41–46.

Huang, A. and Tanbonliong, T. (2015). Oral sedation postdischarge adverse events in pediatric dental patients. *Anesthesia Progress*, 62, 91–99.

Isik, B., Baygin, O., and Bodur, H. (2008). Premedication with melatonin vs midazolam in anxious children. *Paediatric Anaesthesia*, 18, 635–641.

Isik, B., Baygin, O., Kapci, E.G. et al. (2010). The effects of temperament and behaviour problems on sedation failure in anxious children after midazolam premedication. *European Journal of Anaesthesiology*, 27, 336–340.

Iwasaki, J., Vann, W.F., Jr., Dilley, D.C. et al. (1989). An investigation of capnography and pulse oximetry as monitors of pediatric patients sedated for dental treatment. *Pediatric Dentistry*, 11, 111–117.

Jensen, B. and Schroder, U. (1998). Acceptance of dental care following early extractions under rectal sedation with diazepam in preschool children. *Acta Odontologica Scandinavica*, 56, 229–232.

Jensen, B., Schroder, U., and Mansson, U. (1999). Rectal sedation with diazepam or midazolam during extractions of traumatized primary incisors: a prospective, randomized, double-blind trial in Swedish children aged 1.5-3.5 years. *Acta Odontologica Scandinavica*, 57, 190–194.

Jensen, B. and Stjernqvist, K. (2002). Temperament and acceptance of dental treatment under sedation in preschool children. *Acta Odontologica Scandinavica*, 60, 231–236.

Johnson, E., Briskie, D., Majewski, R. et al. (2010). The physiologic and behavioral effects of oral and intranasal midazolam in pediatric dental patients. *Pediatric Dentistry*, 32, 229–238.

Kay, G.G. (2000). The effects of antihistamines on cognition and performance. *Journal of Allergy and Clinical Immunology*, 105, S622–627.

Koirala, B., Pandey, R.K., Saksen, A.K. et al. (2006). A comparative evaluation of newer sedatives in conscious sedation. *Journal of Clinical Pediatric Dentistry*, 30, 273–276.

Kracke, R.R. (1962). Premedication in children undergoing single visit multiple cavity repair. *Journal of Dentistry for Children*, 29, 207–210.

Kupietzky, A. and Houpt, M.I. (1993). Midazolam: A review of its use for conscious sedation of children. *Pediatric Dentistry*, 15, 237–241.

Lam, C., Udin, R.D., Malamed, S.F. et al. (2005). Midazolam premedication in children: a pilot study comparing intramuscular and intranasal administration. *Anesthesia Progress*, 52, 56–61.

Lambert, L.A., Nazif, M.M., Moore, P.A. et al. (1988). Nonlinear dose-response characteristics of alphaprodine sedation in preschool children. *Pediatric Dentistry*, 10, 30–33.

Lampshire, E.L. (1950). Premedication for children. *Journal of the American Dental Association*, 41, 407–413.

Leelataweedwud, P. and Vann, W.F., Jr. (2001). Adverse events and outcomes of conscious sedation for pediatric patients: study of an oral sedation regimen. *Journal of the American Dental Association*, 132, 1531–1539; quiz 1596.

Leelataweewud, P., Vann, W.F., Jr., Dilley, D.C. et al. (2000). The physiological effects of supplemental oxygen versus nitrous oxide/oxygen during conscious sedation of pediatric dental patients. *Pediatric Dentistry*, 22, 125–133.

Levy, J.H., Brister, N.W., Shearin, A. et al. (1989). Wheal and flare responses to opioids in humans. *Anesthesiology*, 70, 756–760.

Lima, A.R.d.A., Costa, L.R.d.R.S., and Costa, P.S.S.d. (2003). A randomized, controlled, crossover trial of oral midazolam and hydroxyzine for pediatric dental sedation. *Pesquisa odontologica brasileira*, 17, 206–211.

Lochary, M.E., Wilson, S., Griffen, A.L. et al.. (1993). Temperament as a predictor of behavior for conscious sedation in dentistry. *Pediatric Dentistry*, 15, 348–352.

Lopez-Munoz, F., Ucha-Udabe, R., and Alamo, C. (2005). The history of barbiturates a century after their clinical introduction. *Neuropsychiatric Disease and Treatment*, 1, 329–343.

Lourenco-Matharu, L., Ashley, P.F. and Furness, S. (2012). Sedation of children undergoing dental treatment. *Cochrane Database of Systematic Reviews*, 3, CD003877.

Lowey, M.N. and Halfpenny, W. (1993). Observations on the use of rectally administered diazepam for sedating children before treatment of maxillofacial injuries: Report of nine cases. *International Journal of Paediatric Dentistry*, 3, 89–93.

Lu, D.P. and Lu, W.I. (2006). Practical oral sedation in dentistry. Part II–Clinical application of various oral sedatives and discussion. *Compendium of Continuing Education in Dentistry*, 27, 500–507; quiz 508, 518.

Lu, J. and Greco, M.A. (2006). Sleep circuitry and the hypnotic mechanism of GABAA drugs. *Journal of Clinical Sleep Medicine*, 2, S19–26.

Malhotra, P.U., Thakur, S., Singhal, P. et al. (2016). Comparative evaluation of dexmedetomidine and midazolam-ketamine combination as sedative agents in pediatric dentistry: A double-blinded randomized controlled trial. *Contemporary Clinical Dentistry*, 7, 186–192.

Martinos, M., Matheson, A., and de Haan, M. (2012). Links between infant temperament and neurophysiological measures of attention to happy and fearful faces. *Journal of Child Psychology and Psychiatry and Allied Disciplines*, 53, 1118–1127.

Mazaheri, R., Eshghi, A., Bashardoost, N. et al. (2008). Assessment of intranasal midazolam administration with a dose of 0.5 mg/kg in behavior management of uncooperative children. *Journal of Clinical Pediatric Dentistry*, 32, 95–99.

McKee, K.C., Nazif, M.M., Jackson, D.L. et al. (1990). Dose-responsive characteristics of meperidine sedation in preschool children. *Pediatric Dentistry*, 12, 222–227.

Meyer, M.L., Mourino, A.P., and Farrington, F.H. (1990). Comparison of triazolam to a chloral hydrate/hydroxyzine combination in the sedation of pediatric dental patients. *Pediatric Dentistry*, 12, 283–287.

Milnes, A.R., Maupome, G., and Cannon, J. (2000). Intravenous sedation in pediatric dentistry using midazolam, nalbuphine and droperidol. *Pediatric Dentistry*, 22, 113–119.

Moore, P.A. and Goodson, J.M. (1985). Risk appraisal of narcotic sedation for children. *Anesthesia Progress*, 32, 129–139.

Moore, P.A., Mickey, E.A., Hargreaves, J.A. et al. (1984). Sedation in pediatric dentistry: A practical assessment procedure. *Journal of the American Dental Association*, 109, 564–569.

Moreira, T.A., Costa, P.S., Costa, L.R. et al. (2013). Combined oral midazolam–ketamine better than midazolam alone for sedation of young children: a randomized controlled trial. *International Journal of Paediatric Dentistry*, 23, 207–215.

Morin, A., Ocanto, R., Drukteinis, L. et al. (2016). Survey of current clinical and curriculum practices of postgraduate pediatric dentistry programs in nonintravenous conscious sedation in the United States. *Pediatric Dentistry*, 38, 398–405.

Musani, I.E. and Chandan, N.V. (2015). A comparison of the sedative effect of oral versus nasal midazolam combined with nitrous oxide in uncooperative children. *European Archives of Paediatric Dentistry*, 16, 417–424.

Musial, K.M., Wilson, S., Preisch, J. et al. (2003). Comparison of the efficacy of oral midazolam alone versus midazolam and meperidine in the pediatric dental patient. *Pediatric Dentistry*, 25, 468–474.

Myers, D.R. and Shoaf, H.K. (1977). The intramuscular use of a combination of meperidine, promethazine and chlorpromazine for sedation of the child dental patient. *ASDC Journal of Dentistry for Children*, 44, 453–456.

Myers, G.R., Maestrello, C.L., Mourino, A.P. et al. (2004). Effect of submucosal midazolam on behavior and physiologic response when combined with oral chloral hydrate and nitrous oxide sedation. *Pediatric Dentistry*, 26, 37–43.

Nathan, J.E. and Vargas, K.G. (2002). Oral midazolam with and without meperidine for management of the difficult young pediatric dental patient: a retrospective study. *Pediatric Dentistry*, 24, 129–138.

Nathan, J.E. and West, M.S. (1987). Comparison of chloral hydrate-hydroxyzine with and without meperidine for management of the difficult pediatric patient. *ASDC Journal of Dentistry for Children*, 54, 437–444.

Needleman, H.L., Joshi, A., and Griffith, D.G. (1995). Conscious sedation of pediatric dental patients using chloral hydrate, hydroxyzine, and nitrous oxide–a retrospective study of 382 sedations. *Pediatric Dentistry*, 17, 424–431.

Okamoto, G.U., Duperon, D.F., and Jedrychowski, J.R. (1992). Clinical evaluation of the effects of ketamine sedation on pediatric dental patients. *Journal of Clinical Pediatric Dentistry*, 16, 253–257.

Padmanabhan, M.Y., Pandey, R.K., Saksena, A.K. et al. (2009). A comparative evaluation of agents producing analgo-sedation in pediatric dental patients. *Journal of Clinical Pediatric Dentistry*, 34, 183–188.

Pandey, R.K., Bahetwar, S.K., Saksena, A.K. et al. (2011). A comparative evaluation of drops versus atomized administration of intranasal ketamine for the procedural sedation of young uncooperative pediatric dental patients: A prospective crossover trial. *Journal of Clinical Pediatric Dentistry*, 36, 79–84.

Poonai, N., Canton, K., Ali, S. et al. (2017). Intranasal ketamine for procedural sedation and analgesia in children: A systematic review. *PloS One*, 12, e0173253.

Poorman, T.L., Farrington, F.H., and Mourino, A.P. (1990). Comparison of a chloral hydrate/hydroxyzine combination with and without meperidine in the sedation of pediatric dental patients. *Pediatric Dentistry*, 12, 288–291.

Primosch, R.E. and Guelmann, M. (2005). Comparison of drops versus spray administration of intranasal midazolam in two- and three-year-old children for dental sedation. *Pediatric Dentistry*, 27, 401–408.

Raadal, M., Coldwell, S.E., Kaakko, T. et al. (1999). A randomized clinical trial of triazolam in 3- to 5-year-olds. *Journal of Dental Research*, 78, 1197–1203.

Reeves, S.T., Wiedenfeld, K.R., Wrobleski, J. et al. (1996). A randomized double-blind trial of chloral hydrate/hydroxyzine versus midazolam/acetaminophen in the sedation of pediatric dental outpatients. *ASDC Journal of Dentistry for Children*, 63, 95–100.

Reinemer, H.C., Wilson, C.F., and Webb, M.D. (1996). A comparison of two oral ketamine-diazepam regimens for sedating anxious pediatric dental patients. *Pediatric Dentistry*, 18, 294–300.

Riekman, G. and Ross, A.S. (1981). A sedation technique for the younger child. *Journal of the Canadian Dental Association. Journal de L'Association Dentaire Canadienne*, 47, 789–791.

Roach, C.L., Husain, N., Zabinsky, J. et al. (2010). Moderate sedation for echocardiography of preschoolers. *Pediatric Cardiology*, 31, 469–473.

Robbins, M.B. (1967). Chloral hydrate and promethazine as premedicants for the apprehensive child. *Journal of Dentistry for Children*, 34, 327–331.

Roberts, S.M., Wilson, C.F., Seale, N.S. et al. (1992). Evaluation of morphine as compared to meperidine when administered to the moderately anxious pediatric dental patient. *Pediatric Dentistry*, 14, 306–313.

Roelofse, J.A. and de V Joubert, J.J. (1990). Arterial oxygen saturation in children receiving rectal midazolam as premedication for oral surgical procedures. *Anesthesia Progress*, 37, 286–289.

Roelofse, J.A. and van der Bijl, P. (1993). Comparison of rectal midazolam and diazepam for premedication in pediatric dental patients. *Journal of Oral and Maxillofacial Surgery*, 51, 525–529.

Rohlfing, G.K., Dilley, D.C., Lucas, W.J. et al. (1998). The effect of supplemental oxygen on apnea and oxygen saturation during pediatric conscious sedation. *Pediatric Dentistry*, 20, 8–16.

Ruble, J.W. (1952). An appraisal of drugs to premedicate children for dental procedures. *Journal of Dentistry for Children*, 19, 22–29.

Sado-Filho, J., Viana, K.A., Correa-Faria, P. et al. (2019). Randomized clinical trial on the efficacy of intranasal or oral ketamine-midazolam combinations compared to oral midazolam for outpatient pediatric sedation. *PloS One*, 14, e0213074.

Sams, D.R., Cook, E.W., Jackson, J.G. et al. (1993). Behavioral assessments of two drug combinations for oral sedation. *Pediatric Dentistry*, 15, 186–190.

Sams, D.R. and Russell, C.M. (1993). Physiologic response and adverse reactions in pediatric dental patients sedated with promethazine and chloral hydrate or meperidine. *Pediatric Dentistry*, 15, 422–424.

Schneider, H.S. (1986). Clinical observation utilizing morphine sulfate and hydroxyzine pamoate for sedating apprehensive children for dental procedures: A nine-year report. *Pediatric Dentistry*, 8, 280–284.

Sehlmeyer, C., Dannlowski, U., Schoning, S. et al. (2011). Neural correlates of trait anxiety in fear extinction. *Psychological Medicine*, 41, 789–798.

Shapira, J., Holan, G., Guelmann, M. et al. (1992). Evaluation of the effect of nitrous oxide and hydroxyzine in controlling the behavior of the pediatric dental patient. *Pediatric Dentistry*, 14, 167-70.

Shapira, J., Kupietzky, A., Kadari, A. et al. (2004). Comparison of oral midazolam with and without hydroxyzine in the sedation of pediatric dental patients. *Pediatric Dentistry*, 26, 492–496.

Sheroan, M.M., Dilley, D.C., Lucas, W.J. et al. (2006). A prospective study of 2 sedation regimens in children: chloral hydrate, meperidine, and hydroxyzine versus midazolam, meperidine, and hydroxyzine. *Anesthesia Progress*, 53, 83–90.

Singh, N., Pandey, R.K., Saksena, A.K. et al. (2002). A comparative evaluation of oral midazolam with other sedatives as premedication in pediatric dentistry. *Journal of Clinical Pediatric Dentistry*, 26, 161–164.

Song, Y.U. and Webb, M.D. (2003). Comparison of the effect of orally versus submucosally administered meperidine on the behavior of pediatric dental patients: A retrospective study. *Anesthesia Progress*, 50, 129–133.

Stetson, J.B. and Jessup, G.S. (1962). Use of oral chloral hydrate mixtures for pediatric premedication. *Anesthesia and Analgesia*, 41, 203–215.

Sullivan, D.C., Wilson, C.F., and Webb, M.D. (2001). A comparison of two oral ketamine-diazepam regimens for the sedation of anxious pediatric dental patients. *Pediatric Dentistry*, 23, 223–231.

Surendar, M.N., Pandey, R.K., Saksena, A.K. et al. (2014). A comparative evaluation of intranasal dexmedetomidine, midazolam and ketamine for their sedative and analgesic properties: A triple blind randomized study. *Journal of Clinical Pediatric Dentistry*, 38, 255–261.

Tafaro, S.T., Wilson, S., Beiraghi, S. et al. (1991). The evaluation of child behavior during dental examination and treatment using premedication and placebo. *Pediatric Dentistry*, 13, 339–343.

Tilliss, T.S. (1993). Behavior management techniques in predoctoral and postdoctoral pediatric dentistry programs. *Journal of Dental Education*, 57, 232–238.

Toomarian, L., Salem, K., and Ansari, G. (2013). Assessing the sedative effect of oral vs submucosal meperidine in pediatric dental patients. *Dental Research Journal*, 10, 173–179.

Torres-Perez, J., Tapia-Garcia, I., Rosales-Berber, M.A. et al. (2007). Comparison of three conscious sedation regimens for pediatric dental patients. *Journal of Clinical Pediatric Dentistry*, 31, 183–186.

Tweedy, C.M., Milgrom, P., Kharasch, E.D. et al. (2001). Pharmacokinetics and clinical effects of sublingual triazolam in pediatric dental patients. *Journal of Clinical Psychopharmacology*, 21, 268–272.

Wan, K., Jing, Q., and Zhao, J.Z. (2006). Evaluation of oral midazolam as conscious sedation for pediatric patients in oral restoration. *Chinese Medical Sciences Journal*, 21, 163–166.

Weerink, M.A.S., Struys, M., Hannivoort, L.N. et al. (2017). Clinical Pharmacokinetics and Pharmacodynamics of Dexmedetomidine. *Clinical Pharmacokinetics*, 56, 893–913.

Wilson, S. (2000). Pharmacologic behavior management for pediatric dental treatment. *Pediatric Clinics of North America*, 47, 1159–1175.

Wilson, S. (1996). A survey of the American Academy of Pediatric Dentistry membership: Nitrous oxide and sedation. *Pediatric Dentistry*, 18, 287–293.

Wilson, S. and Alcaino, E.A. (2011). Survey on sedation in paediatric dentistry: A global perspective. *International Journal of Paediatric Dentistry*, 21, 321–332.

Wilson, S., Easton, J., Lamb, K. et al. (2000). A retrospective study of chloral hydrate, meperidine, hydroxyzine, and midazolam regimens used to sedate children for dental care. *Pediatric Dentistry*, 22, 107–112.

Wilson, S. and Gosnell, E.S. (2016). Survey of American Academy of Pediatric Dentistry on nitrous oxide and sedation: 20 years later. *Pediatric Dentistry*, 38, 385–392.

Wilson, S. and Houpt, M. (2016). Project USAP 2010: Use of sedative agents in pediatric dentistry-a 25-year follow-up survey. *Pediatric Dentistry*, 38, 127–133.

Wilson, S., Matusak, A., Casamassimo, P.S. et al. (1998). The effects of nitrous oxide on pediatric dental patients sedated with chloral hydrate and hydroxyzine. *Pediatric Dentistry*, 20, 253–258.

Wilson, S. and McTigue, D.J. (1989). Survey of conscious sedation practices in pediatric dentistry advanced residency programs. *Journal of Dental Education*, 53, 595–597.

Wilson, S. and Nathan, J.E. (2011). A survey study of sedation training in advanced pediatric dentistry programs: Thoughts of program directors and students. *Pediatric Dentistry*, 33, 353–360.

Wood, M. (2010). The safety and efficacy of intranasal midazolam sedation combined with inhalation sedation with nitrous oxide and oxygen in paediatric dental patients as an alternative to general anaesthesia. *SAAD Digest*, 26, 12–22.

Wright, G.Z. and McAulay, D.J. (1973). Current premedicating trends in pedodontics. *ASDC Journal of Dentistry for Children*, 40, 185–187.

# 14

## Working with a Dentist Anesthesiologist

*Kenneth L. Reed and Amanda Jo Okundaye*

## Introduction

Staying in the dental office is much more convenient for both dentists and patients than going to a hospital operating room. Anesthesia and dental services may be delivered in a dental office at significantly lower costs than in the hospital operating room. With healthcare dollars at a premium, healthcare "reform" well on its way in the United States, and more people paying out of pocket for dental services, hospital operating room use for otherwise healthy pediatric dental patients may decline. There now is a trend toward in-office deep sedation and general anesthetics in some geographical regions (Olabi et al. 2012). This chapter focuses on the reason for that trend, as well as how to work with a dentist anesthesiologist.

As has been described elsewhere in this text, the levels of sedation to anesthesia within medicine and dentistry are minimal sedation, moderate sedation, deep sedation, and general anesthesia. Both minimal sedation and moderate sedation are "conscious" techniques. A hallmark of a conscious technique is that the patient responds to verbal commands or light tactile stimulation. In the case of minimal sedation, the patient responds *normally* to verbal commands or light tactile stimulation. In the case of moderate sedation, the patient responds *purposefully* to verbal commands or light tactile stimulation. If minimal to moderate sedation fails, the next level is deep sedation or general anesthesia. For these levels, the pediatric dentist has to consider whether the patient will be treated in the dental office or in the hospital.

## Educational Requirements for a Dentist Anesthesiologist

Many years ago, there were no formal requirements for dentists to be able to administer any form of sedation or anesthesia. Likewise, there were no guidelines for dentists in the area of sedation and anesthesia. The "Guidelines for Teaching Pain Control and Sedation to Dentists and Dental Students" was first published in 1972 by the American Dental Association (ADA). In the 1985 update of the guidelines, the concept of "deep sedation" was introduced, and training required to perform this level of anesthesia was deemed to be the same as for general anesthesia (Peskin 1993). These documents have been updated many times since the original version and will continue to be updated as needed in the future.

The training to be licensed and permitted to administer minimal to moderate oral sedation may be obtained in almost all pediatric dental residencies or through a variety of continuing education courses. To be licensed and permitted to administer deep sedation or general anesthesia, the training may only be obtained in specific residencies today. The training requirements for deep sedation and anesthesia are the same. For dentists in the United States, the completion of a dental anesthesiology or oral and maxillofacial surgery residency is required in order to obtain a permit to administer general anesthesia. It is not possible to obtain training to administer deep sedation or general anesthesia in a continuing education course. Several pediatric dentists have also completed dental anesthesiology residencies, but the overwhelming majority of pediatric dentists have been trained only to the level of either minimal or moderate oral sedation.

Deep sedation and general anesthesia can be considered equal to one another. Both deep sedation and general anesthesia are "unconscious" techniques in which the patient does not respond to verbal command or light tactile stimulation. The only technical difference is that in deep sedation the patient does respond purposefully following repeated or painful stimulation, whereas in general anesthesia the patient cannot be aroused, even following painful stimulation.

## Hospital-based Versus Office-based Treatment

When minimal to moderate oral sedation fails in the pediatric dental office, deep sedation or general anesthesia may be indicated. Many pediatric dentists currently take these patients to the hospital. Consequently, patients incur extremely high costs and dentists lose productive time in the office. Mass (1993) compared the costs for a typical one-hour dental case of office-based anesthesia versus hospital-based anesthesia. He found that, in the early 1990s, the hospital fee approximated $1,900 while the office-based case would typically cost $150. As of 2009, the Albany Medical Center stated that the cost of office-based anesthesia remained less than 10% of the cost of hospital-based anesthesia for dental procedures.

The spread between hospital-based anesthesia and dental office-based anesthesia pricing still exists today. Rashewsky et al. (2012) determined that the hospital operating room expense for a pediatric dental patient was 13.2 times the expense of office-based anesthesia. At Stony Brook Medicine, dental patients requiring treatment with general anesthesia received dental care in either an outpatient facility at the Stony Brook School of Dental Medicine or in the Stony Brook University Hospital ambulatory setting. Rashewsky examined the time and cost for ambulatory American Society of Anesthesiologists (ASA) Class I pediatric patients receiving full-mouth dental rehabilitation using general anesthesia in these two locations. They reviewed 96 patient records for ASA I patients aged 36–60 months. There were significant differences in cost, total anesthesia time, and recovery room time. The average total time (anesthesia end time minus anesthesia start time) to treat a child at Stony Brook University Hospital under general anesthesia was $222 \pm 62.7$ minutes, and recovery time (time of discharge minus anesthesia end time) was $157 \pm 97.2$ minutes; the average total cost was $7,303. At the Stony Brook School of Dental Medicine, the average total time was $175 \pm 36.8$ minutes, and recovery time was $25 \pm 12.7$ minutes; the average total cost was $414. This study provides evidence that ASA I pediatric patients can receive full-mouth dental rehabilitation using general anesthesia under the direction of dentist anesthesiologists in an office-based dental setting more quickly and at a lower cost than in a hospital operating room. This is very promising for patients with the least access to care, including patients with special needs and those without insurance (Rashewsky et al. 2012). To some extent, the economic barrier is lowered.

So, what are other advantages and disadvantages of treating pediatric dental patients in the hospital operating room versus the dental office? Having provided anesthesia services in both settings, the authors of this chapter know both systems well. To begin, there is a need for both types of treatment. Unfortunately, the choice is often determined by what is available to the practitioner or how the practitioner was originally trained. Many pediatric dentists, especially those trained some time ago, only consider the hospital operating room option.

While the hospital operating room is safe, it is often not the most ideal place to treat many pediatric dental patients. It is a burden for the pediatric dentist to bring all of the drugs, supplies, and equipment needed for an operating room case. In some cases, hospitals charge a facility fee. Hospitals may not have a wide variety of surgical instruments and dental supplies—the dentist has to use what is available. The hospital operating room can also be inefficient. Dental cases are low priority electives in a medical setting, so it is not unusual for a dental case to be "bumped" in order to place a higher priority emergent medical case in the operating room where the dental case was scheduled. Hospital operating rooms also take a significant amount of time to "turn over." Cleaning and replenishing supplies takes much more time compared to the typical dental office.

## The Dentist Anesthesiologist

The anesthesia provider for the vast majority of hospital operating rooms will be either a physician anesthesiologist or, more commonly in the United States, a certified registered nurse anesthetist. There are few dentist anesthesiologists working in hospital operating rooms providing anesthesia services. While physicians and nurses can and do provide safe general anesthesia, they lack an understanding of dentistry compared to a dentist anesthesiologist. Most dentist anesthesiologists will provide intraoral local anesthesia when appropriate for the case, or will at least be available for consultation regarding the feasibility.

Dentist anesthesiologists are comfortable with providing nasally intubated general anesthesia. Some physician anesthesiologists and certified registered nurse anesthetists are less comfortable with nasal intubation and may offer only oral intubation or a laryngeal mask airway (LMA). Neither oral intubation nor an LMA offers the access to the oral cavity, the ability to check occlusion, and the all-around ability to perform ideal dentistry that a nasally intubated pediatric dental case provides. Dentist anesthesiologists are trained as dentists first, acquiring their anesthesia training later. Dentists know dental procedures. Physician anesthesiologists and certified registered nurse anesthetists do not. Dentist anesthesiologists understand that local anesthesia provides post-operative pain control for pediatric dental patients and that longer-acting opioids such as morphine or hydromorphone are not indicated. When physician anesthesiologists and certified registered nurse anesthetists provide deep sedation or general anesthesia for pediatric dentists, they often do not understand this simple concept and sometimes administer large amounts of opioids. This leads to excessively prolonged recovery and unnecessary post-operative nausea and vomiting. Neither of these tends to build patient confidence, nor are they practice builders.

Dentist anesthesiologists are trained to work with patients on whom open airway procedures are performed and are therefore much more comfortable than physician anesthesiologists and certified registered nurse anesthetists who lack such training. Sharing the patient's airway is a normal, daily occurrence for a dentist anesthesiologist, but it is a very foreign concept to most non-dentists performing anesthesia. Most physician anesthesiologists and certified registered nurse anesthetists are not comfortable performing anesthesia outside of a hospital operating room and are unfamiliar with mobile anesthesia practice.

Dentist anesthesiologists understand the private practice of dentistry; they understand the dental environment and strive to maintain a nurturing atmosphere when invited to participate in the care of pediatric dental patients. The atmosphere and expectations in hospital operating rooms are quite different from a private dental office and physician anesthesiologists and certified registered nurse anesthetists often do not understand this distinction. The first dental anesthesia residency was established in 1949, so this is not a new concept. In summary, some have said that when compared to physician anesthesiologists, dentist anesthesiologists are safer, more approachable, less patronizing, and more understanding of the dental process and needs of the dentist.

Additionally, the operating table in an operating room offers fewer options to the pediatric dentist. The ability to place the operating table in an exact location and position is often compromised, unlike a dental chair in a dental office. Room lighting and suction are often more difficult to manipulate in an operating room, and sometimes something as simple as a saliva ejector may not be able to be accommodated.

Pediatric dental patients and their parents or guardians know the pediatric dental office; they know where it is located and they know the office staff. Taking their child to a hospital for dental care can be daunting. Usually, they don't know the system or what to expect. The hospital is generally a less nurturing and less comfortable environment than the private office or clinic. As noted by Rashewsky et al. (2012), patients treated in the hospital spend much more time in non-productive activities, such as prolonged waiting times in a pre-operative holding area or longer times in recovery rooms, in comparison to dental

office treatment. With more and more scrutiny being given to medical expenditures in health care by insurers and governmental agencies, the use of the hospital operating rooms for healthy dental patients may very well become a thing of the past.

While the emphasis so far has been on in-office deep sedation and anesthesia, there still remains a need for some pediatric dental patients to be seen in the hospital operating room. All ASA IV and ASA V pediatric dental patients that require dental treatment should be seen in the hospital operating room, as should most ASA III patients. Only ASA I and ASA II patients would be good candidates for office-based deep sedation or general anesthesia.

## Use of a Dentist Anesthesiologist by Pediatric Dentists

The use of dentist anesthesiologists appears to be an emerging trend in pediatric dental practice (ASDA 2010). A recent paper by Olabi and associates (2012) found that 20–40% of board-certified pediatric dentists currently use a dentist anesthesiologist, and 60–70% would use a dentist anesthesiologist if one were available. The utilization rate appears to be regional. For example, in the northeast United States, only 12% of board-certified pediatric dentists use a dentist anesthesiologist, yet 46% of that same group would use a dentist anesthesiologist if one were available. However, 59% of board-certified pediatric dentists practicing in the western United States currently use the services of a dentist anesthesiologist, and 78% indicated that they would use a dentist anesthesiologist if possible. It is also interesting to note that from a regional perspective, the southwest had the highest percentage of respondents reporting that they administered some form of in-office sedation (88%), employed the services of a dentist anesthesiologist (59%), and would use a dentist anesthesiologist if one were available (78%). Finally, a novel finding of this study was that female board-certified pediatric dentists were more likely to employ a dentist anesthesiologist than their male counterparts.

Based on the data of the foregoing study, it is apparent that dentist anesthesiologist availability is a major impediment to increasing the number of deep sedation and general anesthetics in dental offices. To understand the problem, some understanding of the history is needed. It was realized in the 1950s that a specialty of anesthesia in dentistry would benefit the profession. Concomitantly, the department of dental anesthesiology at the Tokyo Medical and Dental University was created by Dr. Tadashi Ueno (Matsuura 1993). In 1953, the American Dental Society of Anesthesiology was formed (Peskin 1993) and the first application for specialty status was submitted to the ADA (Allen 1992).

The next major event affecting the administration of anesthesia by dentists was in the early 1980s. Physicians drew a metaphorical line in the sand. As a portion of a policy statement in 1982, The American Society of Anesthesiologists (ASA) wrote that "anesthesia care is the practice of medicine." As a consequence, dentists administering anesthesia could be accused by state medical boards of practicing medicine without a license. Fortunately, by 1987, the ASA had published a more reasonable statement: "The ASA recognizes the right of qualified dentists as defined by the American Dental Association to administer conscious sedation, deep sedation and general anesthesia to patients having dental procedures only."

The ASA recognition has allowed the anesthesia specialty to mature. In 2007, the Commission on Dental Accreditation (CODA) published a standards document entitled "Advanced Dental Education Programs in Dental Anesthesiology." Hence, standards now exist for accrediting dental anesthesia residencies. The standards are stringent. Today, dental anesthesiology is a 36-month full time residency, the same duration as physician anesthesiologists and longer than certified registered nurse anesthetists. In addition to many other clinical and didactic requirements, dental anesthesia residents must perform a minimum of 800 deep sedations and general anesthetics, 300 of which must be intubated general anesthetics, and at least 50 of which must be nasotracheal intubations. Also, 25 cases must incorporate advanced airway techniques such as fiber-optic or video laryngoscopy. A minimum of 125 cases must be for children aged seven or younger, and 75 cases must be for patients with special needs.

Physicians and nurses that complete anesthesia training do not have the dental-specific requirements in their training that dentist anesthesiologists do. They may or may not have training in this sub-specialty of anesthesia.

According to a 2007 editorial by Dr. Joel Weaver, three major benefits to the dental profession will be derived from the accreditation of dentist anesthesiologist residency programs. They are as follows.

- Since the demand for dentists to provide advanced sedation and anesthesia services for others has so largely increased, accreditation should provide increased funding opportunities to support more residents and residency programs.
- Accreditation by dentistry helps cement anesthesia at its highest level as being within the scope of dental education and the clinical practice of dentists.
- Finally, accreditation keeps the highest level of anesthesia education within the control of dentistry and maintains our ability to control the quality of anesthesia training that dentist anesthesiologists receive.

State dental boards now have an appropriate measuring stick to judge the adequacy of anesthesia training for dentist anesthesiologists. They should now recognize that future dentist anesthesiologists must be graduates of CODA-accredited training programs to be eligible for anesthesia permits—with, of course, traditional grandfathering for those who completed training prior to accreditation.

Accreditation helped to provide increased support for more residents and residency programs to meet the need and demand. In 2007, there were roughly 200 dentist anesthesiologists in the United States. There were five dental anesthesia training programs in North America that graduated a combined nine residents in dental anesthesia per year. In 2020, there was approximately 400 dentist anesthesiologists in the United States; the number of dental anesthesia training programs in North America has roughly doubled. Currently, approximately 25 residents graduate in dental anesthesia annually.

After many specialty attempts and after CODA accreditation, on March 11, 2019, the ADA recognized Dental Anesthesiology as the 10th specialty of dentistry.

## Clinic Use of a Dentist Anesthesiologist

Dentist anesthesiologists can help pediatric dentists with their more challenging patients by allowing dentistry to be completed safely, efficiently, and in a cost-effective manner in the pediatric dental office. Most dentist anesthesiologists in the United States are "mobile," that is, they bring all of their drugs, supplies, and equipment with them when they travel to a pediatric dental office to provide anesthesia services. Figure 14-1 demonstrates a dentist anesthesiologist's typical "mobile" setup. Figure 14-2 shows the dentist anesthesiologist's drugs, supplies, and equipment in a dental office, providing general anesthesia for a pediatric dental patient.

The usual procedure for involving a dentist anesthesiologist is as follows. The pediatric dentist arranges a day for the dentist anesthesiologist to be in the office. A number of cases are scheduled to make the day more efficient for both doctors. A few days before the treatment day, the office provides a copy of the schedule with patient data to the anesthesiologist, who typically reviews the medical history as collected by the pediatric dentist and phones the parent or caregiver at least one day prior to the anesthetic. Further questioning about the medical history of the child occurs at that time. Contact information for physicians or other healthcare providers may be obtained if consultation with the patient's physician is indicated. Financial arrangements are discussed with the parent. During the preoperative phone call, NPO (*nihil per os*; nothing by mouth)

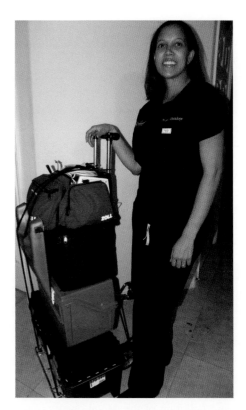

**Figure 14-1** A dentist anesthesiologist's typical "mobile" setup.

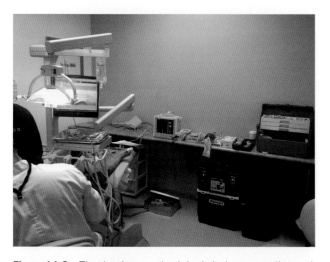

**Figure 14-2** The dentist anesthesiologist's drugs, supplies, and equipment in a dental office, providing general anesthesia for a pediatric dental patient.

requirements are relayed, as well as any other pre-operative instructions, such as which medications to take and which to withhold. The dentist anesthesiologist explains to the parent what to expect. For pre-cooperative pediatric patients or uncooperative patients with special needs, it is especially important to inform the parent or caregiver on the method of induction of general anesthesia and what is expected from them.

### Choice of Deep Sedation or General Anesthesia

Whether deep sedation or general anesthesia is chosen for a particular case is a moot point. The dentist anesthesiologist is trained in both techniques, and there is enough gray area, overlap, and continuum of spectrum between the two techniques that teasing out the exact definition during a given case is nothing but an academic exercise.

### Premedication Before Deep Sedation or General Anesthesia

Premedication before general anesthesia in the pediatric patient is generally not recommended unless it is given in the office by the treating practitioner 30 minutes to an hour before planned anesthetic. Parenteral anxiety is actually the biggest contribution to the anxiety of the child. When a premedication is chosen, the oral route is by far the most common. Furthermore, a benzodiazepine is the most common class of drug for orally administered premedication prior to deep sedation or general anesthesia, and the specific benzodiazepine is most often midazolam. Midazolam provides some degree of amnesia, is an anxiolytic agent, and has a very shallow dose response curve, which translates to a very wide margin of safety.

### Induction of Deep Sedation or General Anesthesia

An IV induction is the safest and most effective method of inducing deep sedation or general anesthesia. Ideally, the patient will allow an IV to be started. Some older children and higher functioning patients with special needs will allow it. If a lack of cooperation precludes starting an IV, there are two primary methods of inducing deep sedation or general anesthesia. Some dentist anesthesiologists prefer an induction with intramuscular (IM) drugs. Most often the IM drug of choice is ketamine, with or without midazolam and/or glycopyrrolate. The other primary method of inducing general anesthesia to an uncooperative dental patient is a "mask" induction. This technique uses an inhaled volatile general anesthetic gas, most often sevoflurane. Many dentist anesthesiologists have both sevoflurane and ketamine available and utilize each technique for different situations, while others exclusively use one technique over the other.

Those that prefer a mask induction understand that it saves the patient the injection experience. Conversely, those who prefer IM induction hold that pediatric patients receive inoculations on a regular basis—this is simply one more "shot," and they will have more in the future. Those that criticize mask inductions say that holding a child down and forcing a mask on them, especially if the patient is claustrophobic, is less than ideal. Others will point out that in the more cooperative pediatric dental patient who participates in holding the mask, the induction can be stress-free. Based on personal experiences, there is no one right or wrong way to induce general anesthesia in the pediatric dental patient.

Once deep sedation or general anesthesia is induced, IV access will be obtained. Having an IV allows administration of additional drugs, if needed, and it provides immediate access should emergency drug administration become necessary.

### Airways

An open or natural airway is defined as an airway that is not intubated or secured with an adjunct such as a naso-endotracheal tube or laryngeal mask. Open airway anesthesia is performed daily for all levels of anesthesia and has been performed safely for many years and taught in many pediatric dental residency programs in the United States. The literature does not provide a sufficient reason for open airway versus intubated anesthetics. Instead, it is left up to the anesthesiologist, whose training and comfort level will dictate the choice. Any level of sedation administered should include a throat pack or oral partition. It is our recommendation that during open airway cases, practitioners should use water judiciously if it is required, as well as a rubber dam to decrease the amount of debris that goes in the throat pack or oropharynx. The throat pack is placed in the oropharynx to (1) protect contents from going down the airway and causing possible complications such as a laryngospasm and (2) prevent or reduce the escape of gases such as nitrous oxide directly into the face of the operator.

When working in a pediatric dental office, the type of airway is often debated by dentist anesthesiologists. Some strongly prefer an "open airway" for all procedures, feeling that the patient can be kept at a lighter plane of anesthesia than with advanced airway manipulation. They contend that induction and recovery are faster in short cases with an open airway. However, a patent airway must be maintained at all times and often the pediatric dentist, dentist anesthesiologist, or dental assistant will manipulate the airway for at least a portion of the procedural time. Fewer supplies and equipment are also necessary in an open airway case than one which requires more aggressive airway manipulation. Both deep sedation and general anesthesia may be accomplished with open airway techniques.

Other dentist anesthesiologists prefer a more secure airway, even though it requires a deeper level of anesthesia. Nasotracheal intubation for general anesthesia is considered by some to be the "gold standard" for dental cases. With experience and good technique, it generally only takes a few seconds to a minute to place the tube. An advantage is that with the secure airway, mandible position and the use of water spray are no concern. If a nasotracheal tube is used, the resultant anesthetic is always general anesthesia, not deep sedation. If the plan is to maintain the anesthetic on a volatile agent such as sevoflurane or isoflurane, some type of advanced airway will be necessary. For a dental procedure in which some degree of airway protection other than an endotracheal tube is desired, a flexible laryngeal mask airway (LMA) may be chosen (Figure 14-3). The LMA offers a more protected airway than a simple throat partition as used in an open airway technique, but it does not offer the same level of protection as an endotracheal tube. Additionally, occlusion may be checked and a variety of other dental manipulations performed in cases of an open airway or nasoendotracheal tube, where these same things may not easily be accomplished under LMA general anesthesia. Technically, deep sedation may be used with an LMA; however, the resultant level if an LMA is used will always be true general anesthesia.

### Maintenance of General Anesthesia

Once the patient is induced, IV access is secured, and the airway of choice is established, the next decision is determining how to maintain general anesthesia. Again, there are two main options. One is to maintain general anesthesia with IV drugs and the other is to maintain general anesthesia with inhaled general anesthetic gas. Maintenance with IV agents has a number of advantages. There is no concern of "gas hygiene" and pollution of the dental operatory with waste anesthetic gases. The equipment used to administer the IV medications is typically a small, light-weight infusion pump, and the drugs used most often are propofol with remifentanil or alfentanil. Each of these drugs have a very short clinical duration of action and, therefore, have a rapid emergence from general anesthesia. Propofol is also a great antiemetic agent when exerting its effects, so post-operative nausea and vomiting are extremely rare. Other agents may be administered through the IV, regardless of whether IV or gas maintenance is desired. Various antiemetics are sometimes administered, as are antibiotics, analgesics, and/or steroids.

If an inhalational maintenance is desired with either an LMA or endotracheal tube in place, that gas may be sevoflurane or, more commonly, isoflurane. Desflurane is rarely used in the mobile environment primary due to the requirement that the vaporizer be heated. Sevoflurane is a good all-around inhalational general anesthetic. It is the most desirable for an inhalational induction, as it is least irritating to the pulmonary system and has an inoffensive odor. It works rapidly and has a relatively quick offset.

Another benefit of inhalational anesthetics is that, generally speaking, there has never been a shortage, nor have prices escalated as they have with most IV drugs. In 2020, every drug used in anesthesia for dentistry has been in short supply or on back order at least once, and the price of most IV drugs used in anesthesia for dentistry has increased from twofold to tenfold over the last decade, but prices of inhalational general anesthetics have been relatively stable or sometimes have fallen.

(a)

(b)

(c)

(d)

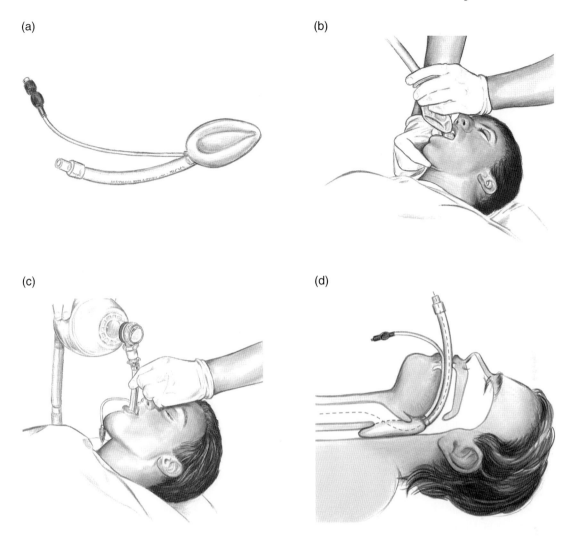

**Figure 14-3** For a dental procedure in which some degree of airway protection other than an endotracheal tube is desired, a flexible laryngeal mask airway (LMA) may be chosen. *Source:* American Heart Association (2000, Figure 3). © 2000, Elsevier.

## Recovery

At the conclusion of the procedure for the pediatric dental patient, the drugs are turned off and the patient is allowed to breathe 100% oxygen. The pediatric patient is allowed to regain consciousness and recover completely. For the patient that had an open airway deep sedation or general anesthetic, the throat partition is simply removed and oxygen continued most often via nasal cannula.

There are different schools of thought on the proper time to extubate those patients that were intubated. Deep extubation has merit, as does light or awake extubation, and each may be used on different patient populations or for different reasons. Deep extubation is performed during emergence when the child is deeply anesthetized and will not respond to the endotracheal tube being removed. Light or awake extubation is when the tube is removed once a patient opens their eyes, lifts their head for five seconds, and breathes spontaneously. It is still debated whether deep extubation versus awake extubation is the preferable technique to reduce the incidence of emergencies on emergence from anesthesia. Regardless of the technique, the overall incidence of adverse events seems to be similar.

Once the patient has regained consciousness, they are observed for a period of time until they may be safely dismissed. For some deep sedation patients, that may be as short a time period as ten minutes, while, for other pediatric dental patients and those who experienced a general anesthesia, the recovery time may exceed one hour. Pediatric dental patients usually recover fairly quickly from deep sedation or general anesthesia in the dental office, and they recover without significant upset or discomfort in the majority of cases. These patients have complete amnesia from shortly after the IM injection or mask induction through part of the recovery period. They generally experience no trauma directly related to the anesthesia.

### Medical Emergencies

Dentist anesthesiologists handle medical emergencies in the dental setting by virtue of their training and by involving the office staff at each individual office where they administer anesthesia. It is the anesthesia provider's responsibility to ensure that the facility meets appropriate standards. Each state or governmental agency's law also mandates minimum levels of equipment and facilities. The anesthesia provider must ensure immediate personal access to emergency drugs and equipment and always ensure that the office staff can provide basic life support and activate EMS. Every patient is monitored as if the patient were in a hospital setting. An ECG is used, and blood pressure, heart rate, respiratory rate, capnography, and oxygen saturation are also monitored. Depending on the practitioner, procedure, and type of airway chosen, a precordial stethoscope may be used. Emergency back-up lighting, oxygen, suction, and monitors are brought to each facility with the anesthesia provider or are already fixed within the facility.

## Summary

There are a variety of locations in which deep sedation and general anesthesia may be safely performed for pediatric dental patients, each with benefits and drawbacks. It is up to the pediatric dentist to make the choice. This chapter was intended to provide background information to facilitate that choice. It has emphasized different cost profiles and availability of both operating room time and mobile dentist anesthesiologists. There are different techniques for inducing and maintaining deep sedation and general anesthesia, different airway adjuncts that may be chosen, different drugs that may be used for maintaining deep sedation and general anesthesia, and different ways of recovering the pediatric dental patient from deep sedation or general anesthesia. The bottom line is that all options are correct. The important thing is not who administers the anesthetic or where, but that there remains the availability of obtaining anesthesia services for pediatric dental patients.

## References

Albany Medical Center, St. Peter's Hospital, Albany, NY. A 2009 hospital statement.

Allen, D.L. (1992). The future of dental education. *Anesthesia Progress*, 39, 1–3.

American Dental Association Council on Dental Education. (1972). Guidelines for teaching the comprehensive control of pain and anxiety in dentistry. *Journal of Dental Education*, 36, 62–67.

American Heart Association (2000). Part (6) advanced cardiovascular life support: Section 3: Adjuncts for oxygenation, ventilation, and airway control. *Circulation* 102, S1, 1–95.

American Society of Anesthesiologists House of Delegates. (1982). Statement regarding the administration of anesthesia by dentists. *October* 26.

American Society of Dentist Anesthesiologists (ASDA). (2010). The necessity for advanced anesthesia services for dental care. http://www.asdahq.org/ DentistAnesthesiologist/About ASDADA.aspx.

American Society of Anesthesiologists Board of Directors. (1987). Statement supporting the right of qualified dentists as defined by the American Dental Association to utilize anesthesia for the management of dental patients. *August* 22.

Mass, R. (1993). Parenteral sedation education. *New York State Dental Journal*, 59, 67–70.

Matsuura, H. (1993). Modern history of dental anesthesia in Japan. *Anesthesia Progress*, 40, 109–113.

Olabi, N.F., Jones, J.E., Saxen. M. et al. (2012). The use of office-based sedation and general anesthesia by board certified pediatric dentists practicing in the United States. *Anesthesia Progress*, 59, 12–17.

Peskin, RM. (1993). Dentists and anesthesia: Historical and contemporary perspectives. *Anesthesia Progress*, 40, 1–13.

Rashewsky, S., Parameswaran, A., Sloane, C. et al. (2012). Time and cost analysis: Pediatric dental rehabilitation with general anesthesia in the office and the hospital settings. *Anesthesia Progress*, 59, 147–153.

# 15

# The Use of General Anesthesia in Behavior Management

*Marcio A. da Fonseca and Travis Nelson*

## Introduction

Most children can receive dental treatment through non-pharmacologic behavior management. However, some may benefit from pharmacologic adjuncts, such as general anesthesia (GA). GA is defined as a controlled state of unconsciousness accompanied by a loss of protective reflexes, including the ability to maintain an airway independently and respond purposefully to physical stimulation and verbal commands (Coté and Wilson 2019). It does not require cooperation from the patient, and thus may be desirable in select cases (Table 15-1). GA allows delivery of dental care in a way that protects the developing psyche and promotes the establishment of a lifelong therapeutic relationship (Nelson 2013).

Dentists feel that today's children exhibit more challenging behaviors than in the past, which has created an increased demand for advanced behavior management techniques, such as sedation and GA, in many countries, such as the United States (Pham et al. 2018; Spera et al. 2017; Young et al. 2018), Canada (Schroth et al. 2014), and Sweden, where the percentage of patients treated under GA has nearly doubled over the past few decades (Klingberg et al. 2010). GA used to be one of the least desirable behavior management techniques in the past, but over time, parents have come to exhibit high levels of acceptance, with most agreeing to have their child treated in the operating room (OR) again if necessary (Patel et al. 2016). However, some parents may struggle to accept GA for their child's dental care, either due to cultural beliefs or blame for placing the child at risk for an adverse event (Amin et al. 2006).

Procedures under GA can now be safely accomplished at an outpatient surgical facility or a dental office, leading to a short recovery period, no overnight stay, and lower costs

than in a hospital (Spera et al. 2017). However, in many countries, GA is not performed outside the OR due to regulatory practices or lack of resources (Wilson and Alcaino 2011). The increased acceptance of dental care under GA may be explained by the public's familiarity with surgery provided on an outpatient basis. To accommodate this shift in practice, it is not uncommon to find medical anesthesiologists, dental anesthesiologists, and nurse anesthetists (i.e., dentists and nurses who have received formal training in anesthesiology) working in dental offices and other outpatient settings in the United States (Pham et al. 2018; Spera et al. 2017; Young et al. 2018). The significant cost savings of office-based GA is a major factor driving this trend (Green et al. 2018). Unfortunately, patients from low- and middle-income countries face significant financial, cultural, and structural barriers to access GA services, including distance to a surgical center; poor roads; lack of transportation; lack of facilities, equipment, and expertise; direct and indirect costs related to surgical care; and fear of undergoing GA (Grimes et al. 2011).

Although the use of GA is mostly uneventful, it is associated with greater morbidity and mortality than provision of dental care under local anesthetic (LA) or minimal sedation. Risk in pediatric anesthesia is divided into minor and major, which includes cardiac arrest, brain damage, and death. Both types of risk occur most frequently in infants and children under three years of age, especially those with co-morbidities (Paterson and Waterhouse 2011). GA-related deaths are as low as 0.1 per 10,000 anesthetics (Somri et al. 2012). Morbidity reported for cases of dental care under GA include coughing and pain (27%), inability to eat (24.8%), psychological changes (24%), and sore throat (21%) (Erkmen Almaz et al. 2019). Sleeping irregularities, vomiting, disruption of bodily functions, diarrhea, sore throat, bleeding, and mild to moderate pain are usually not

*Wright's Behavior Management in Dentistry for Children*, Third Edition. Edited by Ari Kupietzky.
© 2022 John Wiley & Sons, Inc. Published 2022 by John Wiley & Sons, Inc.

**Table 15-1** Indications and contraindications for general anesthesia.

| Indications | Contraindications |
| --- | --- |
| Patients who cannot cooperate due to a lack of psychological or emotional maturity and/or mental, physical, or medical disability | Minimal dental needs in cooperative patients |
| When local anesthesia is ineffective because of acute infection, anatomic variations, or allergy | Predisposing medical conditions that would make general anesthesia inadvisable (e.g., malignant hyperthermia, unstable cardiac condition, and poorly controlled or advanced cystic fibrosis) or contraindicated |
| Patients who are extremely uncooperative, fearful, anxious, or uncommunicative, including language barrier | General anesthesia risk exceeds benefits of proposed procedures |
| Patients requiring significant surgical procedures | Infections of the respiratory tract |
| Patients for whom the use of GA may protect the developing psyche and/or reduce medical risk | Fasting violation |
| Patients requiring immediate, comprehensive oral/dental care | Patients with 5, 10 methylenetetrahydropholate reductase (MTHFR) gene polymorphism or with suspected mitochondrial disease |
| Geographic distance from dental clinic to accomplish multiple operative appointments | |
| Unstable social situation of the family | |

*Sources:* Shay et al. (2007); Matton and Romeo (2017); Turner and Hipp (2018).

significant enough to warrant medical attention (Mayeda and Wilson 2009), with most patients returning to normal behavior within 24 hours (Costa et al. 2011; Mayeda and Wilson 2009; Needleman et al. 2008). In a large cohort study of in-office based anesthesia for dental care, there was no mortality reported, with laryngospasm being the most common (0.5%) pre-discharge adverse event, and nausea and vomiting the most common (5%) post-discharge complication (Spera et al. 2017). Children themselves reported several post-operative complications following dental care under GA, such as nausea, vomiting, bleeding, tiredness, hunger, disturbed eating, being scared/worried, and having discomfort from the intravenous (IV) line (Rodd et al. 2014).

In 2014, the US Federal Drug Administration released a warning based on animal studies that exposure of young brains to anesthetic gases could negatively impact neurologic development (Ganzberg 2017). Recent human studies, however, have provided evidence that anesthesia exposure at an early age was not associated with adverse child development outcomes, even in cases of multiple exposures (Davidson et al. 2016; McCann et al. 2019; O'Leary et al. 2019; Sun et al. 2016).

## Pre-operative Considerations

### Informed Consent

When preparing a family for GA, it is important to ensure that caregivers have enough information to make informed decisions. The dentist can facilitate this process through informed consent (IC). Unfortunately, studies of IC for GA show that parents often feel they are not adequately informed of its risks (Patel 2004; Shahid et al. 2008). In societies with a large influx of immigrants, cultural influences and language fluency must be taken into consideration when obtaining consent. Trained interpreters who have an understanding of cultural norms are very helpful in these situations. Family members, especially children, should not be used as interpreters. When children interpret, there is a reversal of power between them and their caretakers. Family members may also choose not to translate sensitive information, leading to potentially serious misunderstandings. It is crucial that the IC form and the pre-operative instruction paperwork be written in the language spoken by the legal guardians. Although in pediatric dentistry IC must be obtained from an adult, it is important to consider the child's participation ("assent") in the process. Children between the ages of 8 and 13 years have shown a desire to be involved in discussions regarding their care and are highly satisfied with the treatment they receive when they are involved (Adewumi et al. 2001).

### History and Physical Examination

To prevent problems during the delivery of GA, the dentist must gather a detailed medical history for the child and decide which venue is appropriate for the dental procedure, given the patient's health status. For example, if the child is healthy, then dental care under GA can be safely carried out at an outpatient facility or dental office. If the child has moderate to severe or uncontrolled systemic disease, high body mass index, a difficult airway or IV access, or is large and combative, treatment should be done where there is ample and immediate medical care available to support the increased needs of the patient. All patients must undergo a history and physical examination (H&P) within 30 days of the procedure. For healthy children, the exam can be done by the anesthesiologist on the day of the surgery. Given their higher risk for complications, patients with special healthcare needs should have the H&P done by a physician who is thoroughly familiar with their health issues. It is imperative that the dentist discuss concerns related to the delivery of dental care with the physician and the anesthesiologist to anticipate complications (e.g., bleeding in a child with hemophilia). To facilitate comprehensive planning, many hospitals have a pre-anesthesia evaluation service where all stakeholders are consulted so that the patient, family, physicians, anesthesia care team, and dentist understand how the child will be cared for.

## Pre-operative Pain Management

Pediatric patients experience pain with equal or greater intensity as their adult counterparts (Cramton and Gruchala 2012). Dentists should educate themselves on accurate assessment of pain, as well as pharmacologic and non-pharmacologic methods of pain management. When that is not adequate, the child may suffer long-term consequences regarding future pain reactions (Cramton and Gruchala 2012).

Children may experience moderate or severe pain following procedures under GA. Even though post-operative pain is the most common parental concern, many patients do not receive adequate analgesia. Healthcare professionals and parents under-medicate children post-operatively, often due to misconceptions (Cramton and Gruchala 2012; Rony et al. 2010). Socioeconomic status also seems to influence pain perception, with parents who have less education being more likely to report post-procedural pain for their children (Needleman et al. 2008). Therefore, good post-operative pain control starts before surgery. Providing tailored interventions to improve a caretaker's knowledge of analgesia at an earlier stage and allowing ample time for discussion may improve parental attitude (Jensen 2012; Rony et al. 2010).

## Pre-operative Child Anxiety

Although GA is typically a humane and effective way to provide dental care, the surgical experience may have a negative psychological effect on some children. Between 50% and 75% of pediatric patients who undergo ambulatory surgery in the United States each year experience significant fear and anxiety (Tzong et al. 2012). Thus, the anesthesia care team should anticipate and treat anxiety as part of the OR experience.

Pre-operative fear may result from a child's concerns about separation, pain, disfigurement, loss of loved ones, and loss of control or autonomy. Alterations of the family's routine, wearing unfamiliar clothing (i.e., surgical gowns), and experiencing unknown equipment, sights, sounds, and smells also increase stress (Justus et al. 2006). Anxiety frequently causes resistance to the anesthesia mask, prolongs induction, and may require physical restraint of the child. Children may have specific fears of the mask (e.g., inability to breathe, claustrophobia, and concerns about dying or not waking up), aversion (dislike of the feel or odor of the mask), and/or an irrational fear of the mask (Aydin et al. 2008; Przybylo et al. 2005). Furthermore, a complex interplay of genetic and environmental influences determines how each child will respond to the OR experience. Shyness, passive coping style, high baseline anxiety, high parental anxiety, previous upsetting surgical experiences, and male sex are factors associated with anxiety and disruptive behavior in relation to the GA visit (Kain et al. 2000). Age should also be considered, as children between the ages of one and five years appear to be at highest risk for developing significant anxiety before surgery.

Other factors that may contribute to increased levels of anxiety include many people present during induction, a long waiting time between arrival at the facility and induction, having a mother who does not practice a religion, and negative memories of hospital experiences (Wollin et al. 2003).

---

### Case 15.1

Marco is a six-year-old boy with a cleft lip and palate. Over the course of his life, he has had many encounters with healthcare professionals, including a number of surgical procedures. He was referred to your office by the craniofacial team who is managing his care. At his most recent craniofacial visit, the team orthodontist noticed significant caries in Marco's primary molars and canines.

When Marco presents to your office for examination, you note that he is extremely apprehensive. He covers his mouth with his hands, and even with your best communicative behavior management, you are only able to perform a cursory examination. Your clinical findings indicate significant caries in at least four primary teeth; however, you are unable to obtain radiographs. You recommend general anesthesia (GA) for comprehensive dental care. Marco's parents are familiar with the GA process, and they agree to this treatment approach. However, they mention that the last time he had a surgical procedure, he had a very difficult time with mask induction, and he has expressed fears about having additional surgeries in the future.

***Case 15.1, Discussion:*** GA is the optimal way to manage restorative dental care for this child, and it is excellent that the family has informed you of his anxiety. This affords the opportunity to work with the family, child life specialists at your hospital (if available), and the anesthesia team to develop a care plan that takes this into account. Strategies you might consider include implementing a pre-operative preparation program (see below) that teaches Marco coping strategies he can employ during inhalation induction and/or implementing audiovisual distraction such as viewing a preferred television show during the induction, allowing a calm parent to be present, and anxiolytic premedication such as midazolam that will relax the patient and provide some degree of amnesia.

## Pre-operative Pharmacological Interventions to Reduce Anxiety

Induction of anesthesia appears to be the most stressful point of the GA experience. Children may cry, scream, try to avoid the anesthesia mask, and/or require restraint. The principal pharmacological approach to facilitate induction of fearful patients is the use of sedative premedication. While other agents are available, midazolam is the most extensively researched pre-induction sedative, showing an effective anxiety reduction in the 1 to 10-year-old group, especially the most anxious children (Kain et al. 2004). It may also cause amnesia, which is desirable should the induction prove to be difficult (Stewart et al. 2006). However, a paradoxical negative response to midazolam may occur, especially in children with impulsive temperament (Wright et al. 2007). Midazolam may also cause delay in anesthetic emergence, recovery, and discharge as well as an increase in anxiety immediately following surgery (Wright et al. 2007).

## Pre-operative Non-Pharmacological Interventions to Reduce Anxiety

### Parental Presence During Induction

The practice of allowing parents to be present for their child's induction is a highly debated topic. Suggested benefits of parental presence include eliminating separation anxiety, minimizing premedication use, increasing child cooperation, enhancing parental satisfaction, fulfilling parents' perceived sense of duty to be present, and enhancing parental satisfaction with the medical care provided (Kain et al. 2004; Wright et al. 2007). Anesthesia care teams in the United States have increasingly allowed parental presence at induction (Kain et al. 2004). The presence of a calm parent is typically beneficial for an anxious child, whereas an anxious parent does not improve child behavior (Kain et al. 2006). Unfortunately, those who most desire to be present have higher levels of anxiety and tend to have more anxious children than parents who are not as interested in participation at induction (Caldwell-Andrews et al. 2005). A systematic review has shown that presence of parents during induction did not decrease their child's anxiety (Manyande et al. 2015).

## Pre-operative Preparation Programs and Interventions

The goal of these programs is to provide information for the patient and the caretakers about the process (through OR tours, print materials, audiovisual methods, websites, and videos), model the experience (using videos or puppet shows), and teach coping strategies (with Child Life counselors) using age-appropriate language and imagery (Wright et al. 2007). Children who receive these interventions tend to exhibit less pre-surgical anxiety, even upon separation from their parents (Kain and Caldwell-Andrews 2005; Wright et al. 2007). Many factors should be considered when selecting a program, one of the most important being the child's age. According to Piaget's theory of cognitive development, children from three to six years (the pre-operational stage of development) are not able to think logically; thus, pre-operative preparation may have negative effects for them (Brewer et al. 2006). In contrast, children from 7 to 17 years have a strong desire for and benefit from comprehensive information, including details on post-operative pain (Fortier et al. 2009). Timing of preparation is also important—the patient must be allowed to adequately process what was discussed. Children younger than six years should receive preparation no more than one week in advance, while older children benefit most if they are given information more than five days before surgery (Perry et al. 2012). Children with a history of surgical procedures who did not benefit from modeling and play programs should be enrolled in programs that teach coping skills before their next GA procedure (Kain and Caldwell-Andrews 2005).

Parental anxiety is a significant risk factor for child anxiety; thus, caretakers should also receive pre-operative information. Preparation may be even more critical in day surgery than for inpatient procedures. Caretakers who participate in pre-surgical programs exhibit decreased anxiety and show higher levels of satisfaction with the overall quality of care (Chan and Molassiotis 2002; Felder-Puig et al. 2003). Unfortunately, the benefits of these programs do not appear to extend to high-stress periods, such as anesthetic induction, recovery, or even at 2 weeks post-operatively (Kain and Caldwell-Andrews 2005; Wright et al. 2007).

Playing at home with an anesthesia mask was shown to relieve mask-related anxiety, improving its acceptance and shortening the induction period (Aydin et al. 2008). Other contemporary methods that may help reduce pre-operative anxiety include video watching (Kim et al. 2015), video glasses (Kerimoglu et al. 2013), acupuncture, clowns or clown doctors, and low sensory stimulation (Manyande et al. 2015).

## Pre-operative Dental and Surgical Plan

Given the high GA costs, possible complications of GA, and the fact that most children treated in the OR are high caries risk and many experience disease recurrence, an aggressive treatment approach is advocated. For example, using stainless steel crowns (SSC) for full coronal coverage in teeth with extensive decalcification should be considered. In dental care under GA, SSCs have a significantly lower failure rate than amalgams, while composites and composite strip crowns have the highest failure (Amin et al. 2010; Blumer et al. 2017). The tentative treatment plan should consider all potential scenarios, parental compliance with oral care, patient's social history, and longevity of the restorations.

The family must understand the plan may change on the day of the procedure, particularly if no radiographs were available on the day of the initial examination or if there was a long waiting period to schedule the OR visit. Application of silver diamine fluoride (SDF) decreases the odds of children on the waiting list for dental care under GA to need urgent dental care (Yarmarkovich et al. 2019). SDF may also afford time for an uncooperative child to mature psychologically to stand treatment in the dental chair and decrease the high costs of GA (Johhnson et al. 2019). It can also help prevent new carious lesions in primary teeth (Oliveira et al. 2019).

All possible treatments should be discussed in detail, including the appearance of the proposed materials, so as not to take the caretakers by surprise after the procedure is complete. For example, if crowns are planned for the maxillary primary incisors, it is wise to make the family aware that the teeth may need to be extracted if they are found to be abscessed or if too little tooth structure remains after caries removal. Additionally, financial issues, such as the need for pre-authorization from the medical and dental insurance companies, must be addressed before the appointment date. The patient must be tested for COVID-19 within 72 hours of the dental procedure date. If the test is positive and the patient has no medical conditions, he must be rescheduled 4 weeks later if asymptomatic or recovered from only mild, non-respiratory symptoms (American Society of Anesthesiologists 2021). Patients who test positive do not need to be retested within 90 days of a positive result (Centers for Disease Control and Prevention 2019).

## Pre-operative Call to the Family

A few days before the patient's scheduled appointment, a staff person from the surgery center will call the family to discuss the plan for the day. Pre-operative fasting guidelines (Table 15-2) should be discussed in detail both verbally and in writing. Fasting is crucial to reduce the severity of complications related to perioperative pulmonary aspiration of

**Table 15-2**  Pre-operative fasting recommendations for healthy patients undergoing elective procedures.

| Ingested material | Minimum fasting period |
| --- | --- |
| Clear liquids* | 2 hours |
| Breast milk | 4 hours |
| Infant formula | 6 hours |
| Nonhuman milk | 6 hours |
| Light meal** | 6 hours |
| Fried foods, fatty foods, or meat | 8 hours or more |

\* Water, fruit juices without pulp, carbonated beverages, clear tea, and black coffee.
\** Typically consists of toast and clear liquids.
*Source:* American Society of Anesthesiologists (2017). © 2017, Wolters Kluwer Health, Inc.

gastric content, to avoid delays or cancellation of the procedure, to decrease risk of dehydration or hypoglycemia from prolonged fasting, and to minimize perioperative morbidity, such as aspiration pneumonia and respiratory issues (American Society of Anesthesiologists 2017).The time and location of the appointment, payment and surgical pre-authorization information, and COVID-19 test result should also be reviewed. If the H&P was to be performed by a physician prior to the day of surgery, it is important to verify that the documentation clearing the patient for GA has been received. A second change of clothes should be brought in case the child soils those he is wearing. If the parent is planning to drive, a second adult should accompany them to ensure the child's safety on the way home. Patients who have been sedated are at risk for post-procedural airway blockage, loss of head-righting reflex, and re-sedation (Martinez and Wilson 2006). Thus, the child should lie on his side in the car instead of on the back to avoid aspiration of gastric contents in case of vomiting. With a second adult present to watch and assist the child, the driver can focus on the road.

## Perioperative Considerations

Upon arrival at the surgical facility, the child may be given an identification bracelet. Some surgical centers will give the child a surgical gown, while others allow the child to be induced in their own clothes. A staff person, usually a nurse, takes the vital signs, height, and weight, and inquires about fasting, recent respiratory infections, and changes in their health since the H&P was completed, including COVID-19 symptoms in the child and family members. If the patient has a fever, wheezing, cough, or runny nose, or has been exposed to a contagious or infectious disease, the procedure may be canceled. If the patient has violated the fasting recommendations, the procedure may be either canceled or postponed to a later time on the same day to allow for emptying of gastric contents.

Once the admission assessment is complete, the anesthesiologist meets with the family in order to:

1. prepare the patient for anesthesia, determine the child's health status, and prescribe a plan of care;
2. evaluate tonsil size (Brodsky 1989) and potential intubation issues (Mallampati et al. 1985);
3. determine that the fasting requirements have been followed;
4. assess the need for a pre-operative sedative;
5. discuss placement of an IV line for fluid maintenance, route of intubation, anesthetic agents, and the peri- and post-operative pain management plan;
6. review the risks and management of complications related to GA;
7. obtain consent for the procedures;
8. determine whether the caretakers will be allowed to be present during the induction phase and how the separation is to take place. In case their presence is allowed, they must be told the order in which the events will occur, the normal physiological and emotional reactions the child may display, what they will be expected to do, and when they must leave the room.

After the anesthesia evaluation, the pre-operative sedative (if warranted) is ordered for the nurse to administer right away. The dentist then meets with the family and child to review the preliminary treatment plan. Once all questions are clarified, the dental consent form can be signed. Questions about post-operative diet and dental pain management can be deferred until after the treatment is completed. This allows the dentist to provide instructions that are specific to the procedure that was performed (e.g., extractions vs dental restorations). Many parents inquire about whether the dentist will come out to discuss the clinical findings before starting the procedure. To keep the child under GA for the least amount of time to decrease risks and costs, it is better to do so only if there is an unusual finding that may alter the treatment plan significantly or if further consent is necessary. A pre-operative progress note should be written in the patient's chart, documenting the encounter.

## Intraoperative Considerations

The patient is brought into the OR, where identification is checked again. After GA induction is completed (most commonly done with a facial mask), the caretaker is escorted out, padding is placed under pressure points, the patient is secured on the operating bed with safety straps, and an IV line is established for medication infusion and fluid maintenance. The most common calculation used for fluid therapy in pediatrics is the "4-2-1 rule" (Oh 1980)—4 ml for each kg of the first 10 kg of the child's weight, 2 ml for each kg for the second 10 kg, and 1 ml for each remaining kg of the child's body weight. For example, a 25 kg child would receive 65 ml/hr of fluid replacement (40 + 20 + 5 = 65). Administering either normal saline or lactated Ringer's solution is frequently indicated to replace fasting deficits and ongoing losses during the procedure to maintain cardiovascular stability (Bailey et al. 2010; Murat and Dubois 2008). Routine dextrose administration is no longer advised for healthy children (Bailey et al. 2010).

Intranasal endotracheal intubation is preferred in dentistry because it leaves more working room in the oral cavity. However, the anesthesiologist may choose to do an intraoral intubation or laryngeal mask airway due to difficulty passing the tube through the nares (e.g., in cases of nasal atrophy such as seen in epidermolysis bullosa dystrophica), due to a medical concern (e.g., causing intranasal bleeding in a child with hemophilia or rupturing a repaired cleft palate tissue flap) or in case of a very short procedure. Patients who may present cervical spine abnormalities (e.g., Down syndrome and osteogenesis imperfecta) should have minimal manipulation of the neck, avoiding hyperextension during both intubation and dental procedure because of the high risk of fractures and/or spinal cord compression (Belanger and Kossick 2015; Hankinson and Anderson 2010; Russo and Becke 2015). Patients with craniofacial syndromes, macroglossia, and mandibular and/or maxillary hypoplasia may also pose a great challenge for intubation due to their difficult airway (Belanger and Kossick 2015; Russo and Becke 2015).

Following intubation, the patient's body is draped, the eyes are protected, a shoulder roll is placed, and a towel is wrapped around the child's head and eyes to protect them from debris and to secure the endotracheal tube. During the procedure, the dentist must be mindful not to dislodge the endotracheal tube. A time-out should be called to identify the child one more time, introduce all staff assigned to the case and their roles, and review the anesthesia plan, the pain management plan and the dental procedure. The dentist should perform a cursory dental exam to determine the type of radiographs to be obtained, if recent images are not available. A throat pack must be placed, followed by a dental cleaning and a detailed oral and dental exam to define the treatment plan. Rubber dam isolation or Isodry isolation system (https://www.zyris.com/products/isodry/), and a mouth prop should be used throughout the procedure to protect the soft tissues. Treatment sequence should facilitate a clean and dry operating field (e.g., composite restorations prior to extractions) and allow for adequate coagulation of extraction sites prior to extubation. Impressions for oral appliances can be taken at any time during the procedure. It is not uncommon to observe intra- and post-operative angioedema of the oral tissues, including the tongue, due to sensitivity and extensive oral manipulation. In this situation, the anesthesiologist can give the patient IV dexamethasone (0.2–0.5 mg/kg) to reduce inflammation (Belanger and Kossick 2015). Some patients may also produce more saliva under GA. In those cases, the anesthesiologist can inject an antisialagogue (atropine and glycopyrrolate) to help to keep the operating field dry (Belanger and Kossick 2015).

Fifteen minutes before the end of the procedure, the anesthesiologist should be warned to start preparing the patient to emerge from GA. When all dental care is complete, the oral cavity and the face are cleaned, fluids and debris are suctioned out of the mouth, fluoride is applied, the throat pack is removed, and all extracted teeth, needles, sutures, instruments, and gauze used in the case must be accounted for. Another time-out should take place to review the post-operative care plan and any unexpected events that occurred during the procedure. The patient may be extubated in the OR or in the Post-Anesthesia Care Unit (PACU), depending on his status and the anesthesiologist's preference. The anesthesiologist and the dentist must write orders for the PACU staff as well as for home care, including pain management, oral hygiene instructions, diet, follow-up appointment plan, and contact numbers in case of questions or an emergency. The procedure must be documented in detail in the patient's dental or medical chart, including the justification for the procedure, findings, type and number of radiographs, all materials used, which procedures were done per tooth, estimated blood loss, location and amount of LA administered, and complications. The patient is taken to the PACU by the anesthesia care team, who is also responsible for monitoring and supporting the child during transport. Both the anesthesiologist and the dentist must do a verbal transfer of care to a PACU nurse, reviewing what transpired in the OR as well as the post-procedural orders and follow-up plan.

## Post-operative Considerations

It is best to meet with the family in a private area before they are invited to the PACU, where they will focus on the child and not pay full attention to the post-operative discussion. The dentist should start by discussing how the child is doing in the PACU (the anesthesiologist will also visit with the family) and proceed to discuss:

1. the dental treatment performed;
2. location of numbness and expected duration, instructing the family to watch the child carefully to avoid traumatic biting;
3. expected amount and length of bleeding, instructing the family on how to avoid prolonging it (e.g., not sucking through a straw for a few days);
4. suture removal, if necessary;
5. pain management at home;
6. diet—very light meals and lots of fluids on the first day, followed by soft foods for a few more days depending on the treatment;
7. oral hygiene—clarify when to resume toothbrushing and how often;
8. prevention counseling (diet, oral hygiene, frequency of dental visits, and supplemental fluoride);
9. when to return to normal activities (school, sport practices, etc.);
10. common post-operative complications;
11. who and what number to call in case of questions or emergencies; and
12. when the next dental appointment will take place.

The patient may be offered popsicles and liquids in the PACU to enhance the hydration process so that the IV line can be disconnected as soon as possible. The anesthesiologist is responsible for the discharge of the patient; if one is not available, the PACU nurse can make that determination. The most common discharge criteria include the child's ability to hold fluids and light foods without vomiting, to void, to be at least somewhat alert, and to ambulate, even if assisted. It is good practice to have a surgical staff member and the dentist call the family within 12–24 hours for a post-operative check.

### Post-operative Pain Management

Pain tends to be more severe when a high number of dental procedures are performed (Atan et al. 2004; Hu et al. 2018; Needleman et al. 2008; Erkmen Almaz et al. 2019). SSCs and pulpotomies cause more distress than extractions or other types of restorative work (Costa et al. 2011; Mayeda and Wilson 2009). It is important to control pain as rapidly as possible, with analgesic doses titrated according to the patient's response. Early effective treatment is safer and more efficacious than delayed treatment, resulting in improved comfort and possibly less total administered medication. Patients' discomfort tend to be mild and of short duration (Costa et al. 2011; Erkmen Almaz et al. 2019; Jensen 2012; Hu et al. 2018; Mayeda and Wilson 2009), occurring mostly on the day of the procedure or the day after (Erkmen Almaz et al. 2019; Hu et al. 2018). However, in cases of moderate to severe pain, continuous dosing at fixed intervals is recommended. The anesthesia provider may choose to administer pain medications intraoperatively, such as ketorolac, to decrease post-operative pain. Therefore, before prescribing analgesics, it is important to confer with the anesthesiologist regarding the pain management plan to ensure that the child receives the correct amount of medication at the right time.

Oral administration of ibuprofen alone or combined with paracetamol (acetaminophen) decreased the mean pain and distress scores in children compared to paracetamol alone (Gazal and Mackie 2007). In contrast, paracetamol, ibuprofen, and LA used together did not decrease distress in young children who had extractions under GA (McWilliams and Rutherford 2007). Children who receive over-the-counter analgesics the day after the procedures show less pain in the first week (Costa et al. 2011). Sadly, parental adherence to the dentist's analgesic recommendations following extractions under GA is poor (Jensen 2012). The most commonly prescribed analgesics in pediatrics are described in Table 15-3.

Another controversial issue in dental care under GA is the need for LA. In oral surgical procedures, it is not unusual to inject LA (1) to decrease fluctuation of vital signs and anesthesia intervention, (2) to numb the tissues to minimize discomfort at recovery, and (3) to help control bleeding through the action of vasoconstrictors. Evidence suggests that patients who do not receive LA before extractions are more likely to experience changes in heart and respiratory rate, resulting in additional anesthesiologist intervention (Watts et al. 2009). The effect on post-operative discomfort is less clear. Some studies indicate that LA reduces post-operative pain (Atan et al. 2004), while others have shown no difference between LA and control groups (McWilliams and Rutherford 2007; Moness and Hammuda

2019). While LA administration may reduce bleeding in the early recovery period, it may contribute to cheek and lip biting (Townsend et al. 2009). If the decision is made to forgo administration of LA, the use of resorbable hemostatic sponges in the socket and/or sutures may be used to control bleeding.

## Effects of Dental Care Under GA on the Patient and the Family

Dental treatment under GA can improve a child's quality of life (QoL) through reduction of pain, improved eating and sleeping, better acceptance of supervised toothbrushing, improved behavior, and increased concentration at school (Anderson et al. 2004; Amin and Harrison 2007; Klaassen et al. 2009). Families also report improvement in their QoL as a whole because of fewer parental sleep disturbances, less attention required by the child, fewer financial difficulties, and fewer days off work to attend to the child's dental needs (Jankauskiene et al. 2017; Thomson and Malden 2011). On the other hand, parental satisfaction and acceptance of GA for dental care may also lead to more children in the family being treated that way (Edmonds et al. 2019). Patients also reported positive outcomes from the procedure, such as satisfaction with the resolution of their dental issues and receiving attention and rewards from the family (Rodd et al. 2014).

The high levels of parental satisfaction with dental care provided under GA may initially lead to some positive behavioral changes, such as understanding the importance of a healthy primary dentition, improving dental health practices, and reducing sugar consumption and snacking (Amin et al. 2006). However, many caretakers do not follow the preventive advice given before and after the procedure (Amin and Harrison 2007; Jankauskiene et al. 2017;

**Table 15-3** Most commonly prescribed analgesics for children.

| Drug | Route | Dose | Remarks |
|------|-------|------|---------|
| Acetaminophen | Oral | 10–15 mg/kg q4–6 h | Total dose from all sources should not exceed 100 mg/kg for children and 75 mg/kg for infants or 5 doses in 24 hours for all pediatric patients |
| | Rectal | 20 mg/kg q4–6 h | |
| Ibuprofen | Oral | 4–10 mg/kg q6–8 h | Maximum: 40 mg/kg/day |
| Naproxen | Oral | 5–7 mg/kg q8–10 h | |
| Codeine | Oral | 0.5–1 mg/kg q4–6 h | Maximum: 60 mg/dose |
| Acetaminophen with codeine | Oral | 3–6 yr olds: 5 ml (12 mg codeine) q4–6 h | |
| | | 7–12 yr olds: 10 ml (24 mg codeine) q4–6 h | |

*Sources:* Cramton and Gruchala (2012); Sohn et al. (2012); Wilson and Ganzberg (2013).

Olley et al. 2011; Peerbhay 2009). A parental sense of "fatalism" is a major barrier to positive changes. They may feel as though they do not have the ability to control their child's oral health, which may be linked to factors such as their own poor oral care, lack of knowledge about oral health, limited financial resources and time, and lack of access to care (Karki et al. 2011; Olley et al. 2011; Peerbhay 2009). Some do not see the importance of preventive practices at home and fail to keep appointments. Thus, parental readiness to change is an important predictor of whether they will engage in preventive behaviors over time (Amin and Harrison 2007).

A child's pre-operative fear and anxiety may be perpetuated by the GA experience itself. Furthermore, having dental care under GA does not seem to improve the child's previous uncooperative behavior (Amin and Harrison 2007; Klaassen et al. 2009; Savanheimo et al. 2005), although not all studies agree (Al-Malik and Al-Sarheed 2006). Nevertheless, positive experiences and appointments focused primarily on preventive treatment may facilitate the child's acceptance of dental care in the office (Klaassen et al. 2009; Savanheimo et al. 2005).

## Caries Prevention and Recurrence Rates After Treatment Under GA

Most studies report a low follow-up rate, both immediately after the GA appointment and long-term, with many returning only when they have a problem (Kakaounaki et al. 2011; Olley et al. 2011; Peerbhay 2009). Perhaps the dentist contributes to the patient's poor compliance due to a personal sense of fatalism (there is no known effective prevention for early childhood caries (ECC)), misconceptions (these parents are not interested in their child's oral health), and/or unrealistic expectations (counseling low-income families to eat healthy foods, which can be very expensive).

All these factors create a vicious cycle that leads to low oral healthcare support in children with ECC. Many parents complain that the dental team did not offer a plan for continued care after GA (Anderson et al. 2004; Olley et al. 2011), and even those who brought their children regularly reported that preventive advice and interventions were poor (Karki et al. 2011; Olley et al. 2011; Peerbhay 2009). To further complicate matters, dentists seem to prefer operative appointments for uncooperative children with ECC, rather than focusing on prevention (Savanheimo and Vehkalahti 2008). However, children with ECC do not seem to respond to conventional or increased preventive care, which is dependent on regular attendance to the dental office (Amin et al. 2010). Intensive preventive care produced no decrease in new carious lesions in high-risk patients compared to a basic prevention program, which involved less effort and lower costs (Hausen et al. 2000). Dental retreatment was prevalent even for children who complied with follow-up evaluations, despite a statistically significant improvement in plaque, gingival, and mutans streptococci scores (Primosch et al. 2001).

Aggressive dental surgery for ECC may not result in acceptable clinical outcomes, that is, prevention of new carious lesions. It is possible that these patients are affected by more virulent strains of caries-producing bacteria. Caries recurrence is usually evident within a few months of the procedure, with many patients returning for further treatment under GA (Jankauskiene et al. 2017; Olley et al. 2011). Some studies were able to identify predictors for a child's repeat visit to the OR (Kakaounaki et al. 2011; Sheller et al. 2003), but others failed to discriminate influences on predicting compliant behavior (Primosch et al. 2001).

Innovative, family-centered, and evidence-based interventions that address the social determinants of dental caries are needed to prevent dental disease (Amin and Harrison 2007; Olley et al. 2011). Dietary and preventive advice should be provided to the extended family because it is not realistic to expect a change in the diet of one child alone. Furthermore, low-income group children, who comprise the largest share of the population affected by ECC, face many barriers regarding food insecurity, housing instability, and access to dental care (da Fonseca 2012). Moreover, all these issues lead to maternal depression, which is associated with decreased positive parenting behaviors, including dental care (Kavanaugh et al. 2006), and missed dental appointments for their children (Pappas et al. 2020). Oral health programs should be ongoing; they should not only be a snapshot in time. Counseling should be tailored to an individual parent's stage of change and readiness (Amin and Harrison 2007).

## Summary

While most children can receive dental treatment through non-pharmacologic behavior management, some may benefit from GA. The use of GA to provide dental care has dramatically increased in recent decades due to increased access to anesthesia services, child behavioral concerns, and parent preferences. Delivering care safely under GA requires firm adherence to protocol and an appreciation for the strengths and limitations of individual surgical venues. While relatively atraumatic, a significant portion of children who undergo surgery have pre-operative fear and anxiety. By considering child-specific conditions and interventions such as pre-surgery preparation and premedication, it may be possible to limit adverse psychological effects of the surgical experience. While GA allows the dental team to address oral health needs, it does not change the behaviors that caused the conditions. Relapse following GA is common; thus, clinicians should work together with families to improve post-operative outcomes.

## References

Adewumi, A., Hector, M.P., and King, J.M. (2001). Children and informed consent: A study of children's perceptions and involvement. *British Dental Journal*, 191, 256–259.

Al-Malik, M.I. and Al-Sarheed, M.A. (2006). Comprehensive dental care of pediatric patients treated under general anesthesia in a hospital setting in Saudi Arabia. *Journal of Contemporary Dental Practice*, 7, 79–88.

American Academy of Pediatric Dentistry. (2020). Behavior Guidance for the Pediatric Dental Patient. *The Reference Manual of Pediatric Dentistry* (pp. 292–310). American Academy of Pediatric Dentistry, Chicago, IL.

American Society of Anesthesiologists. (2017). Practice guidelines for preoperative fasting and the use of pharmacologic agents to reduce the risk of pulmonary aspiration: Application to healthy patients undergoing elective procedures: An updated report by the American Society of Anesthesiologists task force on preoperative fasting and the use of pharmacologic agents to reduce the risk of pulmonary aspiration. *Anesthesiology*, 126, 376–393.

American Society of Anesthesiologists. (2021). ASA and APSF Joint Statement on Elective Surgery and Anesthesia for Patients after COVID-19 Infection. Available at: https://www.asahq.org/about-asa/newsroom/news-releases/2021/03/asa-and-apsf-joint-statement-on-elective-surgery-and-anesthesia-for-patients-after-covid-19-infection-rv. Accessed on April 6, 2021.

Amin, M.S., Harrison, R.L., and Weinstein, P. (2006). A qualitative look at parents' experience of their child's dental general anaesthesia. *International Journal of Paediatric Dentistry*, 16, 309–319.

Amin, M.S. and Harrison, R.L. (2007). A conceptual model of parental behavior change following a child's dental general anesthesia procedure. *Pediatric Dentistry*, 29, 278–286.

Amin, M.S., Bedard, D., and Gamble, J. (2010). Early childhood caries: recurrence after comprehensive dental treatment under general anesthesia. *European Archives of Paediatric Dentistry*, 11, 269–273.

Anderson, H.K., Drummond, B.K., and Thomson, W.M. (2004). Changes in aspects of children's oral-health-related quality of life following dental treatment under general anaesthesia. *International Journal of Paediatric Dentistry*, 14, 317–325.

Atan, S., Ashley, P., Gilthorpe, M.S. et al. (2004). Morbidity following dental treatment of children under intubation general anesthesia. *International Journal of Paediatric Dentistry*, 14, 9–16.

Aydin, T., Sahin, L., Algin, C. et al. (2008). Do not mask the mask: Use it as a premedicant. *Pediatric Anesthesia*, 18, 107–112.

Bailey, A.G., McNauli, P.P., Jooste, E. et al. (2010). Perioperative crystalloid and colloid fluid management in children: Where are we and how did we get here? *Anesthesia & Analgesia*, 110, 375–390.

Belanger, J. and Kossick, M. (2015). Methods of identifying and managing the difficult airway in the pediatric population. *American Association of Nurse Anesthetists Journal*, 83, 35–41.

Blumer, S., Costa, L., and Peretz, B. (2017). Success of dental treatments under behavior management, sedation and general anesthesia. *Journal of Clinical Pediatric Dentistry*, 41, 308–311.

Brewer, S., Albino, J.E., Tedesco, L.A. et al. (2006). Pediatric anxiety: Child life intervention in day surgery. *Journal of Pediatric Nursing*, 21, 13–22.

Brodsky, L. (1989). Modern assessment of tonsils and adenoids. *Pediatric Clinics of North America*, 36, 1551–1569.

Caldwell-Andrews, A.A., Blount, R.L. , Mayes, L.C. et al. (2005). Motivation and maternal presence during induction of anesthesia. *Anesthesiology*, 103, 478–483.

Centers for Disease Control and Prevention. Interim Guidance on Duration of Isolation and Precautions for Adults with COVID-19. Available at: https://www.cdc.gov/coronavirus/2019-ncov/hcp/duration-isolation.html. Accessed on April 6, 2021.

Chan, C.S. and Molassiotis, A. (2002). The effects of an educational programme on the anxiety and satisfaction level of parents having parent present induction and visitation in a postanesthesia care unit. *Paediatric Anaesthesiology*, 12, 131–139.

Coté, C.J. and Wilson, S. (2019). Guidelines for monitoring and management of pediatric patients before, during, and after sedation for diagnostic and therapeutic procedures. *Pediatric Dentistry* 41, 26E–52E.

Costa, L.R., Harrison, R., Aleksejuniene, J. et al. (2011). Factors related to postoperative discomfort in young children following dental rehabilitation under general anesthesia. *Pediatric Dentistry*, 33, 321–326.

Cramton, R.E.M. and Gruchala, N.E. (2012). Managing procedural pain in pediatric patients. *Current Opinion in Pediatrics*, 24, 530–538.

da Fonseca, M.A. (2012). The effects of poverty on children's development and oral health. *Pediatric Dentistry*, 34, 32–38.

Davidson, A.J., Disma, N., de Graaff, J.C. et al. (2016). Neurodevelopmental outcome at 2 years of age after general anaesthesia and awake-regional anaesthesia in infancy (GAS): an international multicentre, randomised controlled trial. *Lancet*, 387, 239–250.

Edmonds, B., Willimans, T., and Carrico, C. (2019). The prevalence and factors associated with sibling-recurrent dental treatment under general anesthesia at an academic institution. *Pediatric Dentistry*, 41, 40–46.

Erkmen Almaz, M., Akbay Oba, A., and Saroglu Sonmez, I. (2019). Postoperative morbidity in pediatric patients following dental treatment under general anesthesia. *European Oral Research*, 53, 113–118.

Felder-Puig, R., Maksys, A., Noestlinger, H.G. et al. (2003). Using a children's book to prepare children and parents for elective ENT surgery. *International Journal of Pediatric Otorhinolaryngology*, 67, 35–41.

Fortier, M.A., Chorney, J.M., Rony, R.Y. et al. (2009). Children's desire for perioperative information. *Anesthesia & Analgesia*, 109, 1085–1090.

Ganzberg, S. (2017). The FDA warning on anesthesia drugs. *Anesthesia Progress*, 64, 57–58.

Gazal, G. and Mackie, I.C. (2007). A comparison of paracetamol, ibuprofen or their combination for pain relief following extractions in children under general anaesthesia: A randomized controlled trial. *International Journal of Paediatric Dentistry*, 17, 169–177.

Green, L.K., Lee, J.Y., Roberts, M.W. et al. (2018). Cost analysis of three pharmacologic behavior guidance modalities in pediatric dentistry. *Pediatric Dentistry*, 40, 419–424.

Grimes, C.E., Bowman, K.G., Dodgion, C.M. et al. (2011). Systematic review of barriers to surgical care in low-income and middle-income countries. *World Journal of Surgery*, 35, 941–950.

Hankinson, T.C. and Anderson, R.C.E. (2010). Craniovertebral junction abnormalities in Down syndrome. *Neurosurgery*, 66(3 Suppl), 32–38.

Hausen, H., Karkkainen, S., and Seppa, L. (2000). Application of high-risk strategy to control dental caries. *Community Dental and Oral Epidemiology*, 28, 26–34.

Hu, Y.H., Tsai, A., Ou-Yang, L.W. et al. (2018). Postoperative dental morbidity in children following dental treatment under general anesthesia. *BMC Oral Health*, 18, 84.

Jankauskiene, B., Virtanen, J.I., and Narbutaite, J. (2017). Follow-up of children's oral health-related quality of life after dental general anesthesia treatment. *Acta Odontologica Scandinavia*, 75, 255–261.

Jensen, B. (2012). Post-operative pain and pain management in children after dental extractions under general anesthesia. *European Archives of Paediatric Dentistry*, 13, 119–125.

Johhnson, B., Serban, N., Griffin, P. et al. (2019). Projecting the economic impact of silver diamine fluoride on caries treatment expenditures and outcomes in young U.S. children. *Journal of Public Health Dentistry*, 79, 215–221.

Justus, R., Wyles, D., Wilson, J. et al. (2006). Preparing children and families for surgery: Mount Sinai's multidisciplinary perspective. *Pediatric Nursing*, 32, 35–43.

Kain, Z.N., Mayes, L.C., O'Connor, T.Z. et al. (2000). Social adaptability, cognitive abilities, and other predictors for children's reactions to surgery. *Journal of Clinical Anesthesiology*, 12, 549–554.

Kain, Z.N., Caldwell-Andrews, A.A., Mayes, L.C. et al. (2004). Trends in the practice of parental presence during induction of anesthesia and the use of preoperative sedative premedication in the United States, 1995–2002: Results of a follow-up national survey. *Anesthesia & Analgesia*, 98, 1252–1259.

Kain, Z.N. and Caldwell-Andrews, A.A. (2005). Preoperative psychological preparation of the child for surgery: An update. *Anesthesiology Clinics of North America*, 23, 597–614.

Kain, Z.N., Caldwell-Andrews, A.A., Maranets, I. et al. (2006). Predicting which child-parent pair will benefit from parental presence during induction of anesthesia: A decision making approach. *Anesthesia & Analgesia*, 102, 81–84.

Kakaounaki, E., Tahmassebi, J.I., and Fayle, S.A. (2011). Repeat general anesthesia, a 6-year follow up. *International Journal of Paediatric Dentistry*, 21, 126–131.

Karki, A.J., Thomas, D.R., and Chestnutt, I.G. (2011). Why has oral health promotion and prevention failed children requiring general anaesthesia for dental extractions? *Community Dental Health*, 28, 255–258.

Kavanaugh, M., Halterman, J.S., Montes, G. et al. (2006). Maternal depressive symptoms are adversely associated with prevention practices and parenting behaviors for preschool children. *Ambulatory Pediatrics*, 6, 32–37.

Kerimoglu, B., Neuman, A., Paul, J. et al. (2013). Anesthesia induction using video glasses as a distraction tool for the management of preoperative anxiety in children. *Anesthesia Analgesia*, 117, 1373–1379.

Kim, H., Jung, S.M., Yu, H. et al. (2015). Video distraction and parental presence for the management of preoperative anxiety and postoperative behavioral disturbance in children: A randomized controlled trial. *Anesthesia Analgesia*, 121, 778–784.

Klaassen, M.A., Veerkamp, J.S.J., and Hoogstraten, J. (2009). Young children's oral health-related quality of life and dental fear after treatment under general anaesthesia: A randomized controlled trial. *European Journal of Oral Sciences*, 117, 273–278.

Klingberg, G., Lingstrom, P., Oskarsdottir, S. et al. (2010). Specialist paediatric dentistry in Sweden 2008—a 25-year perspective. *International Journal of Paediatric Dentistry*, 20, 313–321.

Mallampati, S.R., Gatt, S.P., Gugino, L.D. et al. (1985). A clinical sign to predict difficult tracheal intubation: A prospective study. *Canadian Anaesthetists' Society Journal*, 32, 429–434.

Manyande, A., Cyna, A.M., Yip, P. et al. (2015). Non-pharmacological interventions for assisting the induction of anaesthesia in children. *Cochrane Database of Systematic Reviews*, 7, CD006447.

Martinez, D. and Wilson, S. (2006). Children sedated for dental care: A pilot study of the 24-hour postsedation period. *Pediatric Dentistry*, 28, 260–264.

Matton, S. and Romeo, G.P. (2017). Behavioral regression in 2 patients with autism spectrum disorders and attention deficit/hyperactivity disorder after oral surgery performed with a general anesthetic. *JADA*, 148, 519–524.

Mayeda, C. and Wilson, S. (2009). Complications within the first 24 hours after dental rehabilitation under general anesthesia. *Pediatric Dentistry*, 31, 513–519.

McCann, M.E., de Graaff, J.C., Dorris, L. et al. (2019). Neurodevelopmental outcome at 5 years of age after general anaesthesia or awake-regional anaesthesia in infancy (GAS): an international, multicenter, randomized, controlled equivalence trial. *Lancet*, 393, 664–677.

McWilliams, P.A. and Rutherford, J.S. (2007). Assessment of early postoperative pain and haemorrhage in young children undergoing dental extractions under general anaesthesia. *International Journal of Paediatric Dentistry*, 17, 352–357.

Moness Ali, A.M. and Hammuda, AA. (2019). Local anesthesia effects on postoperative pain after pediatric oral rehabilitation under general anesthesia. *Pediatric Dentistry*, 41, 181–185.

Murat, I. and Dubois, M.C. (2008). Perioperative fluid therapy in pediatrics. *Pediatric Anesthesia*, 18, 363–370.

Needleman, H.L. et al. (2008). Postoperative pain and other sequelae of dental rehabilitations performed on children under general anesthesia. *Pediatric Dentistry*, 30, 111–121.

Nelson, T. (2013). The continuum of behavior guidance. *Dental Clinics of North America*, 57, 129–143.

Oh, T.H. (1980). Formulas for calculating fluid maintenance requirements. *Anesthesiology*, 53, 351.

Oliveira, B.H., Rajendra, A., Veitz-Keenan, A. et al. (2019). The effect of silver diamine fluoride on preventing caries in the primary dentition: A systematic review and meta-analysis. *Caries Research*, 53, 24–32.

O'Leary, J.D., Janus, M., Duku, E. et al. (2019). Influence of surgical procedures and general anesthesia on child development before primary school entry among matched sibling pairs. *JAMA Pediatrics*, 173, 29–36.

Olley, R.C., Hosey, M.T., Renton, T. et al. (2011). Why are children still having preventable extractions under general anaesthetic? A service evaluation of a high caries risk group of children. *British Dental Journal*, 210, E13.

Pappas, A., Raja, S., da Fonseca, M.A. et al. (2020). Female caregivers' depression risk affects children's attendance to dental appointments – A pilot study. *Pediatric Dentistry*, 42:464–469.

Patel, A.M. (2004). Appropriate consent and referral for general anaesthesia—a survey in the Paediatric Day Care Unit, Barnsley DGH NHS Trust, South Yorkshire. *British Dental Journal*, 196, 275–277.

Patel, M., McTigue, D.J., Thikkurissy, S. et al. (2016). Parental attitudes toward advanced behavior guidance techniques used in pediatric dentistry. *Pediatric Dentistry*, 38, 30–36.

Paterson, N. and Waterhouse, P. (2011). Risk in pediatric anesthesia. *Pediatric Anesthesia*, 21, 848–857.

Peerbhay, F.B. (2009). Compliance with preventive care following dental treatment of children under general anaesthesia. *South African Dental Journal*, 64, 442, 444–445.

Perry, J.N., Hooper, V.D., and Masiongale, J. (2012). Reduction of preoperative anxiety in pediatric surgery patients using age-appropriate teaching interventions. *Journal of Perianesthesia Nursing*, 27, 69–81.

Pham, L., Tanbonliong, T., Dizon, M.B. et al. (2018). Trends in general anesthesia utilization by board-certified pediatric dentists. *Pediatric Dentistry*, 40, 124–130.

Primosch, R.E., Balsewich, C.M., and Thomas, C.W. (2001). Outcomes assessment an intervention strategy to improve parental compliance to follow-up evaluations after treatment of early childhood caries using general anesthesia in a Medicaid population. *Journal of Dentistry for Children*, 68, 102–108.

Przybylo, H.J., Tarbell, S.E., and Stevenson, G.W. (2005). Mask fear in children presenting for anesthesia: Aversion, phobia, or both? *Pediatric Anesthesia*, 15, 366–370.

Rodd, H., Hall, M., Deery, C. et al. (2014). "I felt weird and wobbly": Child-reported impacts associated with a dental general anaesthetic. *British Dental Journal*, 216, E17.

Rony, R.Y., Fortier, M.A., Chorney, J.M. et al. (2010). Parental postoperative pain management: Attitudes, assessment, and management. *Pediatrics*, 125, e1372–e1378.

Russo, S.G. and Becke, K. (2015). Expected difficult airway in children. *Current Opinion in Anesthesiology*, 28, 321–326.

Savanheimo, N., Vehkalahti, M.M., Pihakari, A. et al. (2005). Reasons for and parental satisfaction with children's dental care under general anaesthesia. *International Journal of Paediatric Dentistry*, 15, 448–454.

Savanheimo, N. and Vehkalahti, M.M. (2008). Preventive aspects in children's caries treatments preceding dental care under general anesthesia. *International Journal of Paediatric Dentistry*, 18, 117–123.

Schroth, R.J., Pang, J.L., Levi, J.A. et al. (2014). Trends in pediatric dental surgery for severe early childhood caries in Manitoba, Canada. *Journal of the Canadian Dental Association*, 80, e65.

Shahid, S.K., Godson, J.H., Williams, S.A. et al. (2008). Obtaining informed consent for children receiving dental care: A pilot study. *Primary Dental Care*, 15, 17–22.

Shay, H., Frumento, R.J., and Bastien, A. (2007). General anesthesia and methylenetetrahydropholate reductase deficiency. *Journal of Anesthesia*, 21, 493–496.

Sheller, B., Williams, B.J., Hays, K. et al. (2003). Reasons for repeat dental treatment under general anesthesia for the healthy child. *Pediatric Dentistry*, 25, 546–552.

Sohn, V.Y., Zenger, D., and Steele, S.R. (2012). Pain management in the pediatric surgical patient. *Surgical Clinics of North America*, 92, 471–485.

Somri, M., Coran, A.G., Hadjittofi, C. et al. (2012). Improved outcomes in paediatric anesthesia: Contributing factors. *Pediatric Surgery International*, 28, 553–561.

Spera, A.L., Saxen, M., Yepes, J. et al. (2017). Office-based anesthesia: Safety and outcomes in pediatric dental patients. *Anesthesia Progress*, 64, 144–152.

Stewart, S.H., Buffett-Jerrott, S.E., Finley, G.A. et al. (2006). Effects of midazolam on explicit vs implicit memory in a pediatric surgery setting. *Psychopharmacology*, 188, 489–497.

Sun, L.S., Li, G., Miller, T.L. et al. (2016). Association between a single general anesthesia exposure before age 36 months and neurocognitive outcomes in later childhood. *JAMA*, 315, 2312–2320.

Thomson, W.M. and Malden, P.E. (2011). Assessing change in the family impact of caries in young children after treatment under general anesthesia. *Acta Odontologica Scandinavica*, 69, 257–262.

Townsend, J.A., Ganzberg, S., and Thikkurissy, S. (2009). The effect of local anesthetic on quality of recovery characteristics following dental rehabilitation under general anesthesia in children. *Anesthesia Progress*, 56, 115–122.

Turner, E. G. and Hipp, C.L. (2018). Hospital Dentistry and General Anesthesia. In: A. J. Nowak and Casamassimo, P. S. (Eds.), The Handbook of Pediatric Dentistry, 282–297. American Academy of Pediatric Dentistry, Chicago, IL.

Tzong, K.Y., Han, S., Roh, A. et al. (2012). Epidemiology of pediatric surgical admissions in US children: Data from the HCUP. *Journal of Neurosurgical Anesthesiology*, 24, 391–395.

Watts, A.K., Thikkurissy, S., Smiley, M. et al. (2009). Local anesthesia affects physiologic parameters and reduces anesthesiologist intervention in children undergoing general anesthesia for dental rehabilitation. *Pediatric Dentistry*, 31, 414–419.

Wilson, S. and Alcaino, E. (2011). Survey on sedation in paediatric dentistry: A global perspective. *International Journal of Paediatric Dentistry*, 21, 321–332.

Wilson, S. and Ganzberg, S.I. (2013). Pain perception control. In: P.S. Casamassimo, H.W. Fields, D.J. McTigue, A.J. Nowak (Eds.), Pediatric Dentistry Infancy Through Adolescence, 5th ed., 98–104. Elsevier Saunders, St. Louis.

Wollin, S.R., Plummer, J.L., Owen, H. et al. (2003). Predictors of preoperative anxiety in children. *Anaesthesia & Intensive Care*, 31, 69–74.

Wright, K.D., Stewart, S.H., Finley, G.A. et al. (2007). Prevention and intervention strategies to alleviate preoperative anxiety in children: A critical review. *Behavior Modification*, 31, 52–79.

Yarmarkovich, P. , Alrayyes S., Lee, H.H. et al. (2019). SDF's role in reducing urgent-care encounters while awaiting general anesthesia. *Pediatric Dentistry*, 41, 179.

Young, A.S., Fischer, M.W., Lang, N.S. et al. (2018). Practice patterns of dentist anesthesiologists in North America. *Anesthesia Progress*, 65, 9–15.

# 16

# Management of Emergencies Associated with Sedation for the Pediatric Dental Patient

*Kenneth L. Reed and Amanda Jo Okundaye*

## Introduction

Medical emergencies, sometimes life-threatening, can and do occur in the pediatric dental office. While one generally thinks of these as affecting the patient, many medical emergencies occur to others in the dental office such as parents or caregivers, the pediatric dentist, and dental staff. Additionally, many pediatric dentists treat patients with special needs who tend to be relatively older, with more "adult" types of medical emergencies. However, the focus of this chapter will be management of medical emergencies directly associated with sedation in pediatric dentistry. For all other emergency situations, the reader is referred to textbooks devoted entirely to this subject (Bennet and Rosenberg 2002; Malamed 2014).

In-office sedation to treat children has increased over the past three decades. It is estimated that over 20% of children will require pharmacosedation to safely and efficiently complete dental treatment. Children present the highest risk and lowest error tolerance in patient safety during sedation procedures. Although rare, the most serious adverse outcomes of pediatric sedation are brain damage and death. Precipitating adverse events to these tragic outcomes are primarily respiratory, owing to the child's respiratory and cardiopulmonary physiology and anatomy (Chicka 2012). Prevention of an emergency is much more desirable than managing one once it occurs. Most sedation-related medical emergencies are avoidable. Strict adherence to sedation guidelines does not guarantee that emergencies will not occur, but it will definitely prevent most of them. A recent study of malpractice incidents shows that guidelines were not followed in the majority of cases of adverse outcomes (Chikca 2012). Potential problems also may occur due to poor patient evaluation before treatment, overdoses of sedation and/or local anesthesia agents, improper monitoring, and failure to react properly once an emergency situation has been detected.

The basic algorithm for the management of most medical emergencies is (P) position, (A) airway, (B) breathing, (C) circulation, and (D) definitive care: differential diagnosis, drugs, and defibrillation. The algorithm will be discussed in detail, as it relates to sedation in pediatric dentistry.

## Medical History

Familiarity with the patient's medical history is highly important in preventing medical emergencies. Knowing what to expect of the patient based on his/her medical history is invaluable. Completion of the medical history questionnaire before the start of any dental treatment is mandatory. The questionnaire may be completed by the patient's parent or legal guardian (Malamed 2010b). In recent years, computerized medical history forms have become available, simplifying the history-taking process.

Next, the pediatric dentist reviews the completed form with the patient's parent and questions any medical problems that have been reported. Through this dialog, the dentist seeks to determine any reported medical disorder's significance to the proposed sedation. For example, if a patient has history of asthma, the review of the medical history will include the following questions: "How often does the patient experience attacks?"; "Are there any specific triggers?"; "When was the last attack?"; "Did it require a visit to the emergency room or hospitalization?"; "Has the child ever required intubation in the hospital to manage the asthmatic attack?"; "What medications is the patient taking?"; and "Does the child carry albuterol with them on a regular basis?" Obtaining medical histories for all patients has been discussed in Chapter 7; however, it is of utmost importance when scheduling a patient to receive sedation.

## Physical Examination

The next step is a physical exam. Pediatric dentists actually perform a physical exam on each patient, whether they realize it or not. It may not be as comprehensive or time-consuming, nor is it done in exactly the same fashion as those conducted by physicians, but nevertheless, one is done. The physical exam that pediatric dentists perform is partially formal and partially informal. The informal part consists of things like a simple visual inspection of the patient. By simple observation, the pediatric dentist can determine if a patient has various gross diseases such as obesity, jaundice, exophthalmos, breathing difficulties (asthma or other bronchospastic diseases), or heart defects; possibly, even conditions such as attention deficit hyperactivity disorder (ADHD) may be determined. These two items, history and physical examinations, are referred to as the *H&P*.

The more formal portion of the physical exam consists of things such as recording blood pressure, pulse rate, respirations, height, weight, body mass index (BMI) percentile, Mallampati classification, Brodsky scale, and American Society of Anesthesiology (ASA) Physical Status.

## Body Mass Index Percentile (BMI)

BMI percentile is used as a screening tool to identify possible weight problems for children. The Centers for Disease Control and Prevention (CDC) and the American Academy of Pediatrics (AAP) recommend the use of BMI to screen for overweight and obesity in children beginning at age two years.

BMI for age percentile results are divided into four main groups: children under 5th percentile are considered underweight; those between 5th and 85th percentile, healthy weight; those between 85th and 95th percentile are overweight; and those above 95th percentile are obese, by definition. A recent study examined childhood overweight/obesity as a risk factor for adverse events during sedation for dental procedures (Kang et al. 2012). Overall, weight percentiles were higher in children who had one or more adverse events. Similarly, patients with higher BMI percentiles were more likely to experience adverse events. Although preliminary in nature, these findings suggest that childhood overweight/obesity may be associated with adverse events during sedation for dental procedures. Obese child patients in need of sedation may be referred to a medical center or may be treated together with a dentist anesthesiologist, if appropriate.

## Mallampati Airway Classification

The original Mallampati classification consisted of three classes (Mallampati et al. 1985), but was subsequently expanded into the widely known four-class version (Nuckton et al. 2006), as shown in Figure 16-1.

Mallampati (Samsoon and Young 1987) grading of the upper airway is as follows:

- Class I: everything visible (tonsillar pillars)
- Class II: uvula fully visible, fauces visible
- Class III: only soft palate and base of uvula visible
- Class IV: cannot see soft palate

The Mallampati score is an independent predictor of the presence and severity of obstructive sleep apnea. On average, for every one-point increase in the Mallampati score, the odds of having obstructive sleep apnea increase more than twofold (Nuckton et al. 2006). Patients with obstructive sleep apnea are generally not good candidates for moderate sedation administered by the pediatric dentist, as the perioperative risk to patients increases in proportion to the severity of sleep apnea. The pediatric dentist should consider working with a dentist anesthesiologist potentially utilizing a secured airway to treat these patients (see Chapter 14).

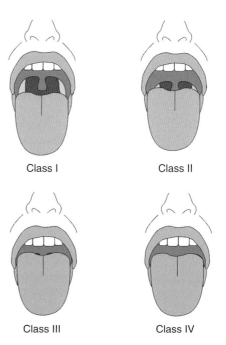

Class I          Class II

Class III        Class IV

**Figure 16-1** Mallampati classification, as modified by Samsoon and Young. Class I: uvula, faucial pillars, and soft palate are visible. Class II: faucial pillars and soft palate are visible. Class III: soft palate is visible. Class IV: only hard palate is visible. *Source:* Baker and Yagiela (2006). © 2006, American Academy of Pediatric Dentistry.

By the age of eight years or so, most children have an airway that resembles that of an adult more than that of an infant or small child. Prior to this point, there are significant anatomical differences compared to adults. Infants have a larynx at C3–4—not C4–5, as in adults—that pushes the tongue, that is larger, superiorly. The epiglottis is also larger, stiffer, and angled posteriorly. Pediatric patients have a large thyroid cartilage and a narrow cricoid cartilage—the narrowest portion of the airway in pediatric patients. Infants may require shoulder or neck rolls in the event that they require facemask ventilation. When evaluating infants, pay particular attention to the chin: if it is posterior to the upper lip, a difficult airway can be expected. Nasal and oral airways can be particularly useful in infants or pediatric patients.

After completion and review of the H&P, the dentist assigns the patient to an ASA physical status category. Most patients, especially pediatric dental patients, are quite healthy. By definition, these are "ASA I" patients with low risk of complications.

## Brodsky Scale

Size 0: The tonsils are absent or have been removed.

Size 1: Barely visible. This is the normal tonsil size. It indicates that the tonsil extends to the pillars.

Size 2: The tongue tissue is not beyond the tonsillar pillars. This is also normal tonsil size. It indicates that the tonsils extend to the pillars.

Size 3: Up to 75% of oropharyngeal airway is taken up by the tonsil. The tonsils are enlarged and seen with infection. It indicates that tonsils extend beyond the pillars but stop short of the midline.

Size 4: More than 75% of airways is taken up by the tonsil. It is seen with significant or almost touching. It indicates that tonsils extend to the midline and are almost touching each other (Brodsky 1989; see Figure 16-2).

## American Society of Anesthesiology (ASA) Physical Status

The American Society of Anesthesiology (ASA) proposed the physical status (ASA PS) classification of preoperative patients for anesthetic risk assessment in 1963. The ASA score is a subjective assessment of a patient's overall health based on five classes (see Table 11-3 in Chapter 11). Only patients with an ASA score of I (a completely healthy, fit patient) or II (a patient with mild systemic disease) should be sedated in a private dental

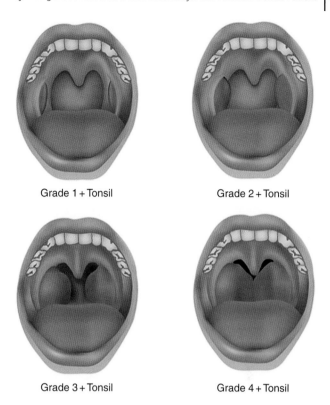

Grade 1 + Tonsil    Grade 2 + Tonsil

Grade 3 + Tonsil    Grade 4 + Tonsil

**Figure 16-2** Grading of palatine tonsils hypertrophy proposed by L. Brodsky. *Source:* Redrawn from Brodsky (1989). Reproduced with permission from Elsevier Co.

setting. Wolters et al. (1996) examined the strength of association between ASA physical status classification and perioperative risk factors and post-operative outcome, concluding that ASA physical status classification was a predictor of postoperative outcome. To summarize, a patient's BMI, airway evaluation and ASA score may all be used to screen out potentially complicated patients.

## ADSA Ten Minutes Saves a Life!®

The Anesthesia Research Foundation of the American Dental Society of Anesthesiology (ADSA) released a "ADSA Ten Minutes Saves a Life!®" application for smartphones and tablets and a dynamic PDF for laptop and desktop computers in November 2018.

Safety checklists originated from the military aviation industry in the 1930s following the crash of the prototype of the B-17 Flying Fortress. Powered flight had become increasingly complex, so much so that it was easy for pilots to overlook or forget critical steps that lead to disasters. Having a checklist eliminated the risk of pilots forgetting one or more of these critical steps and drastically improved aviation safety.

Studies show that memory worsens during periods of stress, and critical steps in the management of rare events often get overlooked. As a result, checklists have become integrated into many industries and professions, such as nuclear power, aviation, and medicine. Checklists serve as cognitive aids during rare crisis events and guide individual actions during the management of that crisis.

The World Health Organization pioneered the use of checklists during surgery more than 10 years ago. Stanford and Harvard Universities have since published emergency cognitive aid manuals for operating room crisis management.

This manual and electronic application is the first cognitive aid resource for dental practitioners providing office-based anesthesia and sedation care and was funded through a grant from the American Dental Society of Anesthesiology's Anesthesia Research Foundation.

The Ten Minutes Saves A Life!® Manual and Application is divided into sections containing common critical events seen during dental office-based anesthesia and sedation. The algorithms vary with the training level of the provider and are meant to guide management of the crisis during the first 10 minutes until emergency medical service (EMS) arrives. Drug doses are taken from multiple sources, including drug package inserts and authoritative texts. They are automatically populated into the algorithms once the weight of the patient is entered.

In addition to use during an actual crisis events, this cognitive aid is also intended for use during office team mock practice drills of crisis resource management. This application is free to all and may be downloaded from the App Store or Google Play. It is automatically updated to the latest version when opening the app while in Wi-Fi or cell service range.

The Anesthesia Research Foundation Working Group sincerely hopes this manual and electronic application will contribute to patient safety in dentistry.

## Medical Emergencies

Early recognition of medical emergencies begins at the first sign or symptom (Norris 1994). The pediatric dentist needs to focus on what is happening second-by-second during a medical emergency. Distractions slow response time, and pediatric patients have physiological and anatomical differences from adults. This causes medical emergencies in pediatric patients to proceed much more rapidly than with adults. When treatment is indicated, the dentist should immediately proceed. Management of medical emergencies in the dental office may be limited to supporting a patient's vital functions until EMS arrives, especially in the case of major morbidity. It may also involve real, aggressive action to address a particular situation such as anaphylaxis. Treatment should at the minimum consist of basic life support and monitoring of vital signs (Fukayama and Yagiela 2006).

The dentist should never administer poorly understood medications. The drugs discussed in this chapter will be limited to those that a pediatric dentist is trained to use and administer. Since there is no venous access during minimal and moderate sedation, drugs given only intravenously will be avoided; however, we will discuss intraosseous access (IO) and drug administration.

### Emergency Kit

A medical emergency kit for a pediatric dental office should consist of three broad categories: equipment, supplies, and drugs. Only equipment and drugs that the pediatric dentist should be able to use confidently will be discussed. However, other components of both equipment and drugs may be required in the dental office. Readers are referred to the AAPD guidelines and to their relevant state or national regulations for other requirements.

### Equipment
- Oxygen E tank with regulator, including pressure gauge and flow adjustment
- Pediatric non-rebreather face mask
- Resuscitation bag, adult 1,000 mL, with pressure manometer and face mask
- Resuscitation bag, pediatric 500 mL, with pressure manometer and face mask
- Stethoscope
- Blood pressure cuff (small and medium) and aneroid sphygmomanometer
- Automatic external defibrillator programmed as per current AHA guidelines with pediatric pads
- Magill forceps. These can be lifesaving in retrieving foreign objects lost in the hypopharynx during dental therapy.

### Supplies
- Yankauer tip. This suction tip is designed to allow effective suction without damaging surrounding tissue. It is used to suction oropharyngeal secretions in order to prevent aspiration.
- Suction tubing, vacuum high volume system adapter
- Nasal cannula
- Nasopharyngeal airways (soft): 4.0, 4.5, 5.0, and 6.0 mm I.D.
- Oral airways (Guedel): 40 mm, 60 mm, and 80 mm
- Laryngeal mask (Supraglottic) airway sizes 1.5 (5–12 kg), 2 (10–25 kg) and 2.5 (25–35 kg)

### Drugs
The following list relates to the limited discussion of this chapter. The basic drug kit for medical emergencies consists at the minimum seven to nine drugs:

- Oxygen (E-Cylinder)
- Epinephrine Pediatric auto-injectors (0.15 mg/actuation), epinephrine adult auto-injector (0.3 mg/actuation), and 1:1000 (1 mg/mL) ampule—quantity two.
- Albuterol (Ventolin) inhalation aerosol (90 mcg/ actuation)
- Diphenhydramine parenteral injection, 50 mg/mL
- Aspirin 325 mg, non-enteric coated
- Nitroglycerin, 0.4 mg tablets
- A form of glucose

Additional medications required if oral sedation using opioids and/or benzodiazepines are used include Naloxone (0.4 mg/mL, 1 mL vial) and Flumazenil (0.1 mg/mL, 10 mL vial). Flumazenil is to be administered **IV/IO only**.

## Management of Medical Emergencies

An emergency management plan, as described by Haas (2010) and Peskin and Siegelman (1995), is of paramount importance. It is recommended that all medical emergencies be managed in the same way by using what is known as the *basic algorithm* (Malamed 2015): (P) position, (A) airway, (B) breathing, (C) circulation, and (D) definitive care: differential diagnosis, drugs, and defibrillation (see Figure 16-3).

The one exception is cardiac arrest, where the currently suggested algorithm is (C) circulation, (A) airway, and then (B) breathing. The basic algorithm for managing all medical emergencies is consistent—that is, one algorithm fits all cases, and all cases are worked through in the same organizational method each and every time. This adds consistency and predictability to a response to a medical emergency. Prevention, prompt recognition, and efficient management of medical emergencies by a well-prepared dental team can increase the likelihood of a satisfactory outcome. Note that drug therapy is always secondary to basic life support. The basic intent in responding to a medical emergency is always the same: ensure that the patient's brain receives a constant supply of blood containing oxygen and glucose with enough perfusion pressure to keep it functioning, and without morbidity.

---

### Pharmacology and Doses of Basic Emergency Drugs

- Albuterol is used in bronchospastic medical emergencies (acute asthmatic attack) as an inhaled beta-2 specific agonist. It causes bronchodilation that increases the lumen size of the bronchioles, leading to better oxygen uptake.
  Dose: Two puffs with deep inspiration.
  [source: drug package insert]
- Epinephrine is the universal agonist; it affects alpha one, alpha two, beta one, and beta two receptors. This is the only drug in the medical emergency kit that must be given rapidly in order to save a patient's life. In case of anaphylaxis, the severe life-threatening allergic reaction, this is the only drug that will help. Alpha one agonistic activity increases blood pressure by causing a vasoconstriction. Beta one effects of epinephrine increase heart rate, force of contraction, stroke volume, and cardiac output. Epinephrine's beta two effects cause bronchodilation, making breathing easier. It may also be used for severe asthmatic attacks unresponsive to albuterol.
  Dose: Pediatric 0.01 mg/kg IM, maximum 0.3 mg/dose. Adult: 0.3 mg/dose
  [source: drug package insert]
- Diphenhydramine is used for mild allergic reactions. Histamine blockers reverse the actions of histamine by occupying H1 receptor sites on the effector cell and are effective in patients with mild or delayed-onset allergic reactions.

  Dose: 2 mg/kg IM up to 50 mg.
  [source: drug package insert]
- Naloxone is required in the medical emergency kit only if sedation using an opioid is used in the pediatric dental office. Naloxone is the specific antagonist for any of the opioids. It may be administered IV, IN, IM or IO and has a duration of action of roughly 45 minutes if administered IV/IO, and four hours if administered IM.
  [source: package insert for Narcan®]
- Flumazenil. Most regulatory jurisdictions will require the immediate availability of flumazenil as a component of the medical emergency kit if sedation using a benzodiazepine is used in the pediatric dental office. While this drug may be legally required, it must be strongly emphasized that the package insert for flumazenil, in no uncertain terms, explicitly says that this drug must be administered IV only. Pediatric Advanced Life Support (PALS) equates IO administration with IV administration of a drug. Therefore, if no one in the pediatric dental office is trained to start an IV or have done so recently, the reality is that flumazenil will not be a valuable drug in a medical emergency unless it is administered IO. IO is, practically speaking, the "go to" route of administration for flumazenil.
  [source: package insert for Romazicon]

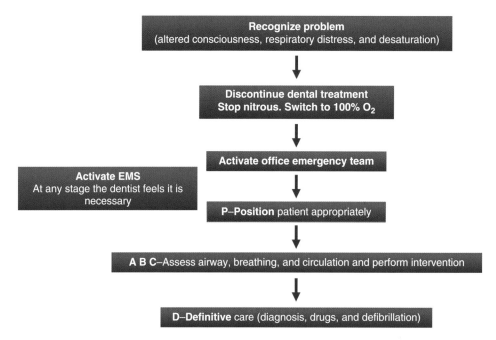

**Recognize problem**
(altered consciousness, respiratory distress, and desaturation)

↓

**Discontinue dental treatment**
**Stop nitrous. Switch to 100% O₂**

↓

**Activate office emergency team**

**Activate EMS**
At any stage the dentist feels it is necessary

↓

**P–Position** patient appropriately

↓

**A B C**–Assess airway, breathing, and circulation and perform intervention

↓

**D–Definitive** care (diagnosis, drugs, and defibrillation)

**Figure 16-3** Dentists should initially manage all medical emergencies in the same way by using what is known as the *basic algorithm. Source:* Based on Malamed (2014).

### Recognize the Problem

Prior to initiating the emergency algorathim protocol, the pediatric dentist needs to recognize that an emergency situation is present. Recognition of the sedated pediatric patient's problem comes about by continuous monitoring, as per AAPD guidelines. The patient's pulse, oxygen saturation, and breathing should always be within age-appropriate normal ranges. Heart rates are typically higher in children and decrease with increasing age. For example, the normal ranges are 80–130 BPM in a two-year-old and 70–110 BPM in a 10-year-old (Haas 2010). Any changes need to be immediately identified and analyzed. The following can be regarded as warning signs:

- **Change in saturation level**: If this occurs, reposition pulse oximeter probe (or, if the extremity is restrained, loosen strap), reposition head, and raise the chin. If level returns to normal, continue treatment.
- **The unresponsive sedated patient**: For the most part, pediatric dentists only administer minimal and moderate sedation. Patients undergoing such sedations should be responsive.

A sedated patient who fails to respond may have advanced to a state of deep sedation, which represents an emergency situation. Therefore, the dentist should cease treatment and evaluate the patient's state. To begin patient evaluation, try to elicit a response. After verifying unresponsiveness by stimulating the patient, including head tilt and jaw lift (Figure 16-4), remove rubber dam.

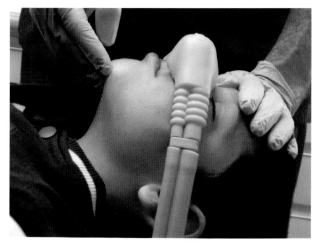

**Figure 16-4** The head-tilt chin-lift maneuver. *Source:* Courtesy of Dr. Ari Kupietzky.

If using nitrous oxide sedation, immediately deliver 100% oxygen. Activate the office emergency team plan/protocol. EMS should be sought as soon as the dentist who is legally responsible for the patient feels it is needed.

Following these steps, proceed immediately to (P) position: place the patient supine in the dental chair with legs elevated slightly (Figure 16-5).

Chest compression, if needed, can be effectively performed in the dental chair. Lepere et al. (2003) demonstrated that the modern dental chair provides firm support for the spinal cord, enabling sufficient blood volume to circulate during cardiac arrest. Most dental chairs are programmable,

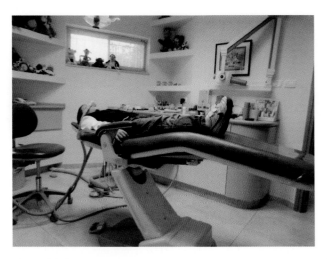

**Figure 16-5** The patient is placed supine in the dental chair with legs elevated slightly. *Source:* Courtesy of Dr. Ari Kupietzky.

allowing the clinician to preset an emergency position option. Pediatric treatment benches are flat and suitable for delivery of all emergency treatments; a pillow may be placed under the child's legs for their elevation. Almost all medical emergencies involving loss of consciousness share the same cause: low blood pressure in the brain. Unconsciousness is defined as the absence of response to sensory stimulation (e.g., verbal or physical stimulation). Making the patient supine will increase blood pressure in the brain and allow the patient to regain consciousness in most cases. If the patient remains unresponsive, proceed to ABC.

### Airway

Practitioners and staff members must ensure patency by tilting the patient's head and lifting the chin immediately. By itself, this maneuver may prevent brain damage, as it moves the tongue away from the back of the pharynx, thereby eliminating the obstruction (the tongue). In turn, this permits oxygenation and ventilation. If the airway is not patent after this maneuver, the clinician should reposition the patient's head once more. If the airway still is not opened, the clinician should perform a jaw thrust maneuver by placing his or her thumbs posterior to the angle of the patient's mandible and advancing them (and the mandible) anteriorly. The two most common emergencies encountered while sedating a pediatric patient are respiratory obstruction and respiratory depression (Haas 2010).

### Respiratory Obstruction

By far, the most common type of medical emergency from an oral sedation overdose is respiratory obstruction. In this case, it is the obligation of the pediatric dentist to stop the dental procedure and "rescue" the patient. While it is

possible that a patient may be sensitive to a drug, the dentists administering more than the recommended dose of a sedation agent causes the overwhelming majority of oral sedation overdoses in pediatric dental offices. Benzodiazepines are most likely to cause respiratory obstruction. They are the most widely used class of drugs for oral sedation in the pediatric dental office today, and when used in recommended doses, they are remarkably safe. Some pediatric dentists, however, are tempted to push the limits of oral sedation in their practices. While it is true that increasing the dose of a sedative agent increases efficacy, it is equally true that increasing doses beyond manufacturer's recommendations leads to decreased safety. The dose in a package insert has been shown to be both safe and efficacious. Beyond that dose, there is no safety data.

The tongue relaxing and obstructing the airway typically causes respiratory obstruction. The treatment is to pull the tongue off of the airway, which has classically been treated as simply a head tilt with a chin lift. More recently, a jaw thrust with less head tilt and chin lift has been demonstrated to be even more effective.

Finally, turning the patient's head approximately 30° to either side opens the airway even more efficiently. Assuming the oral sedation drug was not given in such a large dose as to cause apnea, the patient should regain consciousness with spontaneous ventilation within 1–3 minutes.

Flumazenil, which is in the medical emergency kit, reverses the effects of the benzodiazepines. However, the drug package insert clearly states that this drug must be given IV only. Flumazenil should never be administered IM, subcutaneously, or sublingually, but IO is an acceptable alternative to IV. Flumazenil, therefore, is of little benefit to most pediatric dentists who do not use IV regularly unless they have the ability to utilize an IO device, and this drug should not be relied upon for reversal of a benzodiazepine overdose.

### Respiratory Depression

The second type of respiratory event secondary to an overdose of an orally administered sedative is respiratory depression. This rarely occurs after administration of a benzodiazepine alone. When respiratory depression occurs, it is almost always associated with the administration of an opioid, which is essentially always administered in conjunction with a benzodiazepine (very rarely by itself). Opioids benefit oral sedation and increase efficacy, but they do so at additional risk. Opioids do not have the wide safety profile of the benzodiazepines, and their overdose is not managed as simply as head tilt with chin lift. Again, not exceeding a manufacturer's maximum recommended doses means overdose will rarely occur. However, pushing the limits by adding "just a little bit more" every time will eventually cause overdose. Respiratory depression essentially always follows or is in conjunction with respiratory obstruction, so head tilt with chin lift and/or jaw thrust still needs to be done. In addition to good airway management, respiratory depression requires the delivery of positive pressure oxygen via a bag-valve-mask technique to either supplement or supplant the respiratory effort by the patient. The mask is sealed with the thumbs of each hand, and the mandible is elevated via jaw thrust to open the airway. One person performs the ventilations, while another maintains a patent airway with two hands (Figure 16-6).

Unlike flumazenil, the specific opioid antagonist naloxone may be administered IM. However, IM administration has a significantly longer onset and peak effect than IV administration. Expect 20–30 seconds for an onset of action with IV/IO administration, 2–3 minutes for an onset of action of IM administration, and a peak effect to be achieved 3–5 minutes after IV/IO administration, 10–15 minutes after IM administration.

## Breathing and Circulation

In most unconscious persons, head-tilt chin-lift (A = Airway) provides a patent airway. However, airway patency must still be assessed using the "look," "listen," and "feel"

technique (B = Breathing). If the patient is not breathing, administer two breaths, with each breath lasting one second and only using a volume of air sufficient to see the chest rise. The nitrous nasal mask is removed, and the clinician should use a barrier device such as a pocket mask or the mask from a bag-valve-mask device, if available. The dentist should take care not to ventilate too rapidly or administer excessive volumes. In children younger than the age of adolescence—defined as the age just before the onset of puberty, as determined by the presence of secondary sex characteristics—the clinician should administer rescue breaths at a rate of 20–30 breaths per minute. For teenagers and adults, the rate should be 10–12 breaths per minute. Next, the carotid pulse is palpated. In an unconscious child, adolescent, or adult patient, the carotid is the best artery for assessing the pulse. To locate the carotid pulse, the dentist or team member palpates the patient's thyroid cartilage, then moves the fingers into the "groove" just before encountering the sternocleidomastoid muscle (Figure 16-7).

Although basic life support (BLS, also known as *cardiopulmonary resuscitation* (CPR)) training for laypeople recommends skipping the pulse check, that rule does not apply to healthcare providers, including dentists. Healthcare professionals are expected to be able to detect a pulse (Haas 2010). If no pulse can be palpated after 10 seconds, the dentist or a staff member should assume that the patient has experienced cardiac arrest and begin chest compressions at a rate of 100–120 per minute, consistent with current BLS training.

The dentist should place their hands over the lower half of the patient's sternum between the nipples, and then,

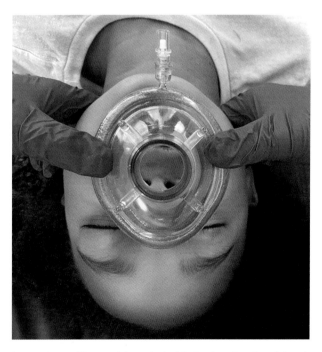

**Figure 16-6** The mask is sealed with the thumbs of each hand and the mandible is elevated via jaw thrust to open the airway. One person performs the ventilations, while the other maintains a patent airway with two hands. Illustration is with the bag-valve-mask removed to better illustrate the mask position.

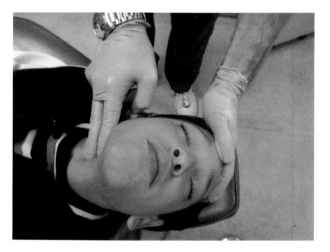

**Figure 16-7** To locate the carotid pulse, the dentist or team member palpates the patient's thyroid cartilage, then moves the fingers into the "groove" just before encountering the sternocleidomastoid muscle. *Source:* Courtesy of Dr. Ari Kupietzky.

push down by using the heel of one hand with the other hand on top. For children older than one year but younger than the age of adolescence, the compressions should depress the chest by one-third or two inches. For older children and adults, each compression should depress the chest 2–2.4 inches (5–6 cm). It is important that the clinician push hard and fast and allow full chest recoil. The compression-to-ventilation ratio for one-person CPR in children is the same as that in adults (30:2), but for two-person CPR in children, the ratio should be 15:2. Four to five sequences are provided in approximately 2 minutes. Coincident with beginning BLS is the administration of oxygen. The next step is to turn on the automated external defibrillator (AED) and follow the voice prompts.

As mentioned, the goal of the steps (P→A→B→C) described thus far is to ensure that the victim's brain and heart are receiving an adequate supply of blood containing oxygen and glucose, the fuels required by the cells of the body to maintain normal function.

## Definitive Care

Definitive care represents the final step of management. Possible components of definitive care include diagnosis, drugs, and defibrillation. When possible, a diagnosis is made and treatment proceeds accordingly. Examples of diagnosed problems are asthma, hypoglycemia, and allergy. Drugs, other than oxygen, which may be administered in any emergency situation, are rarely needed. Notable exceptions are acute bronchospasm (asthma) and allergy.

## Asthma

Probably the most common cause of respiratory distress seen in pediatric dental patients is asthma, also known as *acute bronchospasm* (Malamed 2014). Other possibilities for respiratory distress in pediatric patients include an allergic reaction, tachypnea, hyperventilation, diabetic ketoacidosis, or unconsciousness.

Millions of children in the United States are affected by asthma, a chronic respiratory disease characterized by attacks of difficulty in breathing. An asthma attack is a distressing and potentially life-threatening experience (National Heart, Lung, and Blood Institute 2007). Asthma is one of the leading chronic childhood diseases in the United States (Adams and Hendershot 1996) and a major cause of childhood disability (Newacheck and Halfon 2000). The most current data shows that the challenges of childhood asthma remain, and that asthma persists as a significant public health problem (Akinbami 2006). However, asthma deaths among children are rare. Children most at risk of dying from asthma are those with severe,

uncontrolled disease, a near-fatal attack of asthma, or a history of recurrent hospitalizations or intubation for asthma (McFadden and Warren 1997). Thus, a thorough review of the medical history of an asthmatic child patient is important.

### Management

Patients experiencing asthmatic respiratory distress typically will want to sit upright (P = position). The dentist follows this with an evaluation of the patient's airway. Is it patent? By definition, conscious patients who can talk have a patent airway, are breathing, and have sufficient cerebral blood flow and blood pressure (adequate perfusion pressure) to remain conscious. Definitive care includes administration of a bronchodilator, most commonly albuterol or salmeterol. For conscious patients, this bronchodilator is administered via a metered dose inhaler (MDI). Patients with a history of asthma will have their own inhaler. If the patient loses consciousness or does not cooperate with the administration of albuterol via inhalation due to hypoxia, hypercarbia, or some other reason, or if the bronchospasm is refractory to administration of albuterol, the dentist should contact EMS and administer epinephrine intramuscularly in the appropriate dose based on the child's age and weight.

## Altered Consciousness

As with respiratory distress, altered consciousness or unconsciousness may be present, owing to a variety of precipitating factors including overdose of sedation medication.

Dizziness developing in the dental office may have many origins, but low blood pressure in the brain often is the ultimate cause. The easiest and least-invasive way to increase blood flow to the brain is to place the patient in a supine position. Patients in whom dizziness is the only symptom are conscious and able to talk (airway, breathing, and circulation have been assessed and verified). Definitive therapy consists simply of placing the patient properly in a supine position. The Trendelenburg position is less ideal. In that position, the contents of the lower gastrointestinal tract impinge on the diaphragm, increasing the work of breathing. Once the patient is positioned properly, the pediatric dentist should determine the cause of the dizziness. Was it initiated by vasovagal syncope? Hypoglycemia? Hypovolemia? Although many possible explanations exist, the more common reasons for loss of consciousness in the dental office, assuming no medications have been administered, are syncope and low blood glucose.

### Vasovagal Syncope

Fainting, or vasovagal syncope, is the most common medical emergency seen in the dental office (Findler et al. 2002).

The incidence of syncope is increased in two age groups: young adults (15–24 years) and in those over 65 years of age. However, a lower peak also occurs in older infants and toddlers (Wieling et al. 2004). By far, the most common cause of syncope in young subjects is a reflex syncopal event, and in particular a vasovagal faint.

The basic algorithm is the same as that for dizziness, described earlier. The dentist or a team member should place the patient in a supine position. Most patients with syncope have a patent airway, are breathing, and demonstrate an adequate pulse. Patients who faint typically respond to positional changes within 30 seconds. If the patient does not respond in this time frame, he did not simply faint, and the dentist must consider a differential diagnosis. The responding patient should be kept in a supine position and administered 100% oxygen until full recovery. To allow the body to return to a normal state, the patient should not undergo additional dental treatment for the remainder of the day (Ross et al. 2013).

### Hypoglycemia

Pediatric dentists should consider hypoglycemia in a differential diagnosis of dizziness. Sometimes, but not always, these patients have a history of diabetes. Pediatric dental patients with type-1 diabetes, and some with type-2 diabetes self-administer insulin to lower a high glucose level (hyperglycemia) toward the upper limit of normal (120 milligrams/deciliter or 6 mmol/L). Patients with diabetes must ingest food immediately after administering insulin to prevent the development of hypoglycemia as a result of the insulin injection. The most common cause of hypoglycemia in patients with type-1 diabetes is not eating after administering insulin.

Patients with clinically significant hypoglycemia may be recognizable because they commonly experience diaphoresis and tachycardia, causing them to feel faint. Subsequently, they may be confused and ultimately lose consciousness. As long as the patient retains consciousness, the clinician should allow him/her to remain in a comfortable position. Conscious patients with hypoglycemia have a patent airway, are breathing, and have an adequate pulse. The treatment of choice for patients with hypoglycemia is administration of sugar (specifically glucose, not sucrose). Unconscious pediatric dental patients with hypoglycemia require parenteral administration of sugar. Absolutely never place anything into the mouth of an unconscious patient. Since the use of IM glucagon has generally fallen out of favor, absent proficiency in venipuncture for the pediatric patient, the dentist should activate EMS.

In each of these examples of unconsciousness, the initial management of the emergency situation is the same. The dentist should place the patient in a supine position. If the child has not responded within 30 seconds, the clinician

can rule out syncope. The dentist then should open the airway and assess breathing ("look, listen, and feel") (American Heart Association 2015). If the patient is breathing, the next step is to check circulation. Does the patient have a palpable pulse at the carotid artery (or brachial artery, in infants)? Patients who are breathing spontaneously and normally may be experiencing hypoglycemia or a cerebrovascular accident (CVA), but not cardiac arrest. In cardiac arrest, the patient does not breathe spontaneously; agonal breathing is not normal breathing. A patient with apnea requires positive pressure ventilation with 100% oxygen.

Patients placed in a supine position who do not respond within 30 seconds but are breathing spontaneously are likely experiencing hypoglycemia or a CVA. If the patient's blood pressure is normal, the problem is probably a low blood glucose.

### Seizures

Pediatric dental patients who convulse in the dental office typically have a seizure history and often are characterized as being epileptic (Bryan and Sullivan 2006). The initial treatment for seizures is the same as that for any other medical emergency. The patient experiencing a *generalized tonic-clonic seizure*, the term currently preferred over "Grand Mal," is unconscious and should be placed in a supine position. The dentist should perform a "head tilt, chin lift, and jaw thrust" to the extent possible. Patients who are seizing are breathing and have adequate cardiovascular function, which the pediatric dentist can verify by checking for and finding a strong carotid pulse.

The pediatric dentist or a team member must remove all dental instruments and supplies from the patient's mouth and protect him from harm. No one should place anything into the mouth of a patient who is seizing. The pediatric dentist or a team member should bring the patient's parent into the operatory to help evaluate the patient. The parent may determine that this is a typical seizure for the patient, in which case simple monitoring is sufficient. On the other hand, if a seizure is unusually severe, the pediatric dentist might contact EMS.

### Local Anesthetic Overdose

Many pediatric dentists will not recognize a local anesthetic overdose until a seizure is seen. Of course, prevention is primary. Do not exceed the manufacturer's maximum recommended doses for the local anesthetics chosen, and this problem will essentially cease to exist. Local anesthesia is discussed in depth in Chapter 9 of this textbook. Local anesthetic overdoses are only fatal if the patient's airway is not maintained throughout the episode. Head tilt with chin lift and/or jaw thrust is essential. The administration of oxygen is always recommended in any medical emergency. For the majority of pediatric dentists, this is the entire treatment algorithm for a local anesthetic overdose. However, if a pediatric dentist is trained to start IVs, the IV administration of intralipid is now available. Initial dosing is 1.5 mL/kg of the 20% formulation of intralipid (Brull 2008).

## Allergy

An allergic reaction can be mild or severe. Based on data from Malamed (1993), a "mild allergic reaction" was the second most common medical emergency seen in dental offices after syncope (fainting). Additionally, anaphylaxis was the 11th most common medical emergency. The most common allergen in the dental environment today, of course, is latex (Desai 2007). Penicillin is the most common cause of drug-induced anaphylaxis (Lieberman et al. 2005). Patients can have allergies to penicillin and penicillin-like drugs (amoxicillin, Augmentin®, etc.), as well as other drugs and agents prescribed, administered, and dispensed in dental offices. It should be noted here that a true allergic reaction to an injected local anesthetic in dentistry has an incidence approaching zero. It simply does not occur to any measurable degree (Malamed 1997).

If the allergic reaction presents with itching, hives, or a rash as the only signs and symptoms, the allergy may be considered mild (non–life-threatening). However, if the patient experiences cardiovascular and/or respiratory embarrassment, which are normally seen as dizziness or loss of consciousness due to inadequate blood pressure and/or blood flow to the brain (cardiovascular issues), or difficulty in breathing (respiratory issues), the dental professional must treat the allergy as a life-threatening situation (Reed 2010).

In addition to severity, allergic reactions may also be characterized based on time. Those allergic reactions occurring many minutes to many hours after exposure to the allergen may be termed "delayed onset," while those that occur within a few seconds to a few minutes after contact with the allergen are termed "immediate onset." As a general rule, the faster the signs and/or symptoms occur, the more likely a severe allergy will occur. It is not the purpose of this chapter to review the intricate pathophysiology of allergy involving IgE, IgG, and other antigen-antibodies and other cellular responses, or deal with non-life-threatening mild allergies.

### Severe Allergy (Anaphylaxis)

Anaphylaxis is an acute, life-threatening, systemic reaction with varied mechanisms and clinical presentations. Immediate discontinuation of the offending drug(s) and early administration of epinephrine are the cornerstones of treatment. Epinephrine is the drug of choice in the treatment of anaphylaxis because its alpha-1 effects help support the blood pressure, while its beta-2 effects provide bronchial

smooth-muscle relaxation (Hepner and Castells 2003). Absorption is faster and plasma levels are higher in patients who receive epinephrine intramuscularly in the thigh with an autoinjector (Simons et al. 1998). Intramuscular injection into the thigh (vastus lateralis) is also superior to intramuscular or subcutaneous injection into the arm (deltoid) (Simons et al. 2001). No established dosage or regimen for intravenous epinephrine in anaphylaxis is recognized. Because of the risk for potentially lethal arrhythmias, epinephrine should be administered intravenously only during cardiac arrest, or to profoundly hypotensive subjects who have failed to respond to intravenous volume replacement and several injected doses of epinephrine (Malamed 1997).

If the allergy is severe, the patient has lost (or will soon lose) consciousness. The dentist should place the patient in a supine position, open the airway, and evaluate breathing. Often, breathing is spontaneous and adequate. If the patient is not breathing, the dental professional must administer positive pressure oxygen via a bag-valve-mask device. If the patient has lost consciousness, their cerebral blood pressure is too low. Another dental staff member also must contact EMS, as the patient likely requires treatment in hospital. The appropriate pharmacologic management for anaphylaxis in an outpatient setting is outlined in Figure 16-8.

**Precaution**: When treating patients who may have a history of allergic reactions, the first step is to consult with an allergist to test the patient for allergy to the drug in question. Treatment should be postponed, if at all possible, until this is accomplished. If the allergy is truly to a local anesthetic, another option is the use of general anesthesia, Yet another option is the use of a histamine blocker such as

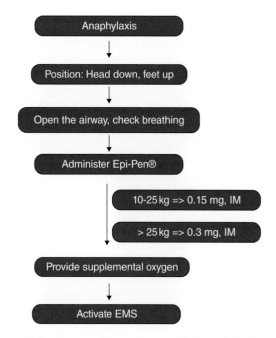

**Figure 16-8** Pharmacologic management of anaphylaxis.

diphenhydramine as a local anesthetic for pain management during treatment. Its efficacy is not great. Most injectable histamine blockers possess local anesthetic properties. Diphenhydramine has been the most commonly used histamine-blocker in this regard (Reed 2010). It should be noted that the drug package insert has the use of diphenhydramine as a local anesthetic listed as a contraindication.

## Foreign Body Aspiration

A common hazard in dental practice that cannot be taken lightly is aspiration of dental instruments and materials (Cameron et al. 1996). Aspiration of foreign objects during restorative procedures, especially under sedation, remains a real threat due to the challenges involved with treating young children and the difficulties of airway management (Adewumi and Kays 2008). Such incidents reinforce the need for prevention. The practicing dentist should routinely employ adequate barrier techniques and high-volume suction. Rubber dams should be used routinely, and cotton rolls or 2 × 2 gauze should never be left in a sedated child's mouth. During handling of stainless-steel crowns, extra precaution is needed if the rubber dam is removed. A 4 × 4 gauze pad with ligature should be used as a throat partition, and the assistant should be prepared with the high-volume suction for instant retrieval of a lost crown.

Following aspiration, most foreign bodies become lodged in the peripheral airways. Large, sharp, or irregular objects may lodge at the laryngeal inlet, especially in children less than one year old (Leith et al. 2008). Foreign bodies may also lodge in the trachea, but in most cases, the inhaled object passes down into one of the main bronchi. In adults, the right bronchus is the most common site for a foreign body to lodge because of its wider diameter and more vertical disposition (Zerella et al. 1998). However, in children, the impaction site of a foreign body is determined by the individual anatomy of the airway. Studies have shown that there is little difference in the distribution of inhaled foreign bodies between the right and left main bronchi in this age group (Black et al. 1994; Ciftci et al. 2003; Zerella et al. 1998). This is generally explained by the relatively symmetric bronchial angles in the pediatric airway until about 15 years of age.

The American Heart Association (2015) has published guidelines for the acute management of foreign body airway obstruction. If the obstruction is mild and the child can cough and make some sounds, it is recommended not to interfere and to allow the victim to clear the airway by coughing or gagging, while observing for more severe signs. These airway reflexes are protective and indicate that the obstruction is incomplete. Complete airway obstruction is recognized by sudden respiratory distress. If the obstruction is complete and the child cannot make sounds, subdiaphragmatic abdominal thrusts (the Heimlich maneuver) are indicated for the child who is one year of age or older. This may be accomplished by lifting the child and delivering the thrusts from behind while standing, or the abdominal thrust may be modified for the patient in the dental chair by delivering the thrust with the heel of the hand from the front of the child (Ganzberg 2013). If the victim becomes unresponsive, CPR should be initiated. It is important to attempt to remove an object from the pharynx with caution, as blind finger sweeps can push obstructing objects further into the oropharynx.

## Summary

Medical emergencies can and do occur in the dental office, and it is important for the entire dental team to be prepared for them. Regardless of the specific type of medical emergency, they all are best managed in basically the same way: position the patient; assess the airway, assess breathing and circulation; and provide definitive therapy.

**DISCLAIMER**: This information is not intended to be a comprehensive list of all medications that may be used in all emergencies. Drug information is constantly changing and is often subject to interpretation. While care has been taken to ensure the accuracy of the information presented, the authors are not responsible for the continued currency of the information, errors, omissions, or the resulting consequences. Decisions about drug therapy must be based upon the independent judgment of the clinician, changing drug information, and evolving healthcare practices.

## References

Adams, P.F. and Hendershot, G.E. (1996). Current estimates from the National Health Interview Survey, 1996. *Vital and Health Statistics*, 10, 200.

Adewumi, A. and Kays, D.W. (2008). Stainless steel crown aspiration during sedation in pediatric dentistry. *Pediatric Dentistry*, 30, 59–62.

Akinbami, L.J. (2006). The State of Childhood Asthma, United States, *1980–2005. Advance data from Vital and Health Statistics* (p. 381). National Center for Health Statistics, Hyattsville, MD.

American Heart Association Guidelines Update for Cardiopulmonary Resuscitation and Emergency Cardiovascular Care Circulation, 2015, 132, S315–S367, November 3, 2015–Volume 132, Issue 18, Suppl. 2.

Baker, S. and Yagiela, J.A. (2006). Obesity: A complicating factor for sedation in children. *Pediatric Dentistry*, 28, 487–493.

Bennet, J. and Rosenberg, M.B. (2002). *Medical Emergencies in Dentistry*. W. B. Saunders, Philadelphia, PA, USA.

Black, R.E., Johnson, D.G., and Matlak, M.E. (1994). Bronchoscopic removal of aspirated foreign bodies in children. *Journal of Pediatric Surgery*, 29, 682–684.

Brodsky, L. (1989). Modern assessment of tonsils and adenoids. *Pediatric Clinics of North America.* 36, 1551–1569.

Brull, S.J. (2008). Lipid emulsion for the treatment of local anesthetic toxicity: Patient safety implications. *Anesthesia and Analgesia*, 106, 1337–1339.

Bryan, R.B. and Sullivan, S.M. (2006). Management of dental patients with seizure disorders. *Dental Clinics of North America*, 50, 607–623.

Cameron, S.M., Whitlock, W.L., and Tabor, M.S. (1996). Foreign body aspiration in dentistry: A review. *Journal of the American Dental Association*, 127, 1224–1229.

Chicka, M.C., Demobo, J.B., Mathu-Muju, K.R. et al. (2012). Adverse events during pediatric dental anesthesia and sedation: A review of closed malpractice insurance claims. *Pediatric Dentistry*, 34, 231–238.

Ciftci, A.O., Bingo¨l-Kologlu, M., Senocak, M.E. et al. (2003). Bronchoscopy for evaluation of foreign body aspiration in children. *Journal of Pediatric Surgery*, 38, 1170–1176.

Desai, S.V. (2007). Natural rubber latex allergy and dental practice. *New Zealand Dental Journal*, 103, 101–107.

Findler, M., Elad, S., Garfunkel, A. et al. (2002). Syncope in the dental environment [in Hebrew]. *Refuat Hapeh Vehashinayim*, 19(1), 27–33, 99.

Fukayama, H. and Yagiela, J.A. (2006). Monitoring of vital signs during dental care. *International Dental Journal*, 56, 102–108.

Ganzberg, S.I. (2013). Medical emergencies. In: P.S. Casamassimo, H.W. Fields, D.J. Mctigue, A.J. Nowak (Eds.), *Pediatric Dentistry Infancy Through Adolescence*, 5th ed. (pp. 126–138). Elsevier Saunders, St Louis, Missouri.

Haas, D.A. (2010). Preparing dental office staff members for emergencies: Developing a basic action plan. *Journal of the American Dental Association*, 141, 8 s–13 s.

Hepner, D.L. and Castells, M.C. (2003). Anaphylaxis during the perioperative period. *Anesthesia and Analgesia*, 97, 1381–1395.

Kang, J., Vann, W.F. Jr., Lee, J.Y. et al. (2012). The safety of sedation for overweight/ obese children in the dental setting. *Pediatric Dentistry*, 34, 392–396.

Leith, R., Fleming, P., Redahan, S. et al. (2008). Aspiration of an avulsed primary incisor: A case report. *Dental Traumatology*, 24, e24-6. doi: 10.1111/j.1600-9657. 2008.00593.x. Epub 2008 Jun 28.

Lepere, A.J., Finn, J., and Jacobs, I. (2003). Efficacy of cardiopulmonary resuscitation performed in a dental chair. *Australian Dental Journal*, 48, 244–247.

Lieberman, P., Nicklas, R., Oppenheimer, J. et al. (2005). The diagnosis and management of anaphylaxis: An updated practice parameter. *Journal of Allergy and Clinical Immunology*, 115, S483–S523.

Malamed, S.F. (1993). Managing medical emergencies. *Journal of the American Dental Association*, 124, 40–53.

Malamed, S.F. (1997). Emergency medicine: Beyond the basics (published correction appears in *Journal of the American Dental Association*, 128, 1070). *Journal of the American Dental Association*, 128, 843–854.

Malamed, S.F. (2010a). *Sedation: A Guide to Patient Management*, 5th ed. Mosby, St. Louis.

Malamed, S.F. (2010b). Knowing your patients. *Journal of the American Dental Association*, 141, 3S–7S.

Malamed, S.F. (2014). *Medical Emergencies in the Dental Office*. 7th ed. Mosby, St. Louis.

Malamed, S.F. (2015). Medical emergencies in the dental surgery. Part 1: Preparation of the office and basic management. *Journal of the Irish Dental Association*, 61(6), 302–308.

Mallampati, S.R., Gatt, S.P., Gugino, L.D. et al. (1985). A clinical sign to predict difficult intubation: A prospective study. *Canadian Anaesthesia Society Journal*, 32, 429–434.

McFadden, E.R., Jr. and Warren, E.L. (1997). Observations on asthma mortality. *Annals of Internal Medicine*, 127, 142–147.

National Heart, Lung, and Blood Institute. (2007). National Asthma Education and Prevention Program Expert Panel report 2: Guidelines for the diagnosis and management of asthma.

Newacheck, P.W. and Halfon, N. (2000). Prevalence, impact, and trends in childhood disability due to asthma. *Archives of Pediatrics and Adolescence Medicine*, 154, 287–293.

Norris, L.H. (1994). Early recognition limits in in-office emergencies. *Journal of the Massachusetts Dental Society*, 43, 19–23.

Nuckton, T.J., Glidden, D.V., Browner, W.S. et al. (2006). Physical examination: Mallampati score as an independent predictor of obstructive sleep apnea. *Sleep*, 29, 903–908.

Peskin, R.M. and Siegelman, L.I. (1995). Emergency cardiac care: Moral, legal, and ethical considerations. *Dental Clinics of North America*, 39, 677–688.

Reed, K.L. (2010). Basic management of medical emergencies: Recognizing a patient's distress. *Journal of the American Dental Association*, 141, 20s–24s.

Ross, P.J., Schneider, P.E., and Helpin, M. (2013). Neurocardiogenic syncope of child dental patient: A case review. *Pediatric Dentistry*, 35, 71–73.

Samsoon, G.L. and Young, J.R. (1987). Difficult tracheal intubation: A retrospective study. *Anaesthesia*, 42, 487–490.

Simons, F.E.R., Roberts, J.R., Gu, X. et al. (1998). Epinephrine absorption in children with a history of anaphylaxis. *Journal of Allergy and Clinical Immunology*, 101, 33–37.

Simons, F.E.R., Gu, X., and Simons, K.J. (2001). Epinephrine absorption in adults: Intramuscular versus subcutaneous injection. *Journal of Allergy and Clinical Immunology*, 108, 871–873.

Wieling, W., Ganzeboom, K.Z., and Saul, J.P. (2004). Reflex syncope in children and adolescents. *Heart*, 90, 1094–1100.

Wolters, U., Wolf, T., Stützer, H. et al. (1996). ASA classification and perioperative variables as predictors of postoperative outcome. *British Journal of Anaesthesiology*, 77, 217–222.

Zerella, J.T., Dimler, M., McGill, L.C. et al. (1998). Foreign body aspiration in children: Value of radiography and complications of bronchoscopy. *Journal of Pediatric Surgery*, 33, 1651–1654.

# 17

## Practical Considerations and the Dental Team

*Jonathon E. Lee and Brian D. Lee*

## Introduction

The foundation for practicing pediatric dentistry is the ability to guide infants, children, and adolescents through their dental experiences. Today, practicing pediatric dentistry is a team effort, with dentists leading and empowering their team members through delegation of responsibilities and projects to their team members: trained dental auxiliaries and administrative office staff. In managing a team, different management styles come into play. Macromanagement leadership style is one where the dentist delegates authority and responsibilities with a hands-off approach; where the dentist trusts their employees to do their jobs as they see best. Macromanagerment dentists are more concerned with overall plans and results than individual styles or day-to-day habits. Micromanagement allows the dentist to focus their attention on developing and executing the overall strategy for the team. This style instills confidence, trust, and professional development and fulfillment of the team. A cohesive and positive pediatric dental teamworking together helps the patient develops a positive attitude toward the dental experience.

The pediatric dental team is an extension of the dentist in that it uses communicative behavior guidance techniques, leading the child patient stepwise through the dental experience. All personnel have a stake in guiding the child through the experience. Dental auxiliaries and reception staff are invaluable when dealing with the pediatric patient (Wright et al. 1983). Therefore, all dental team members are encouraged to expand their skills and knowledge in behavior management techniques. When assembling a team, technical skills are important, but the authors have found that it is more important to hire for positive attitude and passion first.

Happy individuals are much more likely to participate in activities that are adaptive, both for them and the people around them (Fredrickson 2004).

## Six Team Tips for Behavior Management

There are six fundamental tips of behavior management for establishing positive relationships for both the team and the pediatric patient (Wright and Stiger 2011).

1) Have a positive, upbeat approach. Positive attitudes lead to positive outcomes.
2) Have a team attitude and culture. Personality factors, shared values, and commitments to action serve as the basis for relationships and behaviors.
3) Have organized policies, plans, and protocols. Written policies, protocols, and contingency plans with defined roles for each team member are characteristics of a well-organized office. With increased effectiveness and efficiency, there are fewer delays and less indecisiveness.
4) Be truthful and credible. These traits help to build trust with your team members and your patients.
5) Be tolerant and empathic. Cope with different behaviors and situations while maintaining composure and self-control.
6) Be flexible. Team members have to adapt to each situation because children's behaviors are unpredictable.

While nearly everyone would agree with these suggestions, following them is another matter. They are often overlooked. To illuminate the points, Wright applied these tips in context with case scenarios (1983). These updated cases remain applicable today.

*Wright's Behavior Management in Dentistry for Children*, Third Edition. Edited by Ari Kupietzky.
© 2022 John Wiley & Sons, Inc. Published 2022 by John Wiley & Sons, Inc.

---

### Case 17.1   The Positive Approach

Four-year-old Johnny sat in the reception area, awaiting his third dental checkup appointment. Entering the area, the receptionist greeted him: "Hi Johnny, it's your turn now." Johnny withdrew slightly and held his parent's hand firmly. Noticing this, the dental assistant said, "Johnny, don't be afraid. Nothing will hurt you."

---

***Case 17.1, Discussion:*** Both the receptionist and the dental assistant greeted Johnny, and the dental assistant tried to relax him to encourage a smooth patient transfer from the reception area to the dental clinic. Without realizing it, however, the dental assistant's final comment violated a fundamental precept of pediatric patient management: the entire dental team's approach must be positive.

A more positive effect could have been created if the receptionist had simply said something concrete and truthful, such as "Hi Johnny, I like your outfit, it is so colorful and bright. I am glad you came today. We are excited to see you." Then, the dental assistant could have taken the lead and said "Come on Johnny. You were such a good boy last time when you were able to help count your teeth. Dr. J. really wants to see if you can still count to twenty. Let's go quickly."

To achieve success with children, it is important to anticipate success (Wright 1975). Positive statements are far more effective than thoughtless questions or remarks directed mostly to parent figures. When dealing with difficult or challenging pediatric patients, the dental team has to remain positive and mask negative emotional reactions. The dental team member's attitudes or expectation can affect the outcome of an appointment because children are likely to respond with the type of behavior expected of them. In essence, the child fulfills the dentist's prophecy. This theory was advanced by Rosenthal and Jacobson in their book *Pygmalion in the Classroom*, which discusses children and the educational process.

In addition to taking a positive approach, the dental team has to be direct, specific, and confident. Questions that imply choice should be avoided unless the choice will definitely be granted. For example, the dental assistant summoning a child from the reception area will undoubtedly get a better response by saying "Johnny it's your turn to see Dr. J. Please come with me," rather than asking, "Johnny, would you come with me?" The same is true when the dental team member says, "Now I am going to brush and clean your teeth. Please help me by opening nice and big," rather than "I think it is time to clean your teeth now, OK?" Positive and direct communication is easy to learn, and after a short period of time, it becomes automatic. All members of the dental team should be aware of its importance

and help one another to use it with children. Another approach is indeed to give the child a choice, but structure the question and possible choices so that both options will be acceptable and lead to the same outcome. For example, do not ask "Would you like me to clean your teeth?" Instead, ask "Would you like me to clean your top teeth first, or start with your lower ones?" The child is given a choice. Both options will lead to the start of the cleaning. There is actually a benefit to this approach: the child subconsciously realizes that he made the choice to start the cleaning. The following case and discussion were presented in chapter one. It demonstrates the dental team's role in patient management and is repeated here for the reader's convenience.

---

### Case 17.2   Team Attitude and Culture

Mrs. W. brought her six-year-old to the dental office for a recall appointment. As they approached the front desk, the receptionist greeted them: "Hello, Mrs. W. and William. Please fill out a medical update, give me your insurance card so I can copy it, and then have a seat. The doctor will be with you in a few moments.".

---

***Case 17.2, Discussion***: The proper team attitude for dealing with children includes personality factors, such as warmth or patient interest that can be conveyed without a spoken word. A pleasant smile is body language that engages multisensory communication, and it may indicate to a child that the adult cares. In this case, the greeting to the child and his mother was businesslike, matter of fact, and formal. While this may be suitable for some adult patients, a nicer welcoming for the child might be, "Hi Billy, good to see you. How is school these days?" Children are informal. Consequently, they respond best to an attitude that is natural and friendly. Acknowledging Billy's presence first also makes him the center of attention. It places the child at the apex of the pediatric dentistry treatment triangle. At that point, the receptionist can hand out the medical update, which includes a section on insurance, and ask the parent if she needs help filling it out.

An attitude of friendliness can be conveyed to the child patient almost immediately. A casual greeting such as "Hi buddy, how are you today?" usually evokes a smile, whereas "Hello William" does not tend to put a child at ease. A mechanical tone certainly should be avoided, and modulation of voice control should be encouraged. As they famously say in Hawaii, "Hang loose."

It is helpful to make children feel at home in the dental office, and this can be done in many ways. If youngsters have nicknames they prefer, then these should be noted on their patient records and used during future appointments to promote a natural and friendly atmosphere. For example, if William prefers to be called "Billy," it should be noted and used at all times.

The world that we live in today is one that embraces multi-culturalism and diversity. Just look at the authors and contributors in this book. "It is a Small World After All" (Thomas Friedman). Today, it is very common to welcome children in our practices with unique names. For those names that are unfamiliar and difficult to pronounce, it often helps to have the phonetic spelling noted in their charts.

Most children are delighted to share their interests and hobbies. Additionally, having these and other patients' school accomplishments or extracurricular activities noted in the dental record is helpful. Keeping this in mind, and keeping a record of those interests, helps the team initiate future conversations and demonstrate a caring attitude toward child patients. However, care must be taken to prevent matters from getting out of hand. For example, after telling the dental team stories, a child may become excited and difficult to settle down for the dental procedure. While friendliness is fundamental to behavior management, over-permissiveness or an overly affectionate approach should be avoided. Thus, the dental team must project a degree of firm confidence when necessary. Children have to respect the team approach and realize who the leader is. They must be aware of what is expected of them. Sometimes, the behavior guidelines can be re-established by simply saying, "Billy, there is a time for play and a time for work. Now it is time to work." The whole team must embody this attitude and culture.

---

### Case 17.3   Organized Polices, Plans, and Protocols

Five-year-old Tammy had two restorative dental appointments during the previous month and, although not easy to manage, she cooperated adequately to allow the treatment. Now, Tammy requires anterior restorations. At the outset, the dentist invited Tammy's parent into the dental operatory to explain the anterior restorations. While Tammy was seated in the dental chair, the dentist explained the proposed treatment. Since the parent had several questions, the discussion dragged on for 15 minutes. Eventually, Tammy became restless and began to complain, whine, and whimper.

---

*Case 17.3, Discussion*: This case illustrates another fundamental aspect of behavior management. In pediatric dentistry, an organized policy, plan, or protocol is a necessity. A proper, prioritized treatment plan should have been discussed with the parent prior to the appointment, ideally at

the examination and treatment planning appointment. In this case, detailing the procedure at the beginning of the appointment delayed the start of the treatment and was unfair to both the child and the parent. Technical discussions in the presence of a child may build apprehension, and hurrying the conversation does not allow a parent sufficient time to ask questions and make an informed decision.

Organized policy, plans, and protocols in the dental office have many dimensions. For example, begin with the reception area. Who summons the new patient—the dentist, the dental assistant, the dental hygienist, or the receptionist? If a child creates a disturbance in the reception area, who deals with the situation? A plan might stipulate that the dentist be summoned at once, but this may differ from office to office. Each dental office must design its own contingency plans, and the entire office team must know in advance what is expected of them. Such plans can be placed in the office and employment manuals and are a key feature of many pediatric dental offices. Good plans increase efficiency and contribute to successful work environments as well as positive relationships between dental teams and child patients.

---

### Case 17.4   Truthfulness and Credibility

An alert dental assistant has seated a three-year-old patient in the dental chair. While waiting for the dentist, the child looks up and asks, "Am I going to get a shot today?" The dental assistant replies hesitantly, "I'm not sure. Ask when the doctor comes in."

---

*Case 17.4, Discussion*: Many dental assistants have been placed in a position similar to this one. The child asks the question with an apparent concern. If the dental assistant replies affirmatively, the young child might become very apprehensive, and a behavior problem could ensue. If the dental assistant states that the child is not going to have an injection and, in fact, the child needs one, then credibility is lost. Therefore, the assistant adopted an appropriate, "middle-of-the-road" course of action. She deferred to the dentist to inform the child and intercept any adverse behavior if it occurs.

Unlike adults, most children see things as either "black or white." Examples must be concrete. There are no "shades of grey." To them, shades between are abstract and difficult to understand. To youngsters, the dental team is either truthful or not. Therefore, truthfulness is extremely important in building trust and is a fundamental rule for dealing with children.

As the above case exemplifies, the dental team should be careful not to be trapped into being untruthful by circumstances. For example, when a child is told that an appointment is for a checkup, it is wrong to proceed with a restoration without the child's permission. Since children often do not understand the reason for a change in plan, the dentists must take the time to explain. Sometimes, parents coax the dentist to complete the work at the checkup appointment. If this occurs, it seems reasonable to ask the child, "Would you mind having a filling today so that you do not have to come back tomorrow? If I do it today, then Daddy won't have to take more time off work." If the child is agreeable, then the dentist may proceed. If the reply is negative, the child patient's choice should be respected because the youngster was told at the beginning that the appointment was for a "checkup." Parents will accept the explanation that it is wrong to establish one set of expectancies for their child and then suddenly revise them. Remember, parents and caregivers are part of the pediatric dentistry treatment triangle, and most are interested in their children having good working relationships with their dentists. They do not want to see confidence and trust destroyed.

---

### Case 17.5   Tolerance and Empathy

Eight-year-old Paul was undergoing a one-hour restorative appointment. Although he experienced no pain, Paul whined and fidgeted throughout the appointment. Despite the dental team's best efforts, the child's behavior aggravated them. In an attempt to modify the situation, the dentist firmly instructed Paul to stop whining and moving. This proved unsuccessful; the disturbance continued, and the child began to scream. Finally, the dentist felt that she was about to lose control. She decided to take a "time out" and walk away from the dental chair.

---

*Case 17.5, Discussion*: This could happen. Children sometimes whine, fidget, and aggravate, despite the best dental team efforts to minimize disruptive behavior. The important point is that the dentist recognized a potential loss of personal control. This story demonstrates that all people have limitations in dealing with negative behaviors. Recognizing individual tolerance levels and empathizing with the patient and situation is important when dealing with children.

Tolerance level and empathy are seldom-discussed concepts in dentistry, and they vary from person to person. As an illustration, consider the possible effect of Paul's behavior, which might be described as borderline cooperative-uncooperative, on two different dentists. Dr. A. copes with Paul's whining with the attitude that the child will gain confidence and eventually change. She ignores the whining and continues treatment. Dr. B., on the other hand, finds the whining highly irritating. Because it is bothersome and upsetting to the entire dental team, as well as the parent, Dr. B. manages the child by using a firm, reassuring, and positive voice control technique. The dentists tolerated and reacted to the child's behavior quite differently. Yet both provided the treatment successfully, even though their approaches to the problem were dissimilar. Their management of the situation was governed by their individual tolerance levels.

As well as varying from person to person, tolerance levels fluctuate for the individual. For example, an upsetting experience at home can affect the clinician's mood in the dental office. Some people are in a better frame of mind early in the morning, whereas the abilities of others to cope and empathize improve as the day progresses. The important thing is for clinicians to know their tolerance levels. Morning people should instruct receptionists to book behavior problems first thing in the morning. Learning to recognize factors that overtax tolerance levels is one way to avoid loss of self-control.

---

### Case 17.6   Flexibility

Four-year-old Daniel was apprehensive but cooperative for his dental exam one week earlier. Now, he has returned to the office for a restorative treatment. When the dentist entered the operatory and was about to begin treatment, Daniel said, "I have to go to the bathroom." The dentist questioned the boy's necessity and reluctantly acknowledged Daniel's need: "OK, but hurry up!" Then, he added, "Be quick, we are already half an hour behind schedule."

---

*Case 17.6, Discussion*: Daniel may have had an urgent need, or he may have been delaying treatment. The dentist tried to determine the necessity and, failing to do so, allowed Daniel to go to the bathroom. To avoid this situation, patients should be asked to use the restroom before entering the treatment room and be told that during treatment it will be difficult to stop and go to the bathroom. However, Daniel was not prompted before treatment to use the bathroom. In cases such as this, the child has to be given the benefit of the doubt. Sometimes, however, children use this ploy as a means of delaying treatment. The bathroom incident is of secondary importance in this case. It is included here to point out another important principle when dealing with children: the dental team has to be flexible.

Since it was not Daniel's fault that the office was operating behind schedule, there was no reason to be impatient with him.

Children are children. They lack the maturity of adults, and the dental team must be prepared to change its plans at times and as they say, "Go with the flow." A child may begin fretting and squirming in the dental chair after half an hour, and the proposed treatment may have to be shortened. Conversely, a dentist may plan an indirect temporary pulp treatment with final restoration at a second appointment, but because the child is difficult, the plan may have to be altered to complete the treatment in one session. Sometimes, a child may appear for a dental appointment out of sorts, with a low-grade fever and stuffy nose that was unrecognized previously by a parent, and the dental appointment has to be terminated.

The size of children may also demand a change in operating procedure. Many dentists, following accepted four-handed dentistry practices, work at the 11 or 12 o'clock position. This is not always possible with the young child patient. Thus, the dental team has to change with each situation, and flexibility becomes a necessary ingredient in the behavior management of children.

## Keys to Effective Communication in a Pediatric Office

Communications are used universally in pediatric dentistry. Establishing communication with the pediatric patient helps alleviate fear and anxiety; builds a trusting relationship among the dental team, the pediatric patient, and the parent; and aids in promoting the child's positive attitude toward oral health. The dental team must consider the cognitive development of the pediatric patient as well as the presence of other communication deficits, such as hearing disorders, when communicating with them (AAPD 2020). There are keys that help open and guide effective communication with children. These are:

- The first rule is to establish communication. Engage the child in conversation. This enables the dentist and the team to learn about the patient, and may relax the child.
- Be sure that everyone acknowledges the lead communicator. Members of the dental team must be aware of their roles when communicating with a child, and at which point one person takes the lead over the other. For example, the dental assistant starts engaging the child in conversation before the dentist arrives. Then, when the dentist arrives, the dentist takes over the lead, and the assistant becomes an active listener. It is important that

communication comes from one single source. If the parent is in the operatory, this must be explained in advance. When the dentist is conversing with the child, the parent must be a silent observer and active listener. If multiple people try to engage the child in conversation or give directions at the same time, it can be confusing for the child.
- It is important that the message is simple and age-appropriate. When talking with children, use real-life descriptive examples to explain procedures.
- Use the voice appropriately. A controlled alteration of voice volume, tone, or pace to influence and direct the patient's behavior is known as *voice control*. The objectives of voice control are to gain the patient's attention and compliance, avert negative or avoidance behavior, and establish appropriate adult/child roles.
- Use multisensory communication. In addition to spoken messages, nonverbal messages can be used with patients. Body contact such as a simple tap on the shoulder or a smile conveys a friendly feeling of warmth and reassurance. Eye contact is important. Children that avoid eye contact may not be fully prepared to cooperate. When talking with children, every effort should be made to speak at the child's eye level, rather than towering over them. Eye level communication allows for a friendlier and less authoritative or intimidating experience.

The foregoing are keys to communicating with children. There are others as well. All are described in greater detail in the Effective Communication section of Chapter 7.

## Training the Dental Team

The practice of pediatric dentistry is a team effort, with the dentist leading and delegating responsibility to the pediatric dental staff (including trained dental auxiliaries and office personnel). Each pediatric dental auxiliary and office staff member has to be trained and should actively participate in the management of child behavior in the dental office (Wright 1975). The dental auxiliaries and office staff members must support the dentist's efforts to welcome the patient and parent into a child-friendly environment and facilitate behavior guidance and a positive dental visit (AAPD 2020). The responsibility, or role, of individuals varies according to the philosophies and competency of those concerned.

In the pediatric dental team approach, everyone contributes. The pediatric dentist is the leader, but it is important to note that this means giving the team members autonomy and empowerment. As Bill Gates said, "As we look ahead to the next century, leaders will be those who empower others" (Aeker et al. 2010). There are instances where the dental assistant or hygienist may be the "key" person in the control of the child's behavior—instances in which they engage the pediatric patient better than the pediatric dentist. In such instances, it is important to give the dental auxiliary considerable freedom in developing rapport with the child. Research has shown that people working in self-organized teams are more satisfied, resulting in a more positive work environment (Bharat 2007). Research outside of dentistry also has found that happy individuals are much more likely to participate in activities that are adaptive for both them and the people around them. Positive emotions lead people to produce more ideas and think more creatively and flexibly, which in turn encourages imagination and enhances social relationships (Aeker et al. 2010). Auxiliaries need to be encouraged to contribute to this pleasant experience.

Dentistry is often described as an art and a science. Both are important when bringing a team together. Thus, a basic program for training a dental auxiliary to participate in the management of child behavior—a fundamental skill—is important. How each dental office or clinic engages and teaches their auxiliaries will vary, according to the educational background of the auxiliary. There are two types of backgrounds to consider. One type is the person who has been engaged because of a positive attitude and keen interest in children. These persons need to be taught dental assistant skills from the bottom up. The second type is a certified dental assistant who has completed a formal dental assistant program. In this case, begin with a fresh slate and share with them the importance of embracing changes and flexibility. Few dental assisting training programs spend much time teaching behavior management. Additionally, ask the assistants to share ideas that worked well in previous experiences. Foster an open-minded and flexible team culture by implementing the rules of behavior management. The keys to effective team communication not only work with pediatric patients, but also in training the pediatric team member. Personal communication between the dentist and the dental auxiliary is one of the most important and commonly used methods in training the dental auxiliary. Think of it as tell-show-do.

Again, be concrete and have policies, plans and protocols. The dentist must define each auxiliary's role and emphasize that the goal of pediatric dentistry is to positively guide infants, children, and adolescents through their dental experiences. It is absolutely essential to communicate expectations clearly to the auxiliary. The reason many staff members do not achieve their goals or become engaged team members is they have not been given clear or concrete instructions as to their role (Koestner et al. 2002).

While staff roles should be defined, they also need to be tweaked periodically. This is usually based on what is learned while monitoring a staff member's progress (Aeker et al. 2010). Regularly scheduled staff meetings for discussions of the philosophy of child management to which an office subscribes are exceedingly important. Such discussions provide an opportunity for an individual auxiliary to question certain policies and methods and to more clearly understand their application. They also provide an opportunity for the entire staff to share in this understanding, which is absolutely essential. Dental auxiliaries demonstrating a team mentality and loyalty to the practice are important.

## The First Non-Emergent Parent Encounter

The receptionist usually has the first contact with a prospective patient's parent when scheduling an appointment over the telephone. Since parents often do not know how to prepare their children for the first dental visit, it is the role of the receptionist to help "set the stage." The receptionist should provide information that helps the parent understand what to expect prior to an appointment, alleviating anxiety. This is done in several ways, such as a pre-appointment letter or through an office's web page. These strategies are described in detail in Chapter 7. All of these encounters serve as education tools that may answer questions, allay fears, and help the parent and child be better prepared for the first visit (AAPD 2020).

Through this initial contact with a parent, the receptionist can gain important information to prepare the rest of the pediatric dental team for the new patient encounter. For example, is this the child's first dental experience? If not, did the parent indicate that there had been problems in the past? Are other siblings treated in this office? Who referred the patient? It is the responsibility of the receptionist to obtain and record this information and provide it to the team. Figure 17-1 shows a telephone information slip for recording information. (Figure 17-2 is a different telephone information slip that is used for the emergency patient.) A receptionist with a good attitude can gain much information and is extremely important because she is the "preview" of the office staff and the sole contact before the new patient arrives.

## Scheduling Appointments

The parent or caregiver's first direct impression of an office is formed when the pediatric patient's first dental visit is scheduled. This may be the child's first dental experience.

TELEPHONE INFORMATION SLIP NEW PATIENT FORM

New Patient Form

| | |
|---|---|
| Caller Name | City |

| | |
|---|---|
| Patient's Name | Age |

List any family members who are patients

How did you hear about our office

| | | |
|---|---|---|
| Has your child been to the dentist before | Y | N |

| | | |
|---|---|---|
| Name of previous dentist | Date of last visit | |
| Has your child taken any X-rays | Y | N |
| Did the previous dentist find any cavities on the last visit | N | N |
| Did they start the work & have all the work completed | Y | N |
|     How was it done | | |
|     If no, why | | |
| Do you want to have the work done | Y | N |
| Plan on returning to the previous dentist after the work is done | Y | N |
| Is your child having any problems at this time | Y | N |
| Is there pain and for how long | Y | N |

Reason for visit

Describe the problem
If appointment is scheduled then remind parent to contact previous dentist and have them forward the records to our office.

**Figure 17-1** A telephone information slip for recording information.

TELEPHONE INFORMATION SLIP EMERGENCY PATIENT

Patient Emergency Message

Caller Name

| | |
|---|---|
| Date | Time |

Contact Phone Number

| | |
|---|---|
| Patient Name | Age |

| | | |
|---|---|---|
| Name of previous dentist and reason for visit | | |
| Is your child having any problems at this time | Y | N |
| Is there pain and for how long | Y | N |
| Did your child have an injury | Y | N |

Describe the problem

**Figure 17-2** An emergency patient telephone information slip.

Every dental team member should be prepared to make this first significant "one-time" event as pleasant as possible. If a positive first encounter provides a pleasant introduction to dentistry, it is the first stage in building a good dentist–patient relationship.

If a child has not been seen before, it is often difficult to assess the amount of time that will be required for the first visit. Children with special needs may or may not require special consideration. It can be advantageous to schedule these patients where extra time can be allotted if necessary. For most children, a successful first-time scheduling procedure (followed by the authors) is to limit the appointment to an examination and radiographs, if indicated. A second appointment is made for a dental prophylaxis and fluoride treatment. Having two separate visits allows better evaluation of the child's behavior and greater opportunity to engage parents in prevention discussions and the anticipatory guidance aspect of pediatric oral health. By separating into two appointments, the focus is narrowed for each visit and positive experiences are enhanced for the parent and patient. Narrowing the goals and tasks lead to better participation (Latham and Seigjts 1999) and increases the enjoyment of the tasks (Bandura and Schunk 1981; Manderlink and Harackiewicz 1984).

Although many pragmatic factors dictate office procedures, the schedule itself can influence the child's cooperative behavior. Scheduling, appointment length, and time of day are important practical considerations of the child's treatment plan. Further, nobody likes to be kept waiting, including children. A child kept waiting results in a restless patient; thus, there should not be long waiting periods in the reception area. It can have an adverse effect on the child and the parent.

Pediatric dentists have to determine what works best for them and their staff. Many dentists prefer to schedule young patients in the morning. In addition, many dentists feel that, by keeping age groups together (preschoolers in the morning, older children in the afternoon), the peer groups have a positive influence, and the dental office runs more smoothly, with less psychological change of pace for the dental staff. Some pediatric dentists also prefer to see patients with behavior problems first thing in the morning. However, the issue of "tolerance level" must be considered when scheduling. Does the dentist's tolerance level change between 9 a.m. and 5 p.m.? Since tolerance level affects dentist–child interactions, the attitudes of both the patient and the dentist are considered when selecting appointment times. The authors prefer to see behavior problems first in the morning, but a colleague of theirs prefers to wait until he has had his morning coffee. Different strokes for different folks!

Everyone on the pediatric dental team wants the patient to enter the office calmly, progress through treatment easily, and leave the office happy. For this to occur, everything has to go well from beginning to end. The following case scenarios focus on the scheduling of the dental visit and their influence on the behavior of pediatric patients.

---

### Case 17.7 Patient Sequence

Four-year-old Johnny and his mom are contently waiting in the reception room for Johnny's first dental visit. After a brief time, three-year-old Tina storms into the reception room following her treatment. Tina is visibly upset and crying. This has been her history for the past two checkups. Now, Johnny looks up at his mom and starts to tear up.

---

*Case 17.7, Discussion*: Unfortunately, this problem can occur in the dental office. It is termed *behavior contagion*. Johnny was initially sitting beside his mom, waiting calmly. Tina, who was obviously upset by the dental experience, has adversely influenced Johnny, the next patient. If the waiting child is a new patient, the experience likely increases apprehension even more.

To avoid duplicating this type of situation, a good scheduling guideline dictates that a first-time child patient's appointment should follow the appointment of a child with a positive behavioral background. Then, the child who exits happily from the dental operatory can influence the new patient favorably. Perhaps the best way to avoid the problem is an office protocol that instructs receptionists or booking clerks to check the behavior of each patient preceding a new patient. If the exiting child's behavior is positive, it could have a beneficial influence on that of the following child, especially when the children are of the same sex and are closely matched in age.

---

### Case 17.8 Waiting Periods

Mrs. Jones has arrived in the office with her two young children for their dental appointments. After waiting in the crowded reception area for a half hour, the children became restless and began to chase each other around the room. An argument followed, which embarrassed Mrs. Jones and disturbed the other patients.

---

*Case 17.8, Discussion*: Children are bundles of energy. Lacking the patience of adults in an environment that was not designed to occupy their attention, the children

in this case made up their own "game." How unusual is it for children to argue when they are confined in close quarters? The point is that adults may relax and read, but children become restless and tired, especially if there is nothing to occupy them. Beginning an appointment in this way can negatively affect the remainder of an office visit. This is especially true for a new patient, or one who has demonstrated apprehension or uneasiness at earlier appointments.

A good general rule is that a child should not be kept waiting in the reception area, and that every effort should be made to be on time. Years ago, Brauer et al. (1964) pointed out that long waiting periods in the reception area should be avoided because they can have an adverse effect on the child and the parents. This still holds true and emphasizes the importance of staying on schedule and keeping the waiting periods for children as short as possible. The reception area may also be designed as a fun place for kids, with planned activities to avoid problems. Fun is the easiest way to change behavior for the better (Ramos 2009). Many pediatric dentists provide separate areas for children, with activities such as television, video games, or play structures (see Chapter 18). Other suggestions are children's books, toys, fish tanks, blackboards, building blocks, and small chairs and tables.

---

### Case 17.9 Appointment Sequence

Charlene, aged three years, had an appointment for her first dental examination. After entering the operatory, the child screamed and flailed about in the dental chair. With consent from the parent, the dentist used firm positive voice control to manage her behavior. The child ultimately cooperated for the dental examination, but additional treatments were required. At the front desk, the receptionist made Charlene an appointment for a month later.

---

*Case 17.9, Discussion*: This case features a child who misbehaves or is apprehensive and who, by good behavior management, becomes cooperative. After establishing rapport, everything went well, but the scheduling of the next appointment increased the chance of the problem repeating itself. This patient should not have to wait for an extended period for the next office visit. Such a child should be rescheduled as soon as possible to reinforce the newfound positive attitude.

By reducing the time between appointments, the dental team uses a management strategy that can be called the "rapid sequence" appointment technique. It is typically used in the following way for the apprehensive new patient without emergency treatment needs. At the first visit, the dentist expects to perform a clinical examination and to take radiographs, if indicated. The apprehensive child balks or is difficult. Eventually, the child becomes more cooperative through proper management techniques, and the dentist examines the patient without problem. However, the dentist senses that the child is still quite apprehensive. This can be a good place to terminate the appointment and reschedule the patient for the indicated radiographs within two weeks. Delaying the radiographs benefits the clinician as well as the child. It provides the clinician the opportunity to build the child's confidence and reassess the behavior before treatment. The patient leaves the office after the first visit believing that the task was accomplished, which promotes the child's pride and autonomy.

It was previously mentioned that the authors separate the first examination and prophylaxis procedures into two shorter appointments. In this case, children who experience the rapid sequence appointment technique usually perform well upon returning for radiographs. Often, they display little or no apprehension at the second visit. They have been led slowly through the dental experience. Parents usually appreciate the little extra time taken to develop a positive attitude in their children, especially when the situation is explained to them.

The rapid sequence appointment technique is a form of behavior modification that desensitizes the anxious child. From the clinician's viewpoint, this strategy may be too time-consuming and, therefore, impractical. If carried to an extreme, this may be true. However, many first-time child patients exhibiting anxieties accommodate quickly, and they are entitled to be led through initial dental experiences slowly. In the long run, taking time to desensitize the patient offers great dividends to the clinician.

Further, when a long series of restorative appointments have taken place, the final appointment should be brief, and simple procedures should be planned. In this way, the child leaves the dental office awaiting the recall visit with a good feeling.

---

**Case 17.10    Appointment Time**

Alice, aged three years, is apprehensive and very active. She requires considerable dental treatment. The dentist decided to pre-medicate her with an oral conscious sedative. The drug was supposed to relax the child during the lengthy appointment. Despite his knowledge that Alice often naps in the late morning, the dentist recommended an early morning appointment.

---

*Case 17.10, Discussion*: Consider this case carefully. The sedation was supposed to relax and calm the child, facilitating a lengthy treatment. However, the scheduling of the appointment may be in error because children who are accustomed to late morning naps frequently have higher activity levels early in the morning. Thus, both children's behaviors and dentists' management strategies have to be taken into account in the daily office schedule.

If a child is accustomed to napping late in the morning, she is likely to require less sedation, or at least respond better to the sedation prescribed, if her appointment is scheduled near her napping period. Again, the scheduled appointment can influence the behavior management. Although many dentists encourage morning appointments for children, some situations necessitate changes in the office schedule.

---

**Case 17.11    Appointment Duration**

Jeffrey, aged six years, has always been a cooperative dental patient. Returning for a recall appointment, it was discovered that he needed restoration on two of his newly erupted upper first permanent molars and sealants on his two lower permanent first molars. The dentist recommended that Jeffrey have three half-hour appointments—one appointment for each restorative filling and one appointment for the sealants.

---

*Case 17.11, Discussion*: Why was the cooperative patient given three appointments? Would one long appointment (one hour) or two appointments (45 minutes each) be better, or would they be too long? Scheduling appointment length is variable. It often depends on the patient's current behavior and temperament.

Improved technology, the application of time, and motion studies by efficiency experts have altered today's current dental practices. Nowadays, the tendency is to treat the patient quickly and effectively while maintaining concern for patient comfort, health, and time. This change in approach conforms to the definition of behavior management proposed in the introductory chapter of this book. This definition included the terms "effectively" and "efficiently." Given this patient's history, there is little doubt that treatment could be accomplished in one or two sessions. Only a few studies have concentrated on appointment duration. Those few, however, note that appointments lasting one half hour to one hour are not detrimental to a child's behavior.

# Further Considerations for the Dental Team

## Parental Presence/Absence

Parent involvement, especially in their children's health care, has changed dramatically in recent years. It is important to understand the changing emotional needs of parents because of the growth of a latent but natural sense to be protective of their children. Practitioners should become accustomed to this added involvement of parents and welcome their questions and concerns for their children. They should consider parents' desires and wishes and be open to a paradigm shift in their own thinking (AAPD 2020). Currently, many clinicians design operatories to accommodate parents (see Chapter 18).

There is little agreement in practitioner philosophy regarding parents' presence or absence during pediatric dental treatment. Surveys on the topic in the 1970s were almost unanimous in reporting that parents should not accompany their children into the dental operatory. There were, of course, exceptions, such as for the toddler and the special needs patient. However, beginning in the 1980s, surveys found an increasing number of practitioners allowing parents into the dental operatory with their children (see Chapter 4). Nowadays, it is becoming more and more common for the parent–child pairing to remain together.

## Gifts and Tangible Reinforcements

Giving gifts or prizes to children has become a fact of commercial life in North America and almost throughout the world. There is general agreement on the merit of this practice in the dental office, for gift-giving can serve as a reward. If the gift has dental significance (such as a toothbrush kit), it also serves as a reinforcement for dental health.

It is very important that the various trinkets in a toy chest are used as tokens of affection for children—not as bribes. A bribe is a promise to induce positive behavior. A token of affection reward is recognition of good behavior after completion of the operation, without a previously implied promise. What Finn called a *bribe* in 1973, Pink calls a *contingent reward* in his 2009 book, *Drive—The Surprising Truth About What Motivates Us*. This is how a contingent reward sounds: "if you do this, then you will get that." Contingent rewards, or bribes, can have negative effects— they require people to forfeit some of their autonomy (Pink 2009). Studies have shown that when contingent rewards are given to control a person's behavior, they can do long-term damage.

Deci et al. re-analyzed nearly three decades of studies on the subject of rewards. After carefully considering reward effects in 128 experiments, they concluded that tangible rewards tend to have a substantially negative effect on intrinsic motivation when focused short-term to controlling behavior (Deci et al. 1999). Gift-giving practices which are not "contingent" or bribe-based can have spectacular results. Many children who seem tense during operative procedures suddenly perk up upon completion, eager for a gift. These gifts provide a pleasant reminder of the appointment. It is always special when a member of the dental team accompanies the child to the gift box and praises her while she selects her prize (see Figure 17-3).

## Wearing Apparel

When it comes to apparel for the dental team, there has been concern that professional clothing worn by the dentist can increase anxiety in children because fears may be transferable from one situation to another unrelated encounter. For example, if a child had previous poor experiences with a professional in a white coat (who could be a physician or a barber), it is possible that these fears could be generalized to the dental environment. The uniform can be common to all. Similarly, children who have been exposed to prior surgical procedures might be frightened by a face mask. Investigating this potential problem, Siegel et al. (1992) suggested that wearing a mask during dental treatment represents a minimal stressor for the young child, but recommended introducing the child to the dental environment and experience without the use of a protective mask. In 2019, the world experienced the unprecedented event known as the COVID-19 pandemic, which introduced interim infection control guidelines and social distancing protocols in the United States. For example, the recommendation of full-time mask or respirator wear and full-face visors for clinical team members and facial coverings for administrative team members as well as the general public. It has been the authors' experience and opinion that wearing a mask, face shield, or facial covering has not been a significant stressor for the young child. As time goes by and data is collected it, we will be able to gain insight on the effects of personal protective equipment and apparel on patients.

Wearing apparel can conceivably influence both patients and professional staff. Studying the issue in a dental faculty, Mistry and Tahmassebi (2009) found that parents favored traditional dress, as it gives an air of professionalism. Children, however, preferred dental students in casual attire. All are not in agreement with this view. Kuscu et al. (2009) examined the preference in attire of 827 Istanbul school children aged 8–14 years. The children were shown

(a) (b)

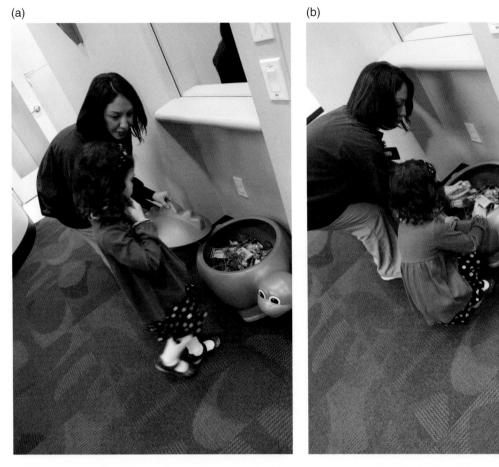

**Figure 17-3** It is always special when a member of the dental team accompanies the child to the gift box and praises her while she selects her prize.

photos of dentists wearing different clothing. Almost half of the children selected formal attire as their choice for dentists' wearing apparel. The study does not support the popular view that white coats raise anxiety levels in children.

An investigation by Austin et al. (1991) surveyed the wearing apparel of women dentists with a questionnaire. Based upon the replies of 928 of 2,000 women, only 51% felt the need to wear a lab coat over their street clothes. Interestingly, women dentists reporting the highest gross incomes were more likely to wear street clothes without a lab coat. The study suggested that dressing for success and infection control was a professional issue.

What to wear in the clinic is not only a dental issue. Truong et al. (2006) reported that physicians wearing standard precautions attire in the pediatric emergency department need to be aware that this apparel may negatively impact their relationship with pediatric patients aged four to eight years. In terms of the effect of physician dress style on patient confidence, patients of all ages who consulted with physicians in a hospital or private practice had the most confidence in a physician who wore a professional white coat (Maruani et al. 2012).

**Taking Radiographs on Children**

In 1987, the FDA developed safe guidelines for the use of dental X-rays. These guidelines were updated in 2004 and again in 2012. The development and progress of many oral conditions are associated with a patent's age, stage of dental development, and vulnerability to known risk factors. Therefore, the 2012 FDA guidelines were presented within a matrix of common clinical and patient factors which may determine the type(s) of radiographs commonly needed. The guidelines are intended to serve as a resource for the practitioner and are not intended as standards of care, requirements, or regulations. While the dentist is responsible for ordering the number and type of X-ray required, auxiliary personnel who take X-rays in a dental office should be aware of the guidelines. They should know how many and what type of films are to be used. Consider the following case.

### Case 17.12    Film Selection

Cora, a lovely four-year-old, was referred to a pediatric dentist as a management problem. While the previous dentist had obtained radiographs, they were of poor quality and the had child refused to have them retaken. The alert dental assistant immediately recognized the problem—the previous dentist used bitewing films, size number 2.

***Case 17.12, Discussion***: Personnel taking radiographs need to know what type of films to use, and it is the dentist's responsibility to ensure that staff members know the procedures. In this case, the child likely was hurt by the type 2 radiographs. Large radiographs also could have caused her to gag. A good rule is to use type 0 films at least until the first permanent molars erupt.

The young patient has to be re-trained. New expectations have to be developed. It is important to point out that "things are different here." In accordance with leaning theory, the stimulus has to be altered to get a different response. One way is to begin by taking an anterior occlusal radiograph (Figure 17-4). This type of film generally does not cause gagging and is easy to obtain. It also allows the clinician to assess the cooperative behavior. An important teaching technique is to begin with an easy task (the occlusal film) and, once successful, increase the difficulty of the tasks (the bitewings). In addition, show the child the size of the radiograph from the former dental office and compare it to the type 0 film that you intend to use. Have the child hold the films. Be sure to keep repeating, "See, things are different here."

If there is difficulty taking a bitewing film, a Rinn holder can help. While it may not provide a good view of the furcation regions, it is adequate for diagnosing proximal caries. In this case, in order to gain Cora's confidence, she needs to be convinced again that "things are different here." A more detailed description of retraining procedures can be found in Chapter 6.

Another consideration should be made when switching over to digital radiography. Two basic techniques are available to obtain digital images: the direct method using an electronic receptor, called a *sensor*, and the indirect method, which uses a semi-indirect sensor called a *photostimulable phosphor plate (PSP)* and scanner (Figure 17-5). The direct sensor may either be cordless or, in many instances, have a fiber optic cable attached. The sensor is quite bulky, and although it may be similar in size to conventional film, its dimensions are not identical. In addition to its increased thickness, the plastic protective cover and cord may be uncomfortable for toddlers and young children. PSP plates are very thin and are available in sizes that match conventional film. The PSP system may be more

(a)    (b)

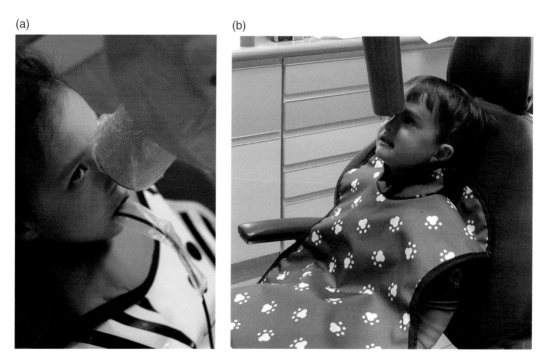

**Figure 17-4**   The anterior occlusal radiograph is the easiest and should be used before taking bitewings. Note the complexity of the sensor system, including plastic barrier sleeve and cable (a) versus the photostimulable phosphor plate (PSP) system (b), which is identical in technique to standard X-ray films. *Source:* Courtesy of Dr. Ari Kupietzky.

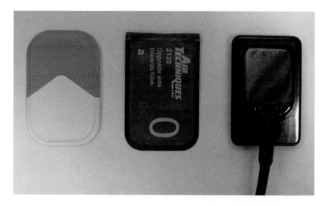

**Figure 17-5** The PSP plate (middle) is almost identical in size and dimension to conventional film (left), unlike the sensor (right), which is bulkier and has a plastic protective sleeve and cord. *Source:* Courtesy of Dr. Ari Kupietzky.

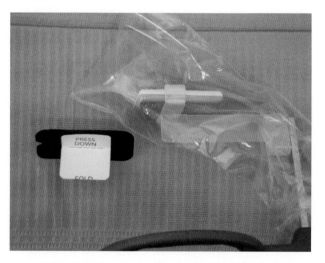

**Figure 17-6** For bitewings, a simple bitewing tab may be used with PSP plates (left) versus the sensor (right), which is used with a bitewing holder or bite block. *Source:* Courtesy of Dr. Ari Kupietzky.

suitable for pediatric dentistry: the thin, flexible plates are almost equal to X-ray films. The protective sleeve covers do not add any bulkiness to the plate. In addition, during bitewing exposures, the conventional bitewing tab may be affixed to the plate (Figure 17-6). The only disadvantage of PSP plates is that when taking occlusal radiographs, the child is asked to bite down on the plate, potentially damaging it. A useful clinical tip is to protect the plate for the occlusal view with a plastic cover found in packages of routine films.

It should be noted that the authors use the direct sensor method successfully, and when switching over to digital radiography, the clinician will ultimately decide which method is best for the dentist's individual style and needs.

Successfully introducing youngsters to radiographic procedures involves both the science and the art of behavior management. Explaining and demonstrating to patients, as well as answering questions and modifying procedures, are all parts of the art of behavior management.

The radiograph introduction is similar to other procedures for the young patient. A child's potential to cooperate should be evident before attempting radiographs. Communication has to be at the child's level of comprehension. Examples, instructions, and explanations should incorporate words and objects familiar to the patient, with as much repetition as necessary to acclimate the child to the procedure. Lengthy, complicated procedures should be broken down into steps for easier communication. When the child performs as instructed, praise is necessary to positively reinforce the desirable behavior. However, the praise should be specific, for example, "You are a good patient. You sat still."

The behavior-shaping procedure, although similar to the tell-show-do method, employs more concepts from learning theory. For instance, the child who is told about the radiographic equipment, shown the equipment, and then looks away may be telling the operator that he is not prepared to cooperate. In this case, attempts to shape behavior by returning to the "tell" portion of the procedure (i.e., the most distant approximation) may be helpful: "Michael, do you remember what I told you? I have a big camera to take pictures of your teeth. Please look over here so that I can show it to you. See it? Good!"

Behavior shaping entails successive approximations of desired behavior. Therefore, the dental assistant would not begin taking radiographs until the child heard, saw, or touched as instructed. Only after the desired behavior has come about should the next approximation occur. Thus, reciprocal interaction is an important feature of any behavior-shaping procedure, and the dental team member has to observe a child patient's reactions closely.

The following description for introducing radiographs begins by placing the protective apron on the child. Radiographs are then placed in the child's hand. Thus, the patient is involved in the procedure. The dentist or dental auxiliary might say: "These are like paper" (if film) or "These are like a memory stick" (if direct hard sensors are used). "They make pictures for your teeth. Can you count them for me to see that I have enough? Can you pick out the biggest ones? Good, you are a smart boy, Mike!"

Every attempt is made to relax the child (patients tend to gag when not relaxed). Since most children like to touch and feel things, the dental assistant may allow them to hold the radiographs. Permitting the youngster to count the films and select the larger ones also helps the clinician estimate a child's developmental level. A four-year-old patient who counts the four films and selects the large ones is probably a capable child.

Again, the child is introduced to the radiographic equipment with explanations from the dental assistant, such as the following: "I use a big camera. Do you ever have your picture taken at home? Yes? Well, my camera is a little different. Look, it has a long neck and a big head." Children have vivid imaginations and like to use them. "Here is its nose" (indicating the cone). Most children will look at the cone carefully. "I see that you are looking at its nose. Look up there. Can you see anything? No? Good! I wouldn't want anything to get in the way of your nice pictures."

Since radiographic technique differs from home photography, a suitable explanation is offered. "When you take tooth pictures, it is a little different from home pictures. The camera moves beside your face (showing the child). It doesn't, but it makes a funny noise (buzz and a beep) as it takes the picture. Also, the picture has to be in your mouth, not in the camera" (pointing to a location in the child's mouth).

In behavior shaping, the "tell" and "show" portions of the technique often go hand in hand. Modeling can be an important part of the showing procedure: "Let me show you how I like the children to do it" (Figure 17-7). The dental assistant can demonstrate film and X-ray machine placement on herself, or a model of a dentition can be used for this purpose. Since an X-ray machine is large and can frighten a young child patient, it should be introduced slowly. Rapid movements or unexpected noises should be avoided. If a specific room is used for radiographs, poster-sized pictures showing children having radiographs can be helpful. The objective of the entire process is to shape the child's behavior, which is brought about by a series of successive approximations.

One common question that preschoolers ask is, "Why do you use the blanket?" (meaning the lead apron). An understandable response might be, "Because I only want to take pictures of your teeth. I don't want your tummy to get in the picture." Another common question is, "Why do you go out of the room (or move away) when you take the picture?"

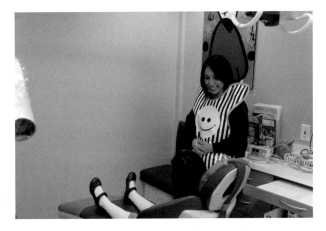

**Figure 17-7** Tell-show-do: The dental assistant is showing the patient the protective apron.

Two logical responses could be "So that I do not get in the picture" or "Because I have to go over here to press the button for the camera." Explanations such as these, made at a level that children can comprehend, usually satisfy curiosity. For older children, these answers will not suffice. They appreciate a brief explanation of radiation hygiene, which also demonstrates the dental team's concern for them.

When it is time to take the radiographs, the child is involved in a potentially pleasant learning situation: "Could you please pick out the biggest picture film and give it to me? Thanks. Mike, first I want to take a picture of your front teeth. Did you know that this picture can show me where your new teeth are? After I take the pictures, I will show you where your new teeth are, and maybe we can tell when they will come in for you."

Taking the X-ray, the dental assistant places the film or sensor in the child's mouth and says, "Close your teeth and hold the picture like a cookie, please." It is important for instructions to be brief, straightforward, and at the child's level of comprehension: "Good, now I will bring the camera nose near your nose to take the picture." The dental assistant, backing away from the camera says, "Hold still and I will take the picture. Don't move. Smile!" Many children grin when told to smile. This also facilitates positioning of the film. The analogy between home photography and radiography is maintained. Following the first film, the child is rewarded socially. The appropriate behavior is reinforced by verbal cues such as "Great!" and smiles from the office staff.

The procedure can move along rapidly. "Can you find the other big picture?" While the child rummages through the films, the operator explains, "We took a picture of your upstairs front teeth. Now I will take one of your downstairs front teeth. Did you know that you had upstairs and downstairs teeth?" While many young children laugh at this dental description, they understand. It is at their level of comprehension.

For a posterior bitewing or periapical view, a film tab or holding instrument is used. This, too, must be introduced to the child: "Look, Mike, when I take pictures of back teeth, I use a holder. It holds pictures. See my holder? I will put it in your mouth now, and you can bite on it. Great, you bit hard! Now I need the holder back" (removing it). "I put the picture in the holder so that it is easy for you to bite on." If you use sensors, you can use the analogy of a sugar-free lollipop. "Now I put the picture in your mouth and take a picture of your other teeth."

## Panoramic Radiography and Extra Oral Bitewings

This procedure presents a different situation for the child patient. While panoramic radiographs or extraoral bitewings are not difficult procedures, some children are alarmed when they first see the equipment. For this reason, the

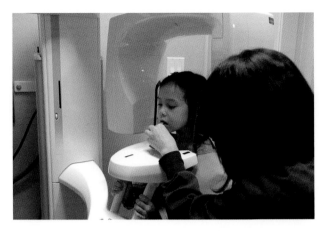

**Figure 17-8** Patient positioning with the dental assistant using the tell-show-do method.

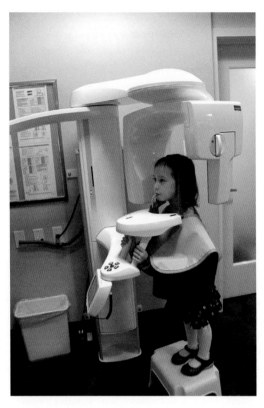

**Figure 17-9** Patient positioning. It is helpful for small children to stand on a stool.

panoramic radiographic equipment should be explained by the dental assistant before it is shown to a child. Children can be told that they are going to have their picture taken in a "space machine" and that they are not to be the space pilots. While positioning children (Figure 17-8), they are told that it is very important to hold still and that the big "space head" will move around them but not touch them. It is helpful to have smaller children stand on a stool (see Figure 17-9). A dry run can be made with the radiation turned off on most machines. Because the length of time that the patient must sit still is considerably greater than with standard radiographic techniques, constant voice contact provides security to the young patient. When taking panoramic, extraoral bitewings or intraoral radiographs on bright, curious children, the dental assistant should expect questions and provide suitable explanations.

## Summary

Dental auxiliaries are an important part of the dental team. Without them, contemporary dental offices would not function as they do. This chapter highlights some of the important aspects of child management in which auxiliaries are involved and hopefully provides information to help them with their work. It also strays somewhat into the area of practice management. That is because, at times, behavior management and practice management are inseparable. Many more aspects could have been added. Indeed, an entire book could be written detailing the work of dental auxiliaries. However, other parts of this book, although written for dentists, also may be applicable to everyone interested in pediatric dentistry.

## References

Aeker, J., Smith, A., and Adler, C. (2010). *The Dragonfly Effect: Quick, Effective, and Powerful Ways to Use Social Media to Drive Social Change.* Jossey-Bass, San Francisco, California.

American Academy of Pediatric Dentistry (AAPD). (2020). *Behavior guidance for the pediatric dental patient. The Reference Manual of Pediatric Dentistry.* Chicago, Ill.: American Academy of Pediatric Dentistry, pp. 292–310.

American Dental Association and US Department of Health and Human Services. (2012). Dental Radiographic Examinations: Recommendations for Patient Selection and Limiting Radiation Exposure. *Revised* 2012.

Austin, G.B., Tenzer, A., and Lo Monaco, C. (1991). Women dentists office apparel: Dressing for success in an age of infection control. *Journal of Law and Ethics in Dentistry*, 4, 95–100.

Bandura, A. and Schunk, D. (1981). Cultivating competence, self-efficacy and intrinsic interest through proximal self-motivation. *Journal of Personality and Social Psychology*, 41, 586–598.

Bharat, M. as told to Julie Bick. (2007). *The Google Way: Give Engineers Room.* New York Times, October 21.

Brauer, J.C., Highley, L.B., Lindahl, R. et al. (1964). *Dentistry for Children*, 5th ed. McGraw-Hill Book Co, New York, USA.

Deci, E.L., Koestner, R., and Ryan, R.M. (1999). A meta-analytic review of experiments examining the effects of extrinsic rewards on intrinsic motivation. *Psychological Bulletin* 125, 627–68; discussion 692–700.

Finn, S.B. (1973). *Clinical Pedodontics*, 4th ed. WB Saunders, Philadelphia, PA, USA.

Fredrickson, B. (2004). The broaden-and-build theory of positive emotions. *Philosophical Transactions: Biological Science*, 359(1449), 1367–1378. doi: 10.1098/rstb.2004.1512.

Koestner, R., Lekes, N., Powers, T.A. et al. (2002). Attaining personal goals: Self-concordance plus implementation intentions equals success. *Journal of Personality and social Psychology*, 83, 231–244.

Kuscu, O.O., Çaglar, E., Kayabasoglu, N. et al. (2009). Preference of dentists' attire in a group of Istanbul school children with related anxiety. *European Journal of Paediatric Dentistry*, 10, 38–41.

Latham, G.O. and Seijt, G.H. (1999). The effects of proximal and distal goals on performance on moderately complex tasks. *Journal of Organizational Behavior*, 20, 421–429.

Manderlink, G. and Harackiewicz, J.M. (1984). Proximal versus distal goal setting and intrinsic motivation. *Journal of Personality and Social Psychology*, 46, 918–928.

Maruani, A., Leger J., Giraudeau, B. et al. (2012). Effect of physician dress style on patient confidence. *Journal of the European Academy of Dermatology and Venereology*, Aug 9. doi: 10.1111/j.1468-3083.2012.04665.x.

Mistry, D. and Tahmassebi, J.F. (2009). Children's and parents' attitudes towards dentists' attire. *European Archives of Paediatric Dentistry*, 10, 237–240.

Pink, D.A. (2009). *Drive: The Surprising Truth About What Motivates Us*. Canongate Books, Edinburgh.

Ramos, K. (2009). Volkswagen Brings the Fun: Giant Piano Stairs and Other "Fun Theory" Marketing. *Los Angeles Times*. October 15. http://latimesblogs.latimes.com/money_ co/2009/10/volkswagen-brings-the-fun-giant-piano-stairs-and-other-fun-theory-marketing.html

Siegel, L.J., Smith, K. E., Cantu, G. E. et al (1992). The effects of using infection-control barrier techniques on young children's behavior during dental treatment. *Journal of Dentistry for Children*, 59, 17–22.

Truong, J., Jain, S., Tan, J. et al. (2006). Young children's perceptions of physicians wearing standard precautions versus customary attire. *Pediatric Emergency Care*, 22, 13–7.

Wright, G.Z. (1975). *Behavior Management in Dentistry for Children*. W.B. Saunders Co., Philadelphia, PA, USA.

Wright, G.Z., Starkey, P.E., and Gardner, D.E. (1983). *Managing Children's Behavior in the Dental Office*. The C.V. Mosby Company, St. Louis, MO, USA.

Wright, G.Z. and Stigers, J.I. (2011). Chapter 3. In J. Dean, D. Avery, and R. McDonald (Eds.), *McDonald and Avery's Dentistry for the Child and Adolescent*, 9th ed., pp. 22–45. Mosby Elsevier, Maryland Heights, MO, USA.

# 18

## The Dental Office

*Jonathon E. Lee, Brian D. Lee, Gerald Z. Wright, and Ari Kupietzky*

## Introduction

When the pediatric dentistry (pedodontic) treatment triangle was first described, one corner of that triangle featured the dentist and his environment. Despite the recognition of its importance, little has been written about the office environment in the pediatric dental literature, yet young pediatric dentists, graduate students, and residents spend countless hours thinking about their future dental offices, dwelling on what should and what should not go into their offices.

One of the first to recognize the importance of the office environment was Dr. Walter Doyle, who teamed up with the architect Sarah Tait to co-author one of the first publications featuring office design in a pediatric dental text. They wrote that designing an office was analogous to planning a city. Two of the innovations that they stressed were an office that would be open and flowing, with few doors and a multi-chair open operatory concept. Tate and Doyle (1975) wrote the following to encourage dentists to think about their office.

> *What is dental environment?.................. A place that allows teeth to grow and change in a healthy way.*
> *What is dental environment?.................. A place that allows the child to grow and change in a healthy way.*
> *What is dental environment?.................. A place that allows the doctor's staff to grow and change in a healthy way individually and collectively.*
> *What is dental environment?................... A place capable of its own growth and change with respect to the life it sustains and maintains.*

Since the "special effects" created within pediatric dental offices can be critical to some patients' attitudes, the office environment can be an important part of behavior management. But it is only the starting point. Behavior management also involves numerous techniques and strategies. It requires skills in communication, empathy, coaching, and listening. Having an office that accommodates these management techniques and strategies is part of the "art" of behavior management. There are many types of pediatric dental offices. Some could be considered basic, while others might be called "glitzy." Some offices are designed for more than one dentist; some might be designed for numerous dentists, hygienists, or expanded-duty dental assistants. The point of this chapter is to identify features that are unique to pediatric dental offices.

Pediatric dental offices are unique. That is why many hours are spent thinking about the office. Be cautious when selecting an office designer or consultant. A traditional dental supply company may suggest a design based upon a standard template. Relatively few office designers appreciate or understand the needs of a pediatric dentist. When designing an office, several important questions need to be asked.

- Does the image that your office projects promote cooperative patient behavior and patient–parent acceptance?
- Is the space provided sufficient for the optimal function of the practice?
- Does the office make it possible to use management techniques appropriately?
- Does the office permit you to practice in the style that most suits you?

Office designers may not focus on these issues. To attract young dentists, the focus is often a financial one. Sales pitches are often along the lines of "We design high-performance offices," or "Let us increase your productivity through a good design." No one denies the importance of earning a good living. However, treating patients properly,

*Wright's Behavior Management in Dentistry for Children*, Third Edition. Edited by Ari Kupietzky.
© 2022 John Wiley & Sons, Inc. Published 2022 by John Wiley & Sons, Inc.

using appropriate management techniques with care and understanding, should lead to that outcome.

*Patients differ. Dentists differ. And, offices differ.*

## Reception, Waiting, and Play Areas

The reception, waiting, and play areas are interconnected, and each requires a great deal of planning. They are critical to the office operation—they are like a store front window. They set the tone for the office and create expectations for both the children and their parents.

Patients should see the receptionist counter as soon as they enter so they don't feel lost. In turn, the receptionist should be able to see all patients, no matter where they are seated, so nobody is forgotten. All pathways should be wide enough, and the receptionist's counter low enough, for children in wheelchairs. When determining how big the waiting room should be, one should take into account that pediatric patients tend to visit the dentist as families. Often, one patient will be accompanied by parents, siblings, and sometimes even friends. For example, a general practice office waiting room size calculation would be:

1) Determine the number of patients expected to be seen during the busiest hour, multiplied by 2.5 to account for accompanying relatives and friends.
2) Subtract the number of exam rooms—that is, how many chairs will be needed.
3) Next, multiply the number of chairs by 20 square feet (1.86 m$^2$).

Accordingly, a solo practice with three exam rooms that peaks at six patients per hour should plan on a 240-square-foot (22 m$^2$) waiting room with 12 chairs. A pediatric dental office would need even more space.

When considering play areas, do not begin with the numbers game. Play can happen intensely in 1 square foot or in 1,000 square feet. Maybe the first question to ask is, "What will the play experience mean within the framework of the child's experience in this dental office?" Is play a diversion from the dental experience, or a simulation? Is it an introduction to the dental experience? What are the limitations of the play experience? Is the noise undesirable? Should the play be segregated from other areas? Is play a potential resource for the pediatric dental office that is vitally concerned with preventive and interceptive dentistry? Are parents involved in the play area? Is the atmosphere of the waiting room one of calmness, or perhaps excitement? Should the child waiting for an appointment be stimulated by a video game—perhaps magnifying hyperactivity—or should their time in the waiting room be relaxing and calming? The play area is a potential resource, for not only play, but for learning and behavior management. Make the most of it.

Excellent products are exhibited at dental meetings for waiting and/or play areas. How will they fit in the dental office? Will they cater to older children and teens, or will they be used by younger children or preschoolers? When thinking about the play area, several considerations are:

- The space has to be developmentally appropriate.
- The safety factor is a prime consideration.
- All toys or products should be hygienic.
- Equipment should be tough and long-lasting.

With these thoughts in mind, consider Figure 18-1. This waiting room area was designed with many of the elements mentioned above and includes a reading section, a toddler/young child play area, and a teenager video game corner. Figure 18-2 is another example of a waiting area that

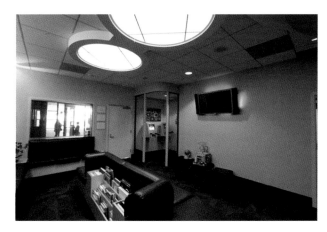

**Figure 18-1** This waiting room area design has many elements mentioned in the text, including a reading section, a toddler/young child play area, and a teenager video game corner, which is isolated by glass.

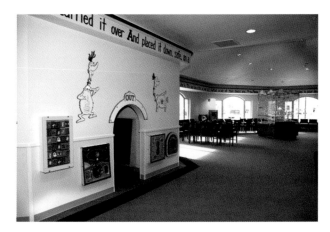

**Figure 18-2** A waiting area that accommodates both children and their parents. The play area is designed for younger children and preschoolers and is separated from the general seating area. *Source:* Courtesy of Drs. Walker, Ritchie, Kutsch, Gill. Richland, WA.

accommodates both children and their parents. The play area is designed for younger children and preschoolers and is separated from the general sitting area. A novel approach to waiting room play areas is a "cave" for children. Toys, games, and magic mirrors all can be contained within the cave (Figure 18-3). The area within the cave may be room-sized or significantly smaller. Its function is to allow a division between the play area and the general waiting area. In addition, it gives the children a sense of privacy and fun. The cave concept can also be used in smaller offices with limited space; prefabricated playhouses are commercially available and serve the same purpose.

Offices shared by multi-disciplinary dentists may have mobile play stations that can be displayed during the pediatric dentist's office hours and removed at other times so as not to label the waiting room as exclusively pediatric in nature. The module shown in Figure 18-4 is designed for small children and can be set anywhere, allowing parents to supervise. Note that it appears hygienic, safe, and tough and long-lasting.

In general, noisy games should be discouraged or used only in separate rooms. Sounds of children playing may not only be a nuisance to other patients in the waiting room but also may disrupt and interfere with the receptionist and front desk. It is also advisable for an office employee to be able to see the play area, since many parents may allow their children to play unsupervised.

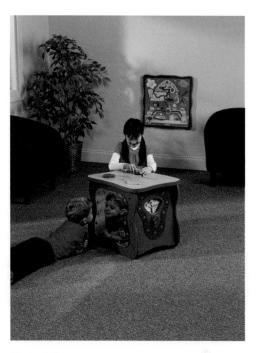

**Figure 18-4** Offices shared by multi-disciplinary dentists may have mobile play stations that can be displayed during the pediatric dentist's office hours and removed at other times so as not to label the waiting room as exclusively pediatric. *Source:* Courtesy of Playscapes. Waunakee, WI.

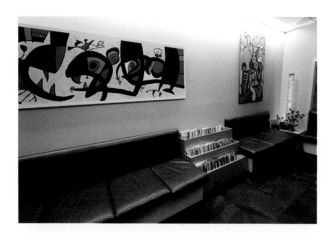

**Figure 18-5** To encourage child–parent interaction, a reading corner may be constructed. The use of bright modern art may be pleasing to both adults and children. It can make the room more energetic.

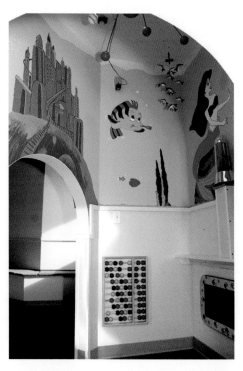

**Figure 18-3** Inside view of "cave" area depicted in Figure 18.2. Toys, games, and magic mirrors all can be contained within the cave. The cave area gives the children a sense of privacy and fun. *Source:* Courtesy of Drs. Walker, Ritchie, Kutsch, Gill. Richland, WA.

Games may be divided into non electronic/electronic, younger/older children-oriented, physically interactive, or passive. Electronic games may be touchscreen or include handheld joy sticks or steering wheels. They may be enclosed in protective casings to prolong their working life. Touchscreens have the advantage of being more user-friendly and less likely to break.

To encourage child–parent interaction, a reading corner may be constructed (Figure 18-5). The use of display shelves

(a)

(b)

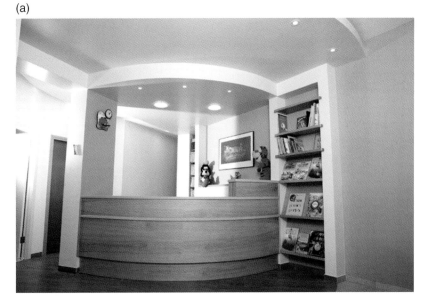
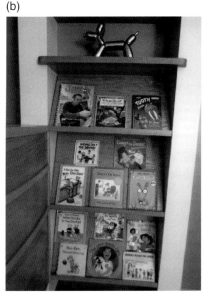

**Figure 18-6** Using shelves similar to bookstore displays makes the books more desirable (a). Among the books are those with dental themes and children's classics familiar to both parent and child (b).

similar to bookstore displays is suggested to make the books more desirable (Figure 18-6). Among the books are ones with dental themes and children's classics familiar to both parents and children (inset). Book set collections are available from vendors, making them easy to purchase.

Another parent–child activity may be a desk station to be used for homework. Siblings may get their homework done while waiting for the other family members' treatments. The same desk may be used by parents as an office in the morning while their child is undergoing a sedation visit. Parents may set up their laptops and phones while waiting. Lastly, a simple drawing corner with old-fashioned crayons and markers can be set up easily. Patients may be encouraged to present their drawing to the dentist and have it proudly displayed on a designated bulletin board.

The waiting room area may also be used for practice management. An informational video may be played constantly played for parents and children. The film may present office policies and services. A computer kiosk can be used to fill out medical history and other forms electronically, which are then submitted directly into the computer network. It goes without saying that Wi-Fi Internet access should be available in this area for the use and benefit of parents and patients.

## The Curbside Check-in Alternative

The 2019 COVID-19 pandemic introduced the concept of social and temporal distancing to prevent crowding and gathering of people in a confined space. With social and temporal distancing protocols, an alternative to the traditional reception, waiting, and play areas has arisen. That alternative is "Curbside Check-In" where patients wait in their cars or an outside public area rather than inside the dental office. With the increasing adoption of electronic health records, patients are sent forms ahead of time to be filled out online instead of in the office reception and waiting areas. The increased use of mobile phones with browsers has given rise to the opportunity where patients can check in for their appointments with a phone call or text message to the dental office that they are here, and the dental office replies as to when they can enter the office. It has been the authors' experience and opinion that curbside check-in works well. It does require clear communication between the dental administrative team, the clinical team, and patients.

## Office Themes

Many modern offices use themes, setting up the waiting room, playroom, and treatment rooms like amusement parks. Many themes, like the jungle, space, or medieval castles, appeal to children of different ages. Using a theme often makes it easier to decorate, since the design has a clear direction. However, a theme can become outdated relatively fast. Some people choose to have a multigenerational and timeless theme, which provides an environment for all age groups, including parents.

## Hallway Designs

Belcher (1898) was the first to write that children should be separated from their parents for the first visit. Parents were told that it was against "office policy" for them to accompany their children into the operatory. Until about 1980, this became an inviolate rule for many. Although the no-parent policy generally has changed (as discussed in Chapter 4), it still continues in some practices. Nonetheless, contemporary practice surveys have shown the trend is for parents to accompany children into the operatory, especially during the first visit. Now, more than ever, they form a greater part of the pediatric dentistry treatment triangle.

Dental offices have to be designed to accommodate current trends. Typical of the open office design is the "Z"-shaped hallway connecting the reception/waiting area with the treatment areas (Figures 18-7 and 18.8).

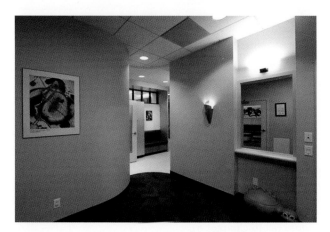

**Figure 18-7** Typical of the open office design is the "Z"-shaped hallway connecting the reception/waiting area with the treatment areas.

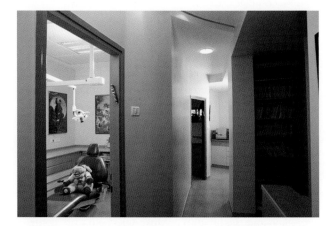

**Figure 18-8** "Z"-shaped hallway: treatment rooms may be color-coded with a predominate color, with the patient, dentist, and dental assistants' chairs matching the walls and/or doors. Patients are asked to go to the green or purple room. Children can easily recognize the room and feel more at ease.

Interestingly, dentists with this type of hallway design notice that children tend to wander into the clinical area by themselves—no coaxing necessary. Parents, too, seem more relaxed and tend to remain in the reception area after one or two visits. They take comfort knowing that their children are not behind closed doors and can often hear their children interacting with the dental team. A writing board may be strategically placed on a wall within the Z hallway. Children are attracted to the writing board. They play, write, or draw (teeth!) before their dental appointment, and sometimes leave messages of thanks to the dental team as they leave the office. In some offices, a pocket door is installed along the hallway. If excessive noise results from an uncooperative child in the treatment area, the door can be drawn closed.

## The Bridging Room

Not so long ago, it was common practice for many dentists to see a new patient in the dental operatory. Entering an operatory and placing a child immediately in the dental chair can be a frightening experience. Pediatric dentists now prefer that the first visit take place in a non-treatment room. Such a room serves as a bridge between the reception/waiting area and the treatment areas (Figure 18-9). A bridging room is much more than the traditional consultation room. It is a multi-purpose room for education and performing:

- the functional inquiry
- examination of very young children in a knee-to-knee position
- implementation of pre-appointment strategies
- demonstration of management techniques
- demonstration of oral hygiene procedures

To accommodate these functions, a bridging room has to be slightly larger than the traditional consultation room and must be equipped properly. If knee-to-knee examinations are performed, then appropriate seating for parent and child as well as examining instruments, a washbasin, and appropriate lighting is needed. If pre-appointment techniques are intended, then audio-visual equipment or modeling dolls have to be available. If oral hygiene instruction is given in this room, then supplies need to be available. It is helpful to have the oral hygiene area nearby (see Figures 18-10 and 18.11) if that is the preferred choice of venue for demonstrations. In summary, a bridging room serves many important functions in the dental office, and some offices have more than one.

An alternative to the bridging room, especially for offices with limited floor space, is the concept of "bridging chairs"

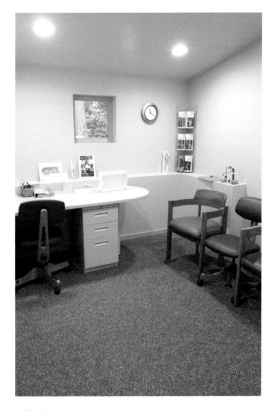

**Figure 18-9** Examples of bridging rooms: Note calming décor, educational aids, and toys for children and appropriate seating for parents and children. A washbasin should also be present. *Source:* Courtesy of Drs. Becker, Hays and Hayes. Bremerton, WA.

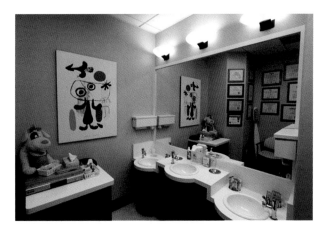

**Figure 18-10** Oral hygiene area: note the age-appropriate counter levels.

(Figure 18-12). Using this concept, two colored chairs are placed in the treatment room opposite the doorway. The patient is invited into the room and immediately asked to choose a chair. The child is pleasantly surprised that she is not asked to sit in the dental chair. The parent sits next to the child in the second chair. The patient is happy to sit on

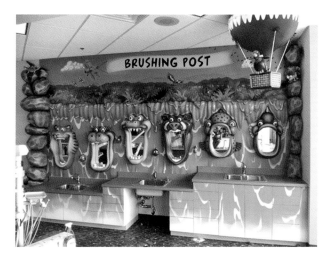

**Figure 18-11** Oral hygiene area for a large "jungle"-themed office. *Source:* Courtesy of Imagination Dental Solutions, Calgary, Alberta, Canada.

the regular chair, eyeing the imposing dental chair. Other children may react by saying they want to sit on the big chair (since they were told not to sit on it). The initial contact and communication is made with the patient by facing the child sitting on the regular chair. Eventually, the child moves on to the dental chair. However, the warming-up period is done with the dental chair in view. This is an advantage over a bridging room, where the child may begin to feel at ease and is then asked to move into another room. This method also works well with infant visits. In such instances, the infant sits on a parent's lap on a regular chair and a knee-to-knee examination is performed (see Figure 6-4 in Chapter 6).

## Treatment Areas

Surveys have shown a change in the parent-accompanying-child trend. Traditionally, US dentists treated children alone and the parent waited in the reception area. However, while surveying southeastern US pediatric dentists, Carr and Wilson (1999) noted that the majority of pediatric dentists allowed parents in the operatory. The main reasons for the change were parental influences and legal and ethical concerns of the practitioners. An AAPD survey of members (Adair et al. 2004) found that parental presence in the operatory appeared to be a common practice for some procedures, but not all. Parental presence in the operatory seems more widespread outside of the United States (Crossley and Joshi 2001). Most UK pediatric dentists (80%) supported parental accompaniment during the course of treatment. Since modern dental operatories need to accommodate parents in a contemporary office, the pediatric operatory will need more floor space than the

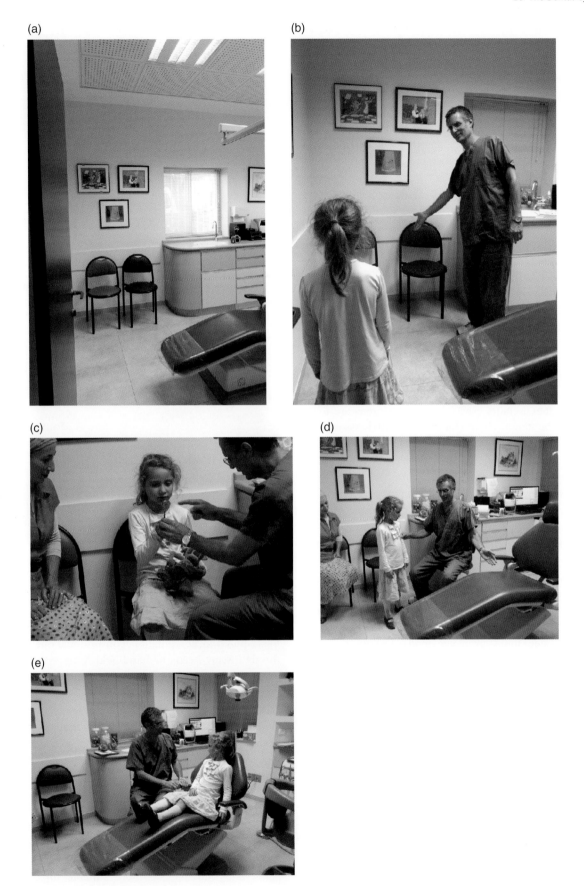

**Figure 18-12** An alternative to the bridging room, especially for offices with limited floor space, is the concept of "bridging chairs."
*Source:* Courtesy of Dr. Kupietzky.

general dentist's treatment room. In addition to the patient, one or two assistants, and the dentist, space will be needed for one or two parents and sometimes an accompanying sibling, and possibly a baby stroller.

Treatment areas have to be designed for children with cooperative behavior, potentially cooperative behavior, and those who lack cooperative abilities. Designs have changed greatly over the past 25 years, and they differ significantly from those of most general dentists in some interesting ways.

Many pediatric dental offices feature open operatories, as opposed to closed operatories. An open operatory contains space for treating several children at one time. Both a dentist and a dental hygienist may be treating patients at the same time. Concomitant treatments offer an opportunity for children to learn from one another, and it can be very efficient. The degree of separation between patient chairs may vary with the practitioner's philosophy and style. Using the six-feet rule in radiography where dental personnel do not stand in the path of the useful beam and must remain behind a protective shield or stand at least six feet away from the patient and at 90°–135° to the direction of the primary beam during an exposure, one should consider a minimum of six-feet social distancing separation between dental chairs especially if radiographs are to be taken at the dental chair. (California Dental Association 2014) Walls between patient chairs may be just high and long enough to screen patients from each other when seated upright, as well as reclined (Figure 18-13). This configuration allows the clinician to monitor the remaining treatment chairs while seated at the head of the patient, and it may be ideal for the pediatric or orthodontic practice (Unthank 2006). Other designs include counters as partitions, or no separation at all (Figure 18-14).

Some have questioned the benefit of the open operatory, suggesting that it may upset children. Indeed, research by Ishikawa et al. (1990) found that children can be bothered by exposure to crying and that the younger age groups (children under four years of age) tend to be bothered more than older age groups. It is incumbent upon a pediatric dentist to recognize that not all children will benefit from an open operatory. If a child cries in an open operatory and could possibly upset a younger patient nearby, the clinician should explain to the observing child what is occurring, and why. Make it a learning experience. Conversely, it is believed that many children benefit from being in the open operatory. It is analogous to a group of children lining up at the school to receive "a shot." Most behave quite well. They do not want to appear apprehensive in front of their peers.

Many offices limit the bay area to recall examinations and dental prophylaxis, orthodontics, and sealant placement. Some dentists also have an issue with taking X-rays in open bay areas. However, as long as patients and staff

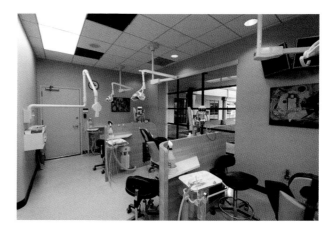

**Figure 18-13** Many pediatric dental offices feature open operatories, as opposed to closed operatories. An open operatory contains space for treating several children at one time. Walls between patient chairs may be just high and long enough to screen patients from each other when seated upright, as well as reclined.

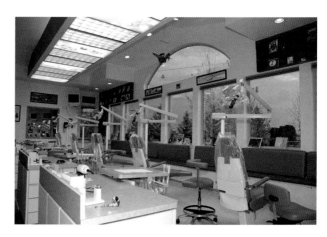

**Figure 18-14** This open bay has no separations at all between patients. *Source:* Courtesy of Drs. Walker, Ritchie, Kutsch, Gill. Richland, WA.

are separated from the X-ray source by at least six feet or the required local regulation, conventional open bay pass-through X-ray heads or hand-held X-ray systems can be used in the open bay operatory (Figure 18-15).

Personal preferences often dictate operatory design. There are dentists who prefer the privacy of an individual, closed operatory. Additionally, some parents do not appreciate what may appear to them to be an assembly-line mode of treatment used in open bay areas. The dentist's attention is seen as being directed more toward the other patients and less toward their own child.

Another point regarding the treatment room is the choice of dental unit delivery system (Figure 18-16). The dental unit can either be supplied as a cart or an over-the-patient arm. Each system has advantages and disadvantages, and one may be more suitable for a pediatric

(a)

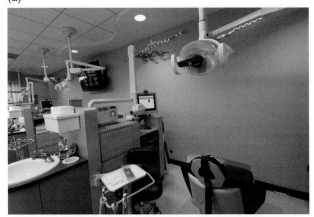

(b)

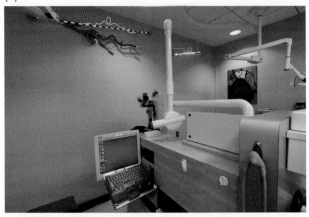

**Figure 18-15** Open bay area with X-ray: As long as patients and staff are separated from the X-ray source by at least six feet or the required local regulation, conventional open bay pass-through X-ray heads or hand-held X-ray systems can be used in the open bay operatory. (Check local regulations.)

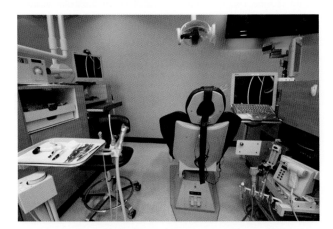

**Figure 18-16** The cart system is most suitable for children. This cart is side-positioned.

practice. The over-the-patient delivery system is the most commonly used in general practice dental clinics today (Georgetown University 2011). It allows for an efficient use of space, and both the dentist and the dental assistant have immediate access to the switches and/or instruments. However, there are drawbacks to this system in a pediatric practice. The array of visible instruments may upset children and make them feel confined, and if a child is aggressive, they could harm themselves with the instruments and the bar over the chair.

The cart system seems most suitable for children. The dental chair is not surrounded by frightening instruments; rather, it is simple and non-threatening. Carts may be either rear-positioned or side-positioned. All of the components can be introduced stage-by-stage. This system can be used with a dental chair, but it is most appropriate for use with the custom bench, described below. In contemporary practices, the cart system is used in conjunction with four-handed dentistry. A dental assistant is required to pass instruments to the dentist. Most cart systems function without a cuspidor. Cuspidors may not be suitable for child patients—they can be used as a delaying tactic when the child constantly asks to sit up and rinse. In addition, a child may become upset when expectorating into the cuspidor and seeing blood. Advantages of the cart system include the fact that: the instruments are less visible to patients, it easily converts to left- or right-handed, it is the least expensive system, and there is open space above the patient, which may be needed if active restraint is required during treatment. Disadvantages include the fact that cords can become tangled and operators or assistants can injure themselves by rubbing against sharp burs if the cart is improperly placed. The cart system is more prevalent in North America, but is less common in Europe.

Another unique feature of many pediatric dental treatment areas is the custom bench. Sometimes referred to as "ironing boards," they have replaced the conventional dental chair in many pediatric dentistry practices. The advantages of the custom bench are:

- They are relatively inexpensive, compared to conventional dental chairs.
- The dentist can lean on it, providing support and relieving pressure on the back.
- There is no tipping back, like a dental chair, which can raise a child's anxiety level.
- The operator can be in close proximity to the child patient.

Unlike conventional dental chairs, custom benches can be designed to contain storage areas (Figure 18-17). They also can hold video sound wiring and contain nitrous oxide lines. Custom benches can also be made adjustable,

(a)

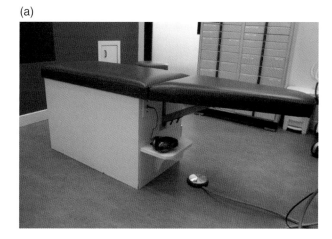

(b)

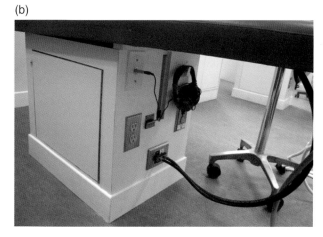

**Figure 18-17** The custom bench can be made adjustable to seat a patient upright (a). It also can be designed with storage areas and can contain video sound wiring and nitrous oxide/oxygen lines (b). Dimensions for the construction are contained in Box 18-1. *Source:* Courtesy of Dr. Weinberger, London, ON, Canada.

---

| **Box 18-1** | **Detailed description of custom bench construction** |
| --- | --- |

It is possible to construct a custom bench from 3/4-inch plywood. The following dimensions can serve as a guide.

- Total length is 66 inches.
- Height is 21 inches to the under-surface of the bench. When seated with the thigh parallel to the floor, the thigh should brush lightly against the under-surface. In offices with multiple clinicians, the stool can be adjusted to compensate for height differences.
- The width for the body is 21 inches.
- From the bottom end, the width begins to taper at 49 inches.
- The tapered portion is 27 inches.

A 3-inch foam covers the plywood, with a vinyl outer covering over the foam. Most benches are constructed so that the top is parallel to the floor. However, some prefer the bench to tip downward slightly, about 7°.

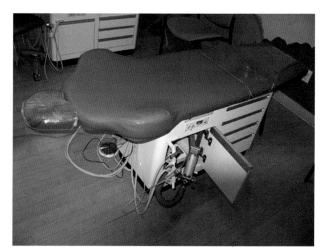

**Figure 18-18** Pediatric dental benches are also available professionally manufactured. The unit and nitrous oxide machine are built into the base of the bench. *Source:* Courtesy of Dr. Sabbadini. Pinole, CA.

---

allowing a patient to sit more upright. Box 18-1 describes the construction of a custom bench. Pediatric dental benches are also available professionally manufactured (Figure 18-18). One advantage of the custom bench is the taper in the design, which makes it more ergonomically favorable. Another advantage is cost. Custom benches can usually be fabricated at a fraction of the cost of their commercial counterparts.

Distracting child patients—diverting their attention from what may be perceived as an unpleasant procedure—can be very important in child management. The dentist may employ the distraction technique by telling a story or choose to use external distraction. External distraction is independent of the dentist or staff. Traditionally, clinicians have employed two types of distractors: audio systems with earphones or video tapes (or television), the advantage of videotapes being that children are able to select their favorite programs. However, with ever-evolving technology,

distractors have drastically changed in their size and content, offering an almost unlimited selection of entertainment. New technological innovations include hand-held music and video players (MP3 and MP4), personal hand-held video games, video glasses, and multimedia viewing monitors.

The effectiveness of distraction techniques has received attention from behavioral science investigators. Hinotsume et al. (1993) studied video film effectiveness and found that 90% of children aged between two and five years exhibited a high degree of interest in videos. There was an overall tendency of better behavior in children watching videos, compared to those without video distraction. The merit of audio devices for distraction was explored by Aitken et al. (2000) with three groups of children aged between four and six years. The children had two visits each and heard relaxed or upbeat music or no music at all. While 90% enjoyed the music, there was no significant difference in their behaviors. Prabhakar et al. (2007) compared audio and audiovisual distraction techniques in managing pediatric dental patients. They studied 60 children, aged four to eight years, and concluded that audiovisual distraction was a more effective procedure than audio distraction for managing the anxious pediatric dental patient.

The effect of distraction on pain threshold has also received attention. Studies have concluded that video distraction is ineffective in reducing pain during cavity preparation (Bentsen et al. 2001) or tooth scaling (Bentsen et al. 2003). Its practical use may lie in reducing general anxiety during less painful medical or dental procedures. Playing video clips during the inhaled induction of children undergoing ambulatory surgery was found to be an effective method of reducing anxiety (Mifflin et al. 2012).

One difficulty in interpreting the results of these studies and comparing them to one another is that no two studies use the same software. A video or film that engages one group of children may have no attraction to another group. Nonetheless, the studies point to a beneficial result using distractors, and they should be part of the behavior management armamentarium in a contemporary dental office.

Proper placement of video screens is important. With the child lying down and facing the ceiling, the monitor should be situated so that the child looks straight up—the line of vision is usually 90° to the ceiling (Figure 18-19). However, it can be more effective to place the monitor slightly farther back so that the child actually has to tip the head backward slightly. This encourages them to open the mouth. In addition, a child with a nitrous oxide nasal mask will be able to view the otherwise blocked monitor. Conversely, placing the monitor at the foot of the bench or chair is discouraged. The patient has to tip the head and chin downward to observe the video. One problem with placing the monitor in the ceiling is that it does not allow patient viewing while sitting up. A third position is approximately two feet to the dentist's side of the long axis of the patient chair and about seven feet above the floor (Unthank 2006). This position aligns with the patient's mid-calf. This placement is ideally suited for patient viewing in a lying or sitting position.

Not everyone likes to have monitors in the operatory. Some dentists limit them to recall examination chairs. They contend it interferes with eye-to-eye communication

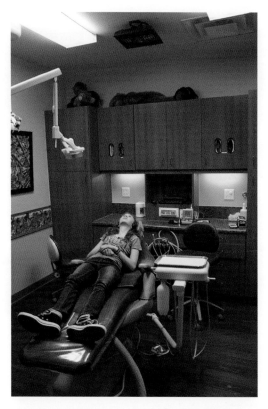

**Figure 18-19** Proper placement of video screens is important. With the child lying down and facing the ceiling, the monitor should be situated so that the child looks straight up—the line of vision usually is 90° to the ceiling. *Source:* Courtesy of Dr. Witkoff, Denver, CO.

with the patient during restorative treatment, making the visit a continuous learning experience. Another consideration is that many children have their own hand-held devices and prefer to entertain themselves. A child holding a device such as an iPod or smart phone may have less hand movement, resulting in less interference with the dental procedures (Figure 18-20).

Careful office planning is required to enable the pediatric dentist to treat an array of behaviors in the treatment area. Therefore, most dentists using open bays will have a designated "quiet" room or soundproof, closed operatory. The most common use of the quiet room is to serve as a treatment area for resistant patients, that is, those who are potentially cooperative or who lack cooperative abilities, and who might create a disturbance in the office. Sedation is primarily the treatment for these children, and it is far better to treat them in the privacy of an isolation room. However, telling a parent that their child will be treated in the "quiet room" rather than in the open bay may cause a "stigma." To overcome this stigma, the office personnel should refer to this multipurpose room as the (1) private operatory, (2) family suite, (3) sedation suite, or (4) orthodontic records room.

(a)                              (b)

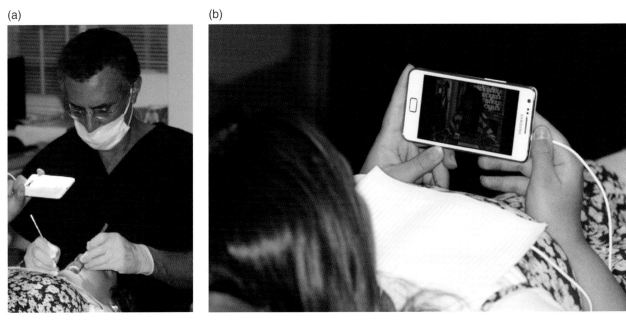

**Figure 18-20** Many children have their own hand-held devices and prefer to entertain themselves. A child holding a device such as an iPod or smart phone may have less hand movement, resulting in less interference with the dental procedures.

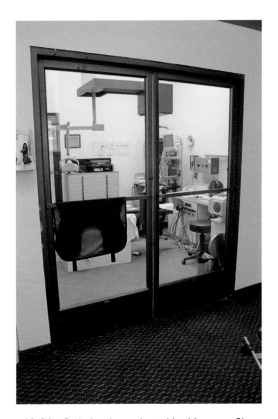

**Figure 18-21** Sedation is conducted in this room. Glass doors offer a sound barrier and allow parents to view from a distance. The double doors accommodate wheelchairs or stretchers. *Source:* Courtesy of Dr. Weinberger, London, ON, Canada.

Parents also can become quite apprehensive if they are unaware of what is transpiring in the room. For this reason, a viewing area for parents is desirable. This can be accomplished with windowed or glass doors (Figure 18-21). They provide an opportunity for parents to observe their children's treatments, and they may increase parents' tolerances for these techniques (Peretz and Zadik 1999). The glass also serves as a sound barrier.

## The Office Décor

Many dentists engage the services of a professional to assist with the decoration in an office. While they may create very tasteful finishing for the new office, they are not dental professionals. Get input from the members of the dental team, who contribute greatly to the success or failure of the office.

While the walls do not need to be shockingly painted in bright blue or bold magenta, the office should consider colors that are warm and welcoming, like yellow or light blue. Carpeting is also an issue. For hygienic reasons, many offices avoid carpeting. However, if considering carpeting, many carpets can be flecked with different colors or include squares or dots of colors without being overwhelmingly busy or too bright. Treatment rooms may be color-coded with a predominate color—the patient, dentist, and dental assistants' chairs match the walls and/or doors (Figure 18-8). Patients are asked to go to the green or purple room. Children can easily recognize the room and feel more at ease.

After the walls have been painted and the flooring is in place, thought has to be given to decorating the walls. Consider the ages of the patients in the practice. Many pediatric dentists err by decorating only for young children. Think of the older children, too. Colorful decorations, such as vintage posters or bright modern art, can be pleasing to both adults and children and can make the room more energetic (Figure 18-5). Animation cells are appealing to all ages. Placing a stuffed animal in a "hiding" spot, such as in the corner of an exam office, can be fun for children to discover and can easily be removed when treating adults. Wall space may be created for the older age group. They are encouraged to bring in one of their school banners. They enjoy participating!

Poster decoration is an important part of the office décor. Posters can be purchased from dental societies or associations. However, having the office staff design and create posters for the office is much more personal, and they are appreciated by children and parents. If possible, posters should be user-friendly and impart information such as why we take X-rays, or the need for urgent care following dental trauma.

*Patients differ. Dentists differ. And offices differ.*

# References

Adair, S.M., Waller, J.L., Schafer, T.E. et al. (2004). A survey of members of the American Academy of Pediatric Dentistry on their use of behavior management techniques. *Pediatric Dentistry*, 26, 159–66.

Aitken, J.C., Wilson, S., Coury, D. et al. (2000). The effect of music distraction on pain, anxiety and behavior in pediatric dental patients. *Pediatric Dentistry*, 24, 114–118.

Belcher, D.R. (1898). Exclusion of parents from the operating room. *British Journal of Dental Science*, 41, 1117.

Bentsen, B., Svensson, P., and Wenzel, A. (2001). Evaluation of effect of 3D video glasses on perceived pain and unpleasantness induced by restorative dental treatment. *European Journal of Pain*, 5, 373–378.

Bentsen, B., Wenzel, A., and Svensson, P. (2003). Comparison of the effect of video glasses and nitrous oxide analgesia on the perceived intensity of pain and unpleasantness evoked by dental scaling. *European Journal of Pain*, 7, 49–53.

California Dental Association (2014). Radiation Safety in Dental Practice. https://www.cda.org/Portals/0/pdfs/practice_support/radiation_safety_in_dental_practice.pdf Accessed: 08-02-2020

Carr, G.K., Wilson, S., Nimer, S. et al. (1999). Behavior management techniques among pediatric dentists practicing in the southeastern United States. *Pediatric Dentistry*, 21, 347–353.

Crossley, M.L. and Joshi, G. (2002). An investigation of paediatric dentists' attitudes towards parental accompaniment and behavioural management techniques in the UK. *British Dental Journal*, 192, 517–21.

Georgetown University. (2011). Chapter 2. Facilities and staffing: Equipment and supplies. *Safety Net Dental Clinic Manual*, National Maternal and Child Oral Health Resource Center. Retrieved from: http://www.dentalclinicmanual.com/chapt2/2_1.html

Hinotsume, S., Hinotsume, K., Matsuda, S. et al. (1993). The infeluence of video films on child patient behaviour during dental treatment. *The Japanese Journal of Pediatric Dentistry (in Japanese, English abstract)*, 31, 850–858.

Ishikawa, T., Nakashima, M., and Shitozawa, K. (1990). The emotional reaction on other child patients caused by the crying of the uncooperative child patient. *Shoni Shikagaku Zasshi*, 28, 1066–74.

Mifflin, KA., Hackmann, T., and Chorney, J.M. (2012). Streamed Video clips to reduce anxiety in children during inhaled induction of anesthesia. *Anesthesia & Analgesia*, 115, 1162–1167.

Peretz, B. and Zadik, D. (1999). Parents' attitudes toward behavior management techniques during dental treatment. *Pediatric Dentistry*, 21, 201–204.

Prabhakar, A.R., Marwah, N., and Raju, O.S. (2007). A comparison between audio and audiovisual distraction techniques in managing pediatric dental patients. *Journal of the Indian Society of Pedodontics and Preventive Dentistry*, 25, 177–182.

Tate, S. and Doyle, W. (1975). The office environment. In: G.Z. Wright, *Behavior Management in Dentistry for Children (pp. 246–260)*. W.B. Saunders Co., Philadelphia, PA, USA.

# Index